MEDICINE AND THE FAMILY

A FEMINIST PERSPECTIVE

LUCY M. CANDIB, M.D.

BasicBooks
A Member of the Perseus Books Group

Chapters 1 and 2 draw on material previously published in "Self-in-Relation Theory: Implications for Women's Health," in A. J. Dan, ed., *Reframing Women's Health: Multidisciplinary Research and Practice* (Thousand Oaks, Calif.: Sage Publications, 1994), 67–78.

Chapter 3 draws on material from "Family Life Cycle Theory: A Feminist Critique," *Family Systems Medicine* 7 (1989): 473–87.

Chapter 4 draws on material previously published in the editorial "Violence against Women: No More Excuses," *Family Medicine* 21 (1989): 339–42; and in "Naming the Contradiction: Family Medicine's Failure to Face Violence against Women," *Family & Community Health* 13 (1990): 47–57.

Chapter 7 draws on two previously published articles: "Ways of Knowing in Family Medicine: Contributions from a Feminist Perspective," *Family Medicine* 20 (1988): 133–36; and "The Family Approach at Each Moment," *Family Medicine* 17 (1985): 201–8.

Chapter 8 is based on a previously published article, "What Doctors Tell about Themselves to Patients: Implications for Intimacy and Reciprocity in the Relationship," *Family Medicine* 19 (1987): 23–30.

Chapter 10 draws on material in "Reconsidering Power in the Clinical Relationship," in M. A. Milligan and E. S. More, eds., *The Empathic Practitioner: Empathy, Gender, and Medicine* (New Brunswick, N.J.: Rutgers University Press, 1994), 135–56.

Library of Congress Cataloging-in-Publication Data
Lucy M. Candib
Medicine and the family : a feminist perspective / Lucy M. Candib.
p. cm.
Includes bibliographical references and index.
ISBN 0-465-00825-9
1. Medicine—Philosophy. 2. Feminism. 3. Physician and patient.
4. Medical care. 5. Family medicine. I. Title.
R723.C37 1995   95–7114
610—dc20   CIP

95 96 97 98 ❖/HC 9 8 7 6 5 4 3 2 1

To Richard

Whose brave daily feminism inspires and sustains

CONTENTS

PREFACE

A LTHOUGH I COULD SAY that I have been working on this book for my whole life, it is more accurate to say that it took me six years to write. And it would not have been written at all without the help of the many people who discussed ideas, read drafts, helped with revisions, and provided crucial supports.

I would first like to thank the people who did the essential research for this book: they located resources, taught me to do computer searches, made dozens of library trips, and photocopied innumerable articles and drafts. This book could not have been completed without the skillful help of Jodie Baxter, Melody Cunningham, Jennifer Eddy, Jean Emans, Alex Houck, Nancy Irons, Wanda Merced, Kathy Powers, Stephanie Prior, and Lynn Riza.

Over the years certain people have been essential to my development as a family physician. At different times each of them showed me a kind of clarity about how I needed to change and grow in my work in family medicine to best meet the needs of patients and trainees: Lynn Carmichael, Jerry Commons, Arlene Dorischild, Annette Dula, Warren Ferguson, John Frey, Michael Glenn, Dan Lasser, Lisa Oneto, G. Gayle Stephens, John Stoeckle, Dick Walton, Rachel Wheeler, Midge Williams, and the members of faculty Balint group, especially the long-term members—Roger Bibace, Bill Damon, Steve Earls, and Sam Pickens.

Family medicine when I entered it had few women practitioners and no women faculty members. Much of what I now understand about a feminist approach to family medicine I learned from residents and colleagues who came after me and enabled me to see how family medicine had to change for both women patients and practitioners. Many of these colleagues are now teaching family medicine themselves. Among the many to whom I owe a great deal are: Joyce Alves, Joan Bedinghaus, Libby Bradshaw, Bea Cumby, Krista Farey, Vanessa Gamble, Mary Gutierrez, Anita Kostecki, Meredith Martin, Joy Melnikow, Susan Schooley, Carol Thayer, Randy Wertheimer, Rachel Wheeler, and Janet Yardley.

The Women's Network within the Society of Teachers of Family Medicine offered me the forum and the sounding board for my ideas and supported me in presenting them at times when they were unfamiliar or unpopular. Particular thanks go to Louise Acheson, Beth Alexander, Nancy Baker, Janice Benson, Sandra Burge, Valerie Gilchrist, Marji Gold, Cate McKegney, Betsy Naumburg, Karen Ogle, Denise Rodgers, Beth Stifel, Janet Townsend, and Sheri Wahlen. Other people in the Family in Family Medicine contingent have given me extended support: Terry Davis, Frank deGruy, Kathy Cole-Kelly, Susan McDaniel, Harley Racer, and Don Ransom, who first linked me up with Basic Books.

Some people offered intangible support through their presence: the many friends I have made through electronic mail, particularly on the Women's Studies List (WMST-L), and the women in my women's group: Patti Gould, Laura Myers, Ellen Ruell, and Betsy Wertheimer. Some people just knew I could do it and didn't mind telling me so over and over again: Joan Bolker, my sister Judith Larkin, Debra Luepnitz, and E. J. Stephens. My editor, Jo Ann Miller, encouraged me while allowing me to write at my own pace. At Basic Books, Suzanne Nichols gracefully shepherded the manuscript through the production process. Cindy Buck's thoughtful copyediting improved the book immeasurably. And many readers have offered helpful comments on drafts of various chapters over the years: Roger Bibace, Joan Bolker, Arlene Brewster, Lorraine Code, Arlene Dorischild, Lynn Eckhert, Richard Frankel, John Frey, Valerie Gilchrist, Michael Glenn, Marji Gold, Susan Jhirad, Judith Larkin, Judith Lorber, Jean Baker Miller, Ellen More, Judy Norsigian, Marianne Pita, Paul Rosen, Susan Steinberg, Beth Stifel, Carolyn Swift, Rhoda Unger, and Irving Zola.

Good friends are essential and I can count many. Important over the years in the writing of this book were Stacy Amaral, Frances Anthes, Gene Bishop, Joan Bolker, Judith Bryant, Marjorie Clay, Joanne Cohen, Annette Dula, Sharon Ervin, Richard Frankel, John Frey, Julianne Frey, Valerie Gilchrist, Marji Gold, Kathleen Hardie, Beverly Johnson, Susan Lederer, Luis Malaret, Susan McDaniel, Ann Nemitz, Judy Norsigian, Marianne Pita, Dianne Rocheleau, Joe Stenger, Miriam Torres, Sue Walton, Rachel Wheeler, and Irving Zola. I want to include a special note of remembrance for Irv, whose persistence and exuberance will continue to be lifelong encouragements for me and many others.

Hundreds of people now or formerly at the Family Health and Social Service Center have made this book possible in different ways. They covered my patients the many days I was writing at home: the staff, the nurses, nurse-practitioners, residents, and other faculty family physicians took on my work without complaint so that I could write part-time. Special recognition goes to my current and recent practice partners, who shared with me the work and joy of patient care and teaching: Joyce Alves, Nancy Berubé, Jeff Borkan, Valerie Early, Warren Ferguson, Marsha Lavoie, Steve Putterman, Rick Sacra, Ted Shoemaker, Lise Tardif, and John Wiecha. Residents show me what it is like to face the joy and desperation of entering people's lives as a doctor for the first time. Every day I see how much they care about our patients, and they remind me once again of how important it is that teachers care deeply about those they teach.

Many patients gave me permission to use their stories, and all my patients put up with my part-time schedule and supported my work with their patient waiting and inquiries about the book. They have weathered long stretches of my unavailability at the clinic, in the interest of the book, as well as my two maternity leaves. They are the ones who know firsthand what it means to wait in line at the welfare office, to sit two hours in the doctor's office, and to have your family decimated by drugs and violence. They know that this is not a fair world for women and people of color and poor people. I hope that many of my patients can know that this book is written to serve their interest.

Some people helped keep body and soul together: Nancy Watrous refueled my energy on countless days when I would otherwise have packed it in. Midge Williams helped me to lay the self-accepting psychological groundwork necessary to examine my own ideas and experience and to believe that I could do it. And one person made it emotionally possible to write this book: Debra Keating, who has been the day-care mother for our children for the past eleven years.

Our children, Addie Helen Candib and Eli Julius Schmitt, ate noodles and vegetables more times than they can count, didn't have their own mother on all those field trips, went to day care during school vacation, and let me work when they would much rather have had a mother who had no other ambition. For them, two African sayings tell it clearly. For Addie: The daughter of a lion is also a lion. For Eli: A person is a person because of another person.

Finally, Richard Schmitt read every word, sometimes dozens of times over, helped me focus ideas that were vague, rescued me from the morass of detail, and reminded me that I didn't have to quote everyone else because I had something to say myself. He took care of our children on nights and weekends, did drop-off and pickup at day care and school, schlepped all the groceries, hauled all the firewood, and cooked more than half the meals. Every night and weekend that I was on call for teaching and patient care, whenever I left in the middle of the night for a delivery, Richard was on call for our children. I cannot count all the times he set his own work aside to attend to my computer emergencies or continued single-parenting whenever my clinical work or meetings took me away from home. He carried me off the ice when I broke my kneecap and attended to my emotional and spiritual needs when I didn't even know I had any. He encouraged me in my gloomiest moments. We have a joke about authors who say that the errors are all their own—I can safely say that, while more of the errors are mine, the effort of writing this book has been completely shared with Richard, for he has contributed to every step of the project. For all these reasons, and because we continue to learn together about what it means to be-in-relation, I dedicate this book to him.

INTRODUCTION

MEDICINE OPERATES under the impression that its theory and practice are gender-neutral. But women, both clinicians and patients, are only too aware that the practice of medicine is gendered in a masculine way. In this book I talk about how the theory is male-gendered as well. Criticism of the theory of clinical medicine—of the assumptions underlying everyday practice—has never been articulated from a feminist viewpoint within the profession. This book offers a feminist understanding of the conceptual problems in contemporary medical practice and proposes a feminist view of clinical work. All theory is created by persons who bring their personal experience—of power and disempowerment, of participation and exclusion, of doing and feeling—to bear on their ideas, however abstract. My work, too, is both personal and theoretical. For this book to make sense to the reader, I need to say who I am, and why I wrote this book. I will start with the personal and move on to the theoretical, with full knowledge that they are intertwined.

When I was three years old, according to Helen McSweeney, who looked after me, I used to pick up the phone and say, "Dr. Candib's office." At three I was sure that I wanted to be a doctor, like my father, and many years later I chose to become a family doctor, akin to the general practitioner that he was. Like him, I wanted to write books, and like him I have often acted on behalf of young women in various kinds of trouble. Similarities do end. My father was a physician-addict, a fact that shaped my entire childhood, and his life ended in depression and despair. He was patriarchal, sexist, and, at times, overtly abusive. In the house of my father I learned both the magic and the misery wrought by male medicine.

Generalism runs on both sides of the family. My immigrant Jewish grandparents owned a general store in Danby, Vermont. My mother, the oldest of their three daughters, could cook dinner, run the store, and play the piano in the silent movies. Early on she learned to deny feelings in the face of the bitter winters and brutal family conflicts. Later losses—her childhood home going up in flames while she watched from the school yard, the death of her beloved younger sister at age twelve, the forbidden romance with the Cuban Joaquin—shaped her into the mother I knew: diversely competent, forebearing, and stern. Doctor's wife, addict's spouse—she was a single parent long before the phrase had been coined. She ran my father's practice, typed his writings, drove the family to Vermont for the summers and back to Brooklyn in time for school (changing a flat tire when necessary), and never failed to plant a garden, paint peeling clapboards, and cook balanced meals for her two daughters. She never missed a beat. I can catalog her diverse competencies still, and many I will never attain. The driving forces behind all this energy? The denial of feelings and the need to keep up appearances at all costs.

My father is long dead, and my mother has Alzheimer's disease. My older sister Judy and I often puzzle about what must have been going on during those years of "business as usual" on the surface and rivers of pain beneath. My sister was the oldest and I was the youngest of four girl cousins who spent our summers in Danby where my mother and aunt grew up. My mother's position as shopkeeper's daughter and doctor's wife led her to care deeply about the impression her daughters made. Looking back now, I see how early I took on, in the family constellation, the task of challenging the lies, refusing to keep up false appearances, and naming the evils when I saw them. I was the child who kept trying to tell people that the emperor, and indeed most of the grownups I knew, weren't wearing any clothes.

Today I still see male medicine addicted to power and magic. Abuse and benevolence still twist around the Aesculapian staff, and the forces of that medicine still prefer to be surrounded by women who will keep up appearances and deny painful feelings at all costs. So I came into doctoring as an adult well prepared by family life for what medicine held. As my father's child, I had to know its power. I had to help desperate people. I had to write about it. As my mother's child, I had to do it very well, in many arenas, against great odds. From my mother also came the ability to fall back on denial as the defense, indeed the skill, that made survival possible, but at great cost. Dismantling that denial, brick by brick, was a requirement for me to arrive at a feminist understanding of healing. Denial, I was later able to learn, is a feminist issue.

In recent years I have also come to see how my consciousness was shaped as a white person. I am embarrassed even now to admit that my parents had a maid, a black woman from South Carolina, Addie Epps, who lived with us from 1942 to 1961. At first she worked for us full-time, but as my father deteriorated and finally died, my mother could no longer pay her. From then on she lived at our house and worked for other families. Addie was the central warmth of our house. I now understand that she was the source of nurturing that neither of my parents could provide. She comforted me when my parents fought and cooked for me while my mother worked two jobs to maintain her desired standard of living. When my mother married my stepfather, a salesman and retired Coast Guard officer from Georgia, I had a rude awakening. He had no intention of sharing a bathroom with a black person. Addie accepted this state of affairs far more diplomatically than I did. I sobbed helplessly as my sister and I drove Addie to Penn Station in Manhattan with her accumulated possessions of twenty years in cardboard boxes tied with string. She returned to the home in South Carolina that she had built with her savings. I remain deeply ashamed of the white privilege I was born to, privilege that allowed me to grow up loved and tended by a black woman who received so little recognition for her labor and care. In 1983 I was finally able to honor her, and Helen McSweeney, the other woman who looked after me, by naming my first child Addie Helen.

I am also a child of the 1960s. The war against Vietnam was for me an example writ large of those in power manufacturing appearances to justify their own goals. My ability to recognize lies and dissembling came in handy when college administrators professed no connection to war industries. At last I had found others who did not think it was right to keep your mouth shut and do what was expected of you. The anti-war movement for me flowed directly into the women's movement. It seemed obvious to me that women, poor women, women of color, all had similar stakes in changing a system that made war on Third World countries.

And still I wanted to be a doctor. While my comrades dropped out to do organizing—of students, welfare mothers, factory workers—I struggled with the question: could I be a radical and still become a doctor? I finally concluded that if radicalism, as I understood it, was to endure, it had to be possible for people to have different jobs and keep on doing radical work. Someone would have to bring it to medicine. And I was that someone. While my best friends and comrades marched on the Pentagon, I stayed home and applied to medical school. Ten months later, after spending a summer working in a factory making circuit-boards, I marched into Amphitheater A at Harvard Medical School. Looking at the plush blue seats, I knew from the first day that I had indeed entered the belly of the monster.

Obligingly, Harvard Medical School did everything to reinforce my politics. In my first year the medical campus expanded its territory, destroying even more of the surrounding neighborhood. This urban imperialism became so infamous that during the Harvard Strike of 1969, the Eighth Demand was the end of medical school expansion. That year I also worked as a nurse's aide in admissions at the Boston Lying-In Hospital, right across from the medical school dormitory where I lived. There I saw how black women in labor were treated, and how their care differed enormously from the care given to the white private patients, including the total segregation of private patients from clinic patients. In the classroom the dogmatic, male-driven text of medical knowledge, handed down in precious "pearls" to be collected, rehearsed, and spewed back, replete with slides of women in bathing suits, made it clear that medicine was male-dominated from theory to practice. I had found another emperor whose nakedness needed proclaiming to the world.

My years in medical school, 1968 to 1972, coincided with the rebirth of the women's movement. At night, I went to a consciousness-raising group, to meetings of Boston Bread and Roses, and later to meetings with other women working in hospitals to look at how our roles shaped the way we treated each other. I joined a group of women dedicated to finding out what was known about women's bodies and making that knowledge available to all women; with that group I wrote an analysis of medicine and capitalism that appeared in the first edition of *Our Bodies, Our Selves*. During the day I was being saturated with Harvard's version of male medicine. By the end I was absolutely sure that I wanted to be a doctor and equally convinced that medicine was an institution rooted in sexism and racism and organized to the greater glory of capitalism.

Yes, I was sexually harassed. An endocrinologist at the Peter Bent Brigham Hospital taunted me with anecdotes about bearded women with large clitorises until I stopped attending the elective. (I recently learned that he continues this practice to this day at another medical school). But there *were* good people along the way. Jim Taylor, then chief medical resident at Boston City Hospital and still the backbone of the East Boston Health Center, rescued me during my first year by letting me follow him around the chaotic emergency room on Saturday nights. John Stoeckle, my undergraduate thesis adviser and a mentor for hundreds of medical students interested in primary care, turned my thesis on the history of neighborhood health centers into a publishable article. Imagine my classmates' surprise when in June of our first year their iconoclastic classmate appeared as coauthor of an article in the *New England Journal of Medicine*! Gene Bishop, a longtime friend and college classmate, pulled me into her ambitious plan to set up a free clinic for women and children in Somerville, a working class city next to

Cambridge, Massachusetts. Through Gene's dogged work and the work of many other women, the Somerville Women's Health Project became a reality, a clinic operating on democratic and feminist principles to serve low-income women and children. Gene's vision gave me the faith to believe that I might one day practice according to those principles.

After four years of medical school, I found the decision about specialty to be difficult. I wanted to do women's health, but obstetrics and gynecology, as a field, seemed to have nothing to do with women's health. I knew that I wanted to work with poor women. To sort it out, I opted for a rotating internship at what was then Cambridge City Hospital, a small municipal hospital serving the poor and working-class people of Cambridge and Somerville, a world away from the Harvard I knew but located just down the street. My work there began with two months of every-other-night pediatrics. This schedule meant being on call Monday, Wednesday, Saturday, and Sunday in the first week, and Tuesday, Thursday, and Friday in the second week. Then the sequence repeated. On nights and weekends I was on call alone for the emergency room, the delivery room, the nursery, and the pediatric floor. I used to go to sleep pondering which child from all of Cambridge and Somerville would be the next to wake me up.

At the end of those two months I was sure of two things. One was that I wanted to continue taking care of children. The other was that I didn't want to be a pediatrician. The grueling hours pitted me, in my exhaustion, against the mothers of the children I saw. If the child was not sick, why did they come in? If the child was desperately ill, why didn't they come in earlier? Pediatrics, by taking a child advocacy position, framed the work in opposition to the child's parents, usually the mother. I wanted no part of it. Yet I loved the work. Of my own free will, I chose another month of that awful schedule at the end of the year to do pediatrics again. And by that time it was also clear to me that I wanted to deliver babies as well. There was, and still is, only one specialty that allows you to do both: family medicine. I took a year off and set out to locate a family practice program.

In those years, family practice was just forming as a specialty. There were a few dozen programs around the country. As a fledgling specialty, it appealed to dissidents, mavericks, and generalists at heart like me. Family practice combined crucial elements for me: It was critical of established medicine for dividing patients into body parts, according to specialty. It focused on the doctor-patient relationship. It encouraged taking care of children and their parents, not children in opposition to their parents. It emphasized a low-technology, whole-person, whole-family approach. At that time family medicine identified itself as countercultural (Stephens, 1989); it proposed an alternative way to doctor. From a chance comment in a parking lot, I was referred to John Frey, who was starting a family practice residency in a neighborhood health center in Worcester. I drove out to Worcester, where John and I immediately launched into an hourlong discussion of Michael Balint, the Hungarian-born psychoanalyst who brought British general practitioners together in groups to discuss the doctor-patient relationship. This conversation began my formal career in family medicine and my continuing friendship with John. I joined that residency as a second-year resident with my practice in that urban health center serving mostly women and children. I had found a place to practice the kind of medicine I believed in, with the kind of patients who needed it. I would have paid to do it!

I am still at that neighborhood health center, and many of the patients I see today are people I began to take care of during my residency from 1974 to 1976. With John Frey, I began a faculty Balint group that is still running today. When my residency was over, I stayed on as a staff physician and teacher of residents, with a faculty appointment from the University of Massachusetts Medical School. After four years I became the medical director of the center. Other women family physicians joined me as faculty—Rachel Wheeler, Meredith Martin, Susan Schooley, Joan Bedinghaus—and many women medical students chose to train with us.

But it was far from ideal. The director of the health center was uncomfortably threatened by me. He told dirty jokes to discomfit me and ridiculed the women staff for their commitment to family. In 1985, when I suggested that the health center draw on its expertise in women's health to become a "center for women's health," I was laughed out of the boardroom. (Now, less than ten years later, our city has two women's health centers, one run by a hospital complex, and one by a large health maintenance organization [HMO].) Again, as in pediatrics, I found myself pitted against women with children—my coworkers this time, not the patients. As medical director, I was the official apologist for a sexist system that underpaid women as they struggled to offer good health care to other women. I used my entrenched skill at denial not to hear what my women partners and residents were trying to tell me—that full-time was too much, that every third or fourth night was too much, and that the salary (compared with the private sector and with any salaries offered to men doing comparable work) was unacceptably low. Caught by their feelings of responsibility toward each other and by their commitment to their patients, my colleagues persevered through years of insulting insinuations that because they had families they were unwilling to work hard enough. Unwittingly, I stood for a system that required every doctor to have a wife to care for home and children; I failed to recognize that the doctors I worked with were already caring for home and children. My ability to suppress my own feelings, learned from an expert, turned out to be oppressive not only to me but, more importantly, to the women who had joined me in our chosen work.

I suppose the story could have ended there. I could have kept on going, closing my eyes and ears to what was all around me. But about this time I started a relationship with my life partner, Richard Schmitt, and got pregnant. Once I had entered into all the demands and sharings of raising a child with another thoughtful adult, my skills at denial worked for only so long. Ultimately I had to make a choice—I stepped back from the position of medical director and went part-time. Richard and Addie, and later Eli, taught me what my women partners and residents had been unable to drum into my head. A stiff upper lip is the solution neither to overwork and fatigue nor to the complexity of multiple commitments. Once I accepted the importance of my own need to be in-relation, I was able to see that male medicine was based on ignoring such needs and on refusing to allow them to be met. My self-denial—as well as my denial of the needs of my colleagues, part of my mother's legacy—needed to be disowned. What was for my mother a survival strategy that ultimately deprived her of any sense of herself held the same potential to deny me a full feminist consciousness. Unlike my mother, I had the full support of a loving partner to help me to discard this part of my inheritance. I came to see that if the structures and organization of medicine were oppressive to women, then the medicine practiced in those settings could not be liberatory. Family practice, inner-city medicine, and generalism were still fundamental to my work. But I began to understand that as a feminist I had to recognize and challenge the masculinist assumptions underlying the medicine I loved. It took me another ten years to figure out what is the matter with male medicine and to write it down for others to read. This book is that attempt.

In my own life, my medical colleagues are unfamiliar with feminism, and my feminist friends find my doctoring an anomaly. Likewise, in the academic arena, feminism and medicine have very little overlap. In the past twenty years feminist scholars have transformed activities in the halls of academia. They have developed majors in women's studies, started feminist journals in dozens of fields, reshaped research agendas, and made scathing critiques of traditional male scholarship in the social sciences and humanities. Feminists have also developed a critique of the conduct and social organization of scientific research. Yet despite twenty years of feminist critiques of health care, medicine, broadly speaking, has remained relatively untouched by feminism. Clinicians who otherwise pride themselves on remaining current in medicine are unlikely to be conversant with feminist theory as it applies to women's health or to the organization and conduct of the medical relationship.

On the other side, feminist critiques of medicine have largely been directed at medical practice, and rightly so. Women's experience in the medical care system offers ample grounds for criticism. Historically, women have had their symptoms blamed on their reproductive systems; they have undergone excessive, inappropriate, and experimental surgery; they have been overmedicated with tranquilizers; and to this day they are underrepresented in scientific studies that have a bearing on their health. Yet, with only a few exceptions, feminists have not examined with the same intensity the principles underlying male medicine. Nor have they made themselves familiar with a feminist critique of medicine from the inside. Although feminists in various academic disciplines collaborate through women's studies departments to share scholarly analysis of the academy and build a research agenda, they are unaware of feminists in medicine—or worse, they may construe them as an enemy. And on the personal level, when feminists enter the medical care system as patients, they do not have the benefit of critical insights from feminists on the inside—the critique of the reductionist approach, the relevance of context, the importance of relationships, the interconnection of things physical and psychological, the importance of narrative, to name a few. In the last ten years feminists have made major theoretical and clinical advances in psychotherapy, leading to healing therapist-client relationships that recognize women's oppression. Nevertheless, no one has been asking what a feminist medical relationship would look like.

Instead, at the practical and individual level, feminism has often promoted a consumerist approach to health care. Armed with ample information and prepared for battle, a woman marches into the doctor's office. If she doesn't get what she wants, she can take her business elsewhere. This marketplace mentality, suppported by both "consumers" and "marketers" of health care (as well as by the widespread penetration of commercial language into medicine), results in adversarial clinical relationships and ample ammunition for later litigation. Feminism has not articulated a critique of the capitalist construction of medicine as a product to be marketed and sold. What we have instead in the 1990s is adherence to a capitalist model of health care as a product dictating that whole networks of health care be traded in the corporate marketplace to glean profits for conglomerates. Relationships between doctors and patients are lost in the yearly shuffle of contracts between HMOs. Consumers may have the appearance but not the reality of choice of clinician in this maze dominated by the jargon of the bottom line.

I have been fortunate until now that market forces have ignored health care for poor people. For years the private sector was uninterested in providing health care to uninsured patients and those with public assistance. This lack of interest, and at times deliberate neglect, ensured that the patients in our practice would be able to continue care at our health center without interruption. Only when patients landed steady jobs with guaranteed health insurance from an HMO did they leave the practice for good. In recent years such success has become a source of mutual loss. For instance, I worked for eight years with one young woman, first as a teen mother, later as a mother of asthmatic children, and finally as a battered woman. With great determination, she recovered from many setbacks and married her second husband, a serious man with a regular job and benefits. She was forced to transfer her care and that of her three children to the largest local HMO. I still take care of her mother, sister, and brother, and she occasionally brings her mother for visits. She has now finished two years of college and passed the entrance exam to become a respiratory therapist. We both miss the chance to reminisce about the hard road she has traveled and to celebrate the enormous leaps she has been able to make. We try to make up for our loss of contact around the edges of her mother's visits. This sustaining clinical relationship was amputated because her family was finally doing well enough to become a desirable commodity in the medical marketplace. A feminist critique of such "managed" competition must recognize the destructive effect of the market on healing relationships.

Within family medicine, my home within medicine, I have found a small group of feminist family doctors who join me in developing a feminist approach to our work. But family medicine as a field is unclear in its writings about the relevance of feminism to health care. In reality, family medicine and feminism are strange bed partners. Although it benefited from the reform energy of the 1960s and 1970s, family medicine evolved from a masculine predecessor, general practice. Family medicine training programs sprang up around the country directed by male general practitioners who had seen the need for a new specialty to address widespread dissatisfaction over the increasing subspecialization and depersonalization of medical care. These program directors were as baffled by the needs of women students and residents as were men in any other field of medicine. At the same time family medicine did share a number of assumptions with feminism: that we all should be cared for as persons, not as body parts; that the body and the mind cannot be split off from each other; that persons should be seen in context, not as isolated organisms; that persons have a right to understand and make decisions about their bodies. I use the word *persons* because, though family medicine would champion all these statements, if the word *women* were substituted, many family medicine leaders would balk at the apparent feminism of these assumptions.

Claiming standard academic neutrality, family physicians are likely to believe that good health care for families combines thoughtful caring and scientific practice for all family members regardless of gender. Many male family physicians are likely to believe that feminist concerns about health care have been addressed by the increasing number of women health professionals and the heightened consciousness about women's health in the last twenty years. Yet if we examine feminism's active concerns, we find that family medicine as a discipline is unlikely to agree wholeheartedly with certain feminist tenets:

- Women have been and continue to be exploited and oppressed.
- A commitment must be made to change this condition.
- A critical perspective on the intellectual traditions that support the oppression of women must be developed (Walker & Thompson, 1984; Acker, Barry, & Esseveld, 1983).

My goal in writing this book is twofold: to show how traditional male medicine continues to be an intellectual tradition that is oppressive to women, and to show how a medicine transformed by feminism would require a change in how we look at persons and at the relationships between persons. I have drawn on writings across medical disciplines, since all medicine, not just family medicine, derives from an oppressive intellectual tradition. The first part of the book addresses the first goal through an examination of bias in the theoretical groundings of modern medical care. The second half is devoted to a feminist reconsideration of the clinical relationship.

In the first two chapters I look at how writings about infant, child, and adult development in medicine assume that men's outlooks and experiences are representative of the viewpoints and experiences of women. In other words, medicine applies the template of male development to all of human development. Careful scrutiny of the conceptual framework underlying common health care teachings about infants, children, adolescents, and adult women reveals a preoccupation with separation and autonomy, key themes in male identity. This view exemplifies the assumption that all mature adults are fundamentally separate. In this construction, women's adult development appears as a limited or truncated version of male development: women are viewed primarily in terms of their family commitments and reproductive status (chapter 2). In these two chapters I also begin to sketch the outlines of another way of looking at human beings—not as separate and autonomous units but as beings-in-relation, each connected in increasingly complex ways to others, from infancy on (Jordan, Kaplan, Miller, Stiver, & Surrey, 1991). The clarification of the themes of relatedness rather than separateness in women's vision of adulthood permits a reframing of development theory for both women and men and offers an alternative to conventional understandings of family life cycle theory.

In chapter 3, I show how family medicine's unquestioning adherence to the family life cycle turns on another set of assumptions about women: that they are essentially heterosexual and reproductive figures whose role revolves around their assumed complementarity with men.

Another favorite family medicine belief, the notion of the family system, interferes with the examination of women's health and safety in the family. Chapter 4 examines how family systems theory, the reigning model of family interaction, fails to provide an adequate explanatory or treatment framework for the problems women experience in families. In dealing with violence against women in families, systems theory promotes the clinician's stance of neutrality and objectivity, thus supporting the status quo in violent families. Moreover, the language of systems theory obscures the reality of violence against women. Both family life cycle theory and family systems theory lock women into unchanging positions and prevent the possibility of viewing women in-relation. When applied to incest and sexual abuse of children, widespread secrets of family life, family systems theory obscures the crucial power inequalities that allow and perpetuate sexual misconduct across generational lines. Family systems theory thus exonerates men for their role in violence against women and the sexual abuse of children by blaming the system or by obscuring the power differential between men and women.

Violence against women is not only a matter of battering. When I began this book, child sexual abuse was considered an occasional crisis in pediatrics. It had not been linked to battering or to rape, not even in the textbooks that addressed these problems. But rape crisis centers and battered women's shelters were making the connection. Women in consciousness-raising groups were making the connection. Women bringing sexual harassment suits were making the connection. When the director of the health center sat down across from me at the annual picnic and jokingly said to the male intern next to him, "I'd like to date my secretary's daughter [age ten], but she won't let me,"—I finally made the connection. Chapter 5 outlines the traditional medical and psychiatric interpretations of childhood sexual abuse and confronts these self-serving accounts with the ever-growing evidence of the universality of male sexual violence toward children. I draw on survivors' accounts to link battering, rape, and sexual abuse as manifestations of the patriarchal abuse of power.

The second half of the book is a feminist reexamination of the doctor-patient relationship. It is fashionable in contemporary medical literature to consider the doctor-patient relationship as a contract, a notion that implies equality between separate and autonomous persons and ignores the enormous power differential between doctor and patient. Contracts, made between separate persons who are assumed to have conflicting interests, require negotiation skills. The contractual approach thus excludes from consideration relations of trust between persons of unequal power (mother-infant, teacher-student, caregiver-sick person). Chapter 6 details how the idea of contract exemplifies the subtlety, at a theoretical level, of the male bias in medicine.

Feminist reconsiderations of persons caring and being-cared-for prompt alternative ways of looking at *what* we know and *how* we know when we are in-relation. Chapter 7 fleshes out the idea of connected knowing (Belenky, Clinchy, Goldberger, & Tarule, 1986) as it relates to clinical work. I contrast the medical tradition of separate knowing with connected knowing in four areas—context, time span, believability, and empathy—and show in detail my use of connected knowing in considering the life history and family context of my patients. Clinicians, too, are in-relation. Chapter 8 takes up the touchy area of what doctors tell about themselves to patients, setting these disclosures within the theme of mutuality in clinical work. Mutuality exemplifies involvement (rather than neutrality) and subjectivity (rather than rationality). Such disclosures offer an opportunity to examine one example of a potentially feminist practice in the doctor-patient relationship.

The theme of mutual self-realization, the height of what Whitbeck calls "core feminist practice" (1983), is an important one in the last two chapters, on caring and power. A being-in-relation approach allows caring to take center stage in clinical work, in contrast to the masculinist emphasis on rationality, objectivity, and rules for responsibility within relationships. In chapter 9 I look at what it means to care for patients in long-term clinical relationships. Even the idea of caring suffers from contamination by the language of separateness; it is necessary to talk about "connected caring" and "connected empathy" and "care respect" to move beyond the usual medical meanings of these terms. I draw on writings in nursing, mothering, and teaching to show that caring-in-relation is a feminist understanding drawn from the skilled work of women in many fields who have discovered similar themes simultaneously.

These understandings lead to the realization that a feminist view of clinical relationships requires us to think about power in a new way. Placing caring at the center of the relationship supplants the conventional negative understanding of power between doctor and patient with a redefinition of the enabling and growth-promoting nature of power within the healing relationship. Such enabling is only possible when caring is the context of clinical work.

Chapter 10 takes up the requirement that we arrive at a new formulation for clinical work that makes empowerment—long the watchword of the battered women's movement—the goal. Being-in-relation offers a theoretical and practical basis for a transformation of medical power relations, grounded in the reality of the connectedness of patients and clinicians, in their lives and with each other.

This book is both personal and theoretical. I start from my own life and my own work in family medicine. I draw on stories of patient care from my own practice and from the work of my colleagues. I have tried to be faithful to the clinical events while changing names and other particulars to protect patients' privacy. Some of our patients have read these accounts and agreed to have their stories included (Mrs. Rodriguez, Mrs. Santana and her daughter Jessica, Mr. Powers, Mrs. O'Donnell, Sheryl Sharmat). Because many years have passed since I began collecting these stories and some patients have long since left Worcester, others have not done so. My rendering of these events comes from a clinical standpoint and necessarily reflects the position of someone who has done relational work in medicine for twenty years.

Even though family medicine is my anchor in medicine, I do not see it as the only clinical possibility for patients and clinicians seeking a feminist perspective. Among those patients who choose to go to doctors, many will elect other kinds of specialists besides family practitioners. Among clinicians, those with feminist ideals will not always find themselves suited by interest or temperament to the work of family practice. And physicians are not the only important clinicians. Nurse-practitioners and physician's assistants provide health care in innumerable settings, including our health center, where they care for patients and families in the offices next door to family doctors and family practice residents. All kinds of patients and all kinds of clinicians can examine health care from a relational perspective. The medicine I write about is a broad spectrum of clinical work as conducted by a variety of practitioners.

Women need health care to change. I am not arguing for the creation of a women's health specialty; such a course would affect health care only for a privileged minority. Real change would make a difference to those women who perform the vast majority of caring work for the dependent and ill, young and old, and who, in the course of this work, arrange most medical care for children and for their families. Doing this work, women have innumerable encounters with a variety of health care professionals. All of these interactions need to be informed by a feminist approach both to the identified patient and to the woman who brings in that patient. If only a minority of practitioners are trained to care for women, then all the other clinicians whom women will meet in the course of their caring work for their families will follow the traditional medical approach emphasizing the separateness of persons rather than their relatedness. This is inadequate. All clinicians need to change.

Doctors, of course, are going to be regarded by many patients and by many of the other clinicians in health care as the most powerful, most important, and most influential of the practitioners they see. And doctors do see large numbers of patients and form relationships with these patients over the years and throughout the course of various illnesses as well as of ordinary health care. A few doctors are explicitly committed to the goals of feminist practice. Others who may have had little exposure to feminist thought are nevertheless implicitly committed to these goals. Through personal experience of prejudice or oppression, or such experiences of loved ones, they have become open to feminist ideas. Many can understand that the privilege and power that characterize their status and practice are sources of oppression to others and are looking for ways to transform their practice. These physicians may find my perspective helpful.

A being-in-relation approach makes it possible to bring a coherent feminist perspective to clinical work in health care. Despite the enormous power inequities, I believe that clinical practice can be transformed, that the experiences of those out of power can be brought to bear on medical practice. Perhaps only a minority of practitioners of various kinds will be open to this viewpoint. Nevertheless, relationships with these practitioners will be crucial for their patients. Whether a nurse, a therapist, a doctor, or a social worker, each practitioner can examine his or her work as a person in relation to patients and can work to make that relationship healing for the patient and transformative for self. Such a transformation is my goal in writing this book.

PART I

CHAPTER 1

Infant and Child Development

> Whether boy or girl, the 2-year-old is especially prone to dramatize the mother-baby relationship through dolls and otherwise. In a dim way he is beginning to understand this relationship which means that he himself is becoming somewhat detached from his mother. Only by increasing this detachment can he achieve an adequate sense of self.
>
> Arnold Gesell, *The First Five Years of Life* (1940)

> It must be difficult for a mother to see why a child needs to be punished or rejected to establish himself as a separate person, but perhaps it is as simple as that—when he is intensely loved, it is even more difficult to separate. When his behavior creates even a temporary ambivalence in his parent, then he can more easily feel his separateness.
>
> T. Berry Brazelton and Bertrand G. Cramer,
> *The Earliest Relationship* (1990)

T HE THEME OF SEPARATENESS has dominated descriptions of child development for at least fifty years. Since this idea of personhood, which has long shaped prevailing ideas about infants, children, and adolescents, has been so durable, it is difficult to see that it is a cultural construct. Instead, we believe that these contemporary accounts of development are based on scientific facts or self-evident truths. Feminists have uncovered the bias against women in medical texts (Scully & Bart, 1973) and in medical practice (Barrett & Roberts, 1978), but they have made no comparable scrutiny of the medical approach to infant and child development. An examination of the approach to development in medicine and related fields shows that the pervasive theme of separateness reflects a characteristically male image of development.

Although the study of development does not comprise a large part of training in most health care disciplines, certain assumptions about infant, child, and adolescent development are central to the fields that deal with children and families. Here we will reconsider the widely held view that autonomy and independence are the goals of infancy and adolescence. An investigation of the meaning of autonomy for developmentalists reveals an underlying viewpoint about the nature of human beings. The goals of development, which initially appear gender-neutral, under scrutiny emerge as highly gendered—specifically, as strongly influenced by concepts of male identity. This examination of a pervasive theme in teachings about infant and child development provides a first step toward understanding how male concerns about identity have shaped our notions of what it means to become a human being.

INFANCY

Much of the contemporary view of infant development finds its origin in Freud's description of the child's capacity to form relationships; his analysis later evolved into object relations theory. Freud imagined the infant, initially seen as fused in a primitive union with the mother, gradually separating from the inchoate enormity of the mother. The path of infant development led from fusion to independence. Lingering fusion with the female figure was thought to be the source of pathology. Herein lies the notion that dependence is synonymous with what is pathologic, not manly; independence is the goal. Autonomous, separate is healthy; dependent, coupled is childish, or worse, sick. One pediatrics text thus portrays toddlerhood as the time when autonomy and dependence clash: "The child's feeling of power and sense of omnipotence are disabused by increasing parental demands and by his ability to recognize his dependence and relative helplessness. His aggressive urges and his need for love and approval are in conflict with each other. He is ambivalent, aggressive, independent, negativistic, and helpless and clinging" (Vaughan & McKay, 1975, p. 61).

Erik Erikson, following Freud, proposed the "epigenetic principle" (1968, p. 92), by which he meant the "prescribed sequence" of development that unfolds in invariate stages, each in its own time. Each stage is an advance over previous stages, and unresolved themes from previous stages indicate regression or delay. Erikson's stage theory, which continues to dominate popular ideas about human development, consists of the "Eight Ages of Man": basic trust, autonomy, initiative, industry, identity, intimacy, generativity, and ego identity (1963, p. 247). He describes the separation from the mother as occurring during the stages of basic trust and autonomy; this separation is the first of three crises of "wholeness" in the formation of human identity (1968, p. 86). More positive about the initial fusion with the mother than Freud, but no less definite about the need for separation, Erikson locates the timing of the first primordial separation in the mother's response with pain or anger to the infant's biting. Her reaction produces in the child a sense of "basic loss, leaving the general impression that once upon a time one's unity with a maternal matrix was destroyed. . . . This stage seems to introduce into the psychic life a sense of division and a dim but universal nostalgia for a lost paradise" (1968, p. 101).

Next Erikson defines autonomy as the stage when maturation of motor control permits the child to hold on to or let go of bowel movements. If the parent mismanages this stage, shame and self-doubt in the child are the result. As with each stage, Erikson makes a link between the stage in human development and a basic element in society, because "the human life cycle and man's institutions have evolved together" (1963, p. 250). He ties the autonomy of the period of toilet training to the principle of law and order in institutional contexts and to the development of a sense of justice in economic and political life. I will return to this connection between the notions of autonomy and law and order in chapter 6, but at present it is enough to note the centrality of autonomy in Erikson's view of persons.

Eriksonian notions of infant development continue to dominate traditional pediatric teachings. One pediatrics text (Hoekelman, Friedman, Nelson, & Seidel, 1992) uses the term "psychosocial development" as synonymous with Eriksonian development, with basic trust occupying the first year of life, and autonomy the second year, beginning in infancy but usually not "fully realized " until toddlerhood (p. 531). Separation and independence from the mother occupy center stage in the rendering of development offered to students of medicine. The following passages are typical of the view of infancy that has dominated pediatric training for the past twenty years:

> The demands on mother and infant during the first year are for the development of comfortable interactions which will lead to the infant's movement from a position of dependency to one of independent activity.

> The ego of the mother complements and supplements the ego of the child. As the child's ego and initiative develop, however, she must gradually turn over to the child an increasing amount of responsibility for himself until he is able to function relatively autonomously and independently. (Vaughan & McKay, 1975, pp. 24, 56)

A decade later, the fourteenth edition of the same text promotes the same understanding:

> When the infant begins to walk and talk, the emerging ability to separate from the parent and to display individuality is established. The

infant must become comfortable with an optimal balance of dependence and independence to promote the emerging sense of self. Many parents feel uneasy as the infant struggles to gain increasing control over the environment. (Behrman, Kliegman, Nelson, & Vaughan, 1992, p. 46)

Here is the parallel section from a leading family medicine text:

The early symbiosis must give way rapidly to individuation and autonomy. The healthy family is well able to nurture this growth and enjoys the oppositional quality of the toddler. "No!" is frequently one of the early words learned and practiced. "Pick-it-up" is played daily around high chair and play pens. Both activities serve to reinforce the separateness of the child from his or her parents and to test the ability of the child to influence the parents' behavior and the ability of the parents to be influenced by the child. The underlying issues are autonomy and power. (Taylor, 1983, p. 18)

These authors use the commonsense understandings of the terms "separateness," "autonomy," and "independence" to mean "self-sufficiency and distance from others"; I believe this sense of the term "autonomy" is closest to their intentions. But as we have seen, the force behind the perception of a need for separateness is a psychoanalytic interpretation of infancy. If we can set aside this underlying schema, we find that infants are born with abilities to manage their physical separateness and to shape relationships.

Empirical research shows that infants are born with fabulous capacities to manage and respond to their environment. Daniel Stern, in *The Interpersonal World of the Infant* (1985), argues that the subjective world of the infant has been ignored by both the psychoanalysts and the developmentalists.[1] Psychoanalysts in particular are responsible for the "adultomorphizing" of infant behavior. Stern points out that theorists pin the timing of autonomy and separation at different points in infant development: at the time of stranger anxiety, at the time of being able to wander away, at the time of saying no, at toilet training, and so on. In contrast, research on infant eye movement shows that within the first two months of life an infant shows the ability to initiate, maintain, and break off social interactions through the control of gaze. This finding means that from the very beginning infants can actively shape their relationships through engaging or disengaging in eye contact. Responsiveness to high-pitched voices and close faces is further evidence that the infant can elicit the complex responses in parents that serve to stimulate and nurture the infant. The persistence of the qualities of infant temperament, such as rhythmicity and excitability, from early infancy into later childhood further confirms that infants are distinct persons who bring their own unique attributes into relationships from the outset (Birns, 1985; Thomas & Chess, 1977). Thus, infants do not "separate"; they shape their relationships.

Over the past decade, pediatrics texts have begun to acknowledge infants' early ability to engage in and disengage from social interactions (Behrman et al., 1992). Despite this change, the standard pediatric and family medicine references continue to view infant separateness as a developmental stage. Anatomical separateness is not at issue. Once born, the infant begins a life that is bodily its own, with feelings and perceptions that no other can ever experience in the same exact way. But the infant is no more separate at a year or two years than at birth. Childhood is, of course, characterized by increasing competence: the two-year-old wanders off in the store to grab a candy bar; the seven-year-old takes her allowance to the same store, selects a candy bar, pays, and counts her change. We can see these capacities as moves toward separateness or as expanding skills that allow children to shape and reshape their relationships. The inability to see these skills as relational competencies reflects a bias—a central preoccupation with separateness and independence as the core of development.

The bias in this view of development is ideological as well. Janet Surrey identifies this bias in the underlying belief "that the person must first disconnect from relationship in order to form a separate, articulated firm sense of self or personhood" (1991b, p. 36). The prerequisite of disconnection probably originates in the Freudian notion of the Oedipus complex: boys relinquish their mothers out of fear of castration by their fathers, and girls relinquish their mothers out of rage over castration (Stiver, 1991a). In her feminist reworking of psychoanalytic conceptions of infancy, Chodorow (1978) attributes to "asymmetrical parenting"—parenting by mothers—the gender differences in early experiences of separateness: mothers experience sons as "male opposites" and distance them; in contrast, mothers identify with daughters and regard them as extensions of themselves. Chodorow's contribution to our understanding of development is to show that parenting shapes male separateness and female relatedness. Separateness has different meanings for each gender.

Thus, the idea that separateness must precede identity is not gender-neutral. Identity rooted in sameness may be more typical of girls' experience, and boys may differentiate themselves through separation. Certainly the expectations of adults and their own peers reinforce for children these gendered constructions of what it means to be a girl or boy. Separateness, independence, and autonomy are characteristics stereotypically attributed to male identity. Later these same attributes are linked to prevailing images of mental health for adults in general (Broverman et al., 1970). The bias in the above portrayal of infancy lies in the preferential designation of these gender-identified qualities as the goal of development. These preferred qualities are, in addition, culture-bound. Well-known comparative studies of Japanese and American infants show differences in infant behavior by three to four months of age in response to cultural patterns of mothering (Caudill & Weinstein, 1969). Nevertheless, Western valorization of autonomy in infant development persists as if it were a universal, gender-free standard of infant development.

How can we reshape our ideas about what happens to infants as they grow? It is important to review here what infants actually do. They develop their motor control and their capacity for communication; that is, they can do more and say more. In the cognitive realm, their sense of themselves and of others becomes far more elaborate. Objects, persons, and relationships develop permanence. But do these developing capacities constitute separateness and independence? Take, for example, the observation that the infant of two months can choose to maintain or to break away her or his gaze. This could be construed as the preliminary gestures of separateness; we could also describe it as the infant setting a pace of interaction with the parent and thus taking an active role in shaping the relationship. What is at issue here is the focus: on separateness, or on *being in relation to*. I use this awkward-sounding term to call attention to the fact that the emphasis on separateness ignores the infant's growing ability to be an active participant in creating the connection with parents and others.

If the goals of development are imbued with masculine bias, the development of the female infant child and adult poses a conceptual dilemma. Freud himself foundered on this point, and contemporary developmentalists still struggle to clarify how gender fits into normal development. To address this problem, Chodorow locates separateness as a feature of the male pathway to identity: the mother pushes the son toward a more "emphatic individuation." In contrast, the daughter develops her sense of identity within the context of her primary connection with the mother (1978, p. 167). We begin to see that it is difficult to discuss the question of infant identity without immediately addressing the formation of gender identity.

Feminist object relations theory attributes gender differences to the differential behaviors of a mother toward male and female infants. Empirical behavior-based studies lend support to the idea that mothers treat boys and girls differently in ways that may foster the separateness thought typical of male infant development (Aries & Olver, 1985). Of course, such a focus on maternal-infant behavior excludes from consideration the myriad family and social influences that reinforce gender distinctions. Yet even if object relations theory could clarify the origins of gender identity, it does not explain why the masculine template of separation has become the standard for the medical understanding of all infant development. It appears that stereotypical male attributes—

autonomy, separateness, and independence—are translated backward onto infant development. Thus, the notion of separateness as a goal of development derives from a gendered construction of what develop- ment means.

A FEMINIST PERSPECTIVE

"Being-in-relation" theory (also called self-in-relation theory) is an emerging theoretical perspective on development that emphasizes the condition of connectedness and relatedness. A group of feminist psy- chologists and psychotherapists at the Stone Center for Developmental Services and Studies at Wellesley College has proposed this alternative way of thinking about development. They note that being-in-relation theory

> makes an important shift in emphasis from separation to relationship as the basis for self-experience and development. Further, relationship is seen as the basic goal of development: i.e. the deepening capacity for relationship and relational competence. The self-in-relation model assumes that other aspects of self (e.g. creativity, autonomy, assertion) develop within this primary context. . . . There is no inherent need to disconnect or to sacrifice relationship for self-development. (Surrey, 1991c, p. 53)

In this way of thinking, the bond between mother and infant is viewed as an increasingly rich articulation between two individuals; as the infant develops, the ties evolve further. The already intricately inter- woven responses between parent and infant in the newborn period become an ever more complex web of interdependency during the first year of life.

In the example of the toddler games of "no" and "pick-it-up" cited earlier, Taylor identifies parent-infant interaction as central, but he con- cludes by choosing autonomy and power as the crucial infant attrib- utes. From a being-in-relation perspective, we can reframe these games as further unfolding of the relationship. A power-based interpretation of these interactions uses the fashionable term of "testing limits" to describe such toddler activities; a relational model sees the infant ask- ing, "What kinds of things can I do to keep this going?" One theory calls this independence; another, the development of a highly intricate dance between two differentiated human beings or a moment in the evolving process of attachment (Lerner & Ryff, 1978). The capacity for self-direction is present almost at the outset; this capacity is exactly what is required for relating to another person.

Being-in-relation theory begins with the recognition of human relat- edness and places empathy at the center of the relationship. Surrey, in explaining the origins of girls' and women's greater capacity for emotional closeness and relatedness, identifies the continuation of the infant's capacity for empathy as essential to the later ability to feel emotionally connected to others.

> The mother's easier emotional openness with the daughter than with the son, and her sense of identification with this style of personal learning and exploration probably leave the daughter feeling more emotionally connected, understood and recognized. . . . The mutual sharing process fosters a sense of mutual understanding and connection. For boys, the emphasis on early emotional separation and the forming of an identity through the assertion of difference fosters a basic relational stance of disconnection and disidentification. (Surrey, 1991c, p. 56)

This disconnection emerges in the language of separation and independence in the medical texts cited earlier, revealing what happens "when the principles of male development are cast as universal principles of human development" (Surrey, 1991c, p. 52). Casting infant activity in the language of autonomy reflects the centrality of separateness in the masculine worldview and implicitly presents a male image of infant development. The patterns of interdependence, or relatedness, considered typical of girls and women either appear aberrant or go unrecognized. Moreover, the possibility that interdependence and connectedness characterize all human beings disappears. Thus, the language of development excludes what might be girl-like from its imagery while at the same time cutting boys off from connection. As we turn to look at adolescence, we can see how the privileged themes of separateness and independence continue to structure the medical belief system accepted as the science of development.

CHILDHOOD AND ADOLESCENCE

Turning again to Erikson, we find that highly gendered language continues to dominate his description of later development in childhood. After the infant stages of basic trust and autonomy, Erikson described two further stages called initiative and industry. During the initiative stage, the child goes through a second "crisis of wholeness," during which the superego, or "guardian of conscience," develops. Erikson chooses male imagery and military metaphor to describe the superego: "While at one time answering to a foreign king, this governor-general now makes himself independent, using native troops (and their methods) to combat native insurrection" (1968, p. 86). Here a military and imperialist metaphor perpetuates the masculine construction of conscience. Where are the peacekeepers, the tenders of children, the farmers, the teachers in this internal landscape? And what about ambassadors, emigrants, and negotiators?

Not only the conscience but also the activities of the stage of initiative are strongly gendered: initiative "adds to autonomy the quality of undertaking, planning and 'attacking' a task for the sake of being active and on the move" (Erikson, 1963, p. 255). Erikson describes this kind of initiative as "being on the make," with an emphasis "on phallic-intrusive modes" in the boy. "In the girl it turns to modes of 'catching' in more aggressive forms of snatching or in the milder forms of making oneself attractive and endearing" (p. 255). He locates "man's aggressive ideals" in this initiative stage where he finds "a latent and often rageful readiness in the best and the most industrious to follow any leader who can make goals of conquest seem both impersonal and glorious enough to excite an intrinsically phallic enthusiasm in men (and a compliance in women) and thus to relieve their irrational guilt" (1968, pp. 121–22).

Although gender-stereotyped behaviors may be well established in children by school age, to define "intruding" for boys and "snatching" and "catching" for girls as inevitable stage-related activities is highly sexualized projection. The implication for a girl's development is that by this stage her socialization is "closed off, internalised, and consigned to the unconscious long before she ever reaches adulthood" (Enders-Dragaesser, 1988, p. 583). The determinism implicit in stage theory thus contains an "unadmitted devaluation of girls' and women's later experience" (p. 583).

Eriksonian stages face an additional challenge from research. Empirical work with latency-age boys casts doubt on the centrality of "industry" for this age group and suggests the importance of "relational competence" in the development of boys' self-esteem; boys with behavior problems responded better to a program that fostered emotional sharing and empathic inquiry with each other and their teachers than to a task-oriented program based on making a project to bring home (Wenston & Jarratt, 1988). In the arena of academic mastery, boys' reading difficulties, usually thought to be due to biological predisposition, may actually reflect their response to social exclusion by other boys (Best, 1989). These findings conflict with Erikson's emphasis on activity over relationship for school-age boys and suggest that his focus may have obscured the role of relationships in both boys' and girls' development.

Drawing on Erikson, descriptions of adolescence offer different pathways for boys and girls. For instance, one medical textbook claims that achievement and independence are boys' tasks in midadolescence, best worked through in a group, while girls are "developing interpersonal skills and love," best achieved in dyadic relationships (Behrman et al., 1992, p. 31). The same text collapses Erikson's stages of identity and intimacy into adolescence, with identity occupying early adolescence and intimacy the later part with the beginning of sexual relations.

The generic description of adolescence in medical texts again emphasizes the tasks of separation and independence.

> The major psychosocial developmental task of early adolescence is that of initiating independence from the FAMILY, and it is at this time that earlier familial homeostasis may be most evidently disrupted. . . . The adolescent's unspoken wish for limit-setting is in conflict with his or her need for autonomy. (Behrman et al., 1992, pp. 30–31)

> The issue of independence in the adolescent family is of a complementary nature and stems from the extension of the growing autonomy of the child from infancy onward. . . . During [the launching] stage, the family must give up ties of dependence of the child on the parents, and replace them with the more mature ties of interdependence between adults. (Taylor, 1983, p. 18)

We can ask: Is this focus on independence in adolescence, like the construction of autonomy in infancy, a view of adolescent growth that is biased from the male perspective? Is it also possible that this focus describes adolescence from the position of whiteness? Might not African-American adolescents and other teenagers from communities of color face a set of social realities that impose different requirements on their development? We are just beginning to learn about the complex set of recognitions about adversity, leadership, and community that adolescents of color must make in the course of their development. Independence may have little to do with it (Ward, 1990).

The work of Carol Gilligan illuminates the masculinist bias of standard development teachings. Her book *In a Different Voice* (1982) identifies the male bias underlying Kohlberg's (1981) moral development theory, according to which six stages form a progression from concrete to more abstract levels of moral reasoning. In this schema, girls and women often appear less developed because of their concern with feelings and relationships, a concern that Kohlberg places at a middle stage in moral development. The application of universal rules constitutes the highest stage.

Gilligan argues that relationships take precedence over rules in girls' moral thinking: "For women, the moral problem arises from conflicting responsibilities rather than from competing rights. . . . This conception of morality as concerned with the activity of care centers moral development around the understanding of responsibility and relationship just as the conception of morality as fairness ties moral development to the understanding of rights and rules" (1982, p. 19). Although feminists and nonfeminists alike have hotly debated the empirical validity of

Gilligan's work (Auerbach, Blum, Smith, & Williams, 1985; Friedman, Robinson, & Friedman, 1987; Kerber, Greeno, Maccoby, Luria, Stack, & Gilligan, 1986; Walker, 1984), one contribution of hers is clear: she tackled the assumptions in moral development stage theory and showed how patterns considered typical of male development were assumed, without supportive evidence, to be more highly developed than women-identified patterns, which were regarded as less adult, less complex, less mature.

Even in the rather abstract realm of moral development, pediatrics texts continue to reflect a male perspective. Over the past twenty years, this perspective has evolved: "Man not only plays, but is also uniquely capable of creative activity. As a social being he has had to develop a system of values for guiding behavior. He makes laws and concerns himself with religion and philosophy. In so doing he develops a conscience or superego" (Vaughan & McKay, 1975, p. 56). Two editions later (Behrman & Vaughan, 1983), the authors have modernized their discussion of moral development in childhood by replacing the superego with Kohlberg's six stages of moral development (pp. 54–55). Today pediatric texts adopt the work of Kohlberg as standard (Behrman et al., 1992; Hoekelman et al., 1992; Sahler & Kreipe, 1991). Gilligan's work may be mentioned, but only in the service of making generalizations about gender differences between adolescent girls and boys (Sahler & Kreipe, 1991). And even though the latest *Nelson Textbook of Pediatrics* admits that the applicability of Kohlberg's theory to girls may be limited, that disclaimer does not alter the adherence to a male model of moral development as the standard by which to judge all development.

A FEMINIST PERSPECTIVE

Privileging autonomy *as separateness* in our construction of adolescence prevents us from seeing how deeply adolescents cherish their connections to their parents. This possibility is just starting to enter the description of adolescence in medical texts (Rudolph, Hoffman, Rudolph, & Sagan, 1991). A revised construction of individuation in adolescence sees it as a dimension of relationships. In fact, the interplay between individuality and connectedness in a family can serve as a measure of both individual and family functioning. Researchers who assigned families the cooperative problem-solving task of planning an imaginary family vacation found that high-scoring families thrived on examining their differences in the context of connectedness (Grotevant & Cooper, 1986).

These researchers view adolescent development as "transformation in the reciprocal patterning of the parent-child relationship rather than in terms of breaking the bond between parent and child. . . . Adolescent identity formation is realized in individuated relationships in which differences are freely expressed within a basic context of connectedness" (Grotevant & Cooper, 1986, pp. 93–94). Teenage career exploration—when socioeconomic conditions do not constrain choice—also occurs within the context of family relations (Grotevant & Cooper, 1988). Autonomy is a feature, but only one feature, of the complex interactions of teenagers with others in their worlds.

The gendered quality of the ideas of separateness and independence are not lost on teenagers. In the interminable verbal dissection of heterosexual relationships, adolescent girls articulate how the relationship, with all its entanglements, is the goal; freedom from constraints, playing the field, and not getting tied down are the boys' lines. Thus, the girls' locker-room folklore teaches them how to make relationships survive while trying to perpetuate boys' illusion of freedom.

Adults may consider heterosexual activity on the part of the teenage girl as rebellious or independent; it can also be seen as part of the search for relatedness and intimacy, occurring within the network of relationships that are important to the girl herself. The cultural context is crucial as well. For instance, a sixteen-year-old Puerto Rican teenager who runs off with her boyfriend may be "eloping," as did her mother and grandmother before her. The relational perspective may seem foreign to parents and health care clinicians who have long interpreted the struggles of the teenage years in terms of Eriksonian autonomy, but teenagers' accounts of their own experience support its usefulness. What follows is a portion of a session in which a counselor helps a young woman explore barriers to using birth control. The text shows the strands of connection as the young woman makes choices about contraception:

Counselor: What does your mother think about sex?

Client: Typical! Honeymoon, marriage, and all that. She really wants me to be a virgin when I get married. When my sister did it at 16, my mother flipped; she didn't stop crying. She kept going around the house saying, "Where did I go wrong?" My sister tried explaining that she didn't go wrong, but she kept crying.

Counselor: So you're saying you don't want to see her upset again, the way she was with your sister.

Client: Yeah, it was awful.

Counselor: Your sister really got to her.

Client: She doesn't understand. She must see it as something dirty and bad. What difference does marriage make? She just wants to pretend that sex doesn't exist.

Counselor: And your feelings about sex?

Client: It's confusing. I love John. I really want to have sex with him. It's okay. I mean, it's good. When I think about her, I get upset. I guess, guilty. But there aren't problems between John and me. Sex is good between us. It's just my mother.

Counselor: It sounds like you like sex and want to continue having it. It's hard to have feelings and values different from your mother's.

Client: Yeah, it's scary. It seems crazy, but I guess I'm supposed to be kind of the same as her. She says things like, "You don't love me anymore," whenever we disagree. I get really upset because I love her.

Counselor: What does all this mean for your decision about contraception?

Client: I have to choose something she won't know about.

Counselor: How do you feel about that?

Client: Okay. A little strange, but so what.

Counselor: How might that strange feeling interfere with using a method?

Client: When I feel weird, I have sex anyway, but I don't use birth control. It's like the birth control makes having sex more real. Like it's really happening.

Counselor: So your feelings towards your mother don't stop you from having sex; it just stops you from using birth control.

Client: Yeah, but it's stupid, because she'd die if I got pregnant. Then she'd definitely know I was having sex.

Counselor: It sounds like you're saying you don't want your feelings about your mother to interfere with your using birth control.

This dialogue, chosen from a text for teaching counseling skills (Spain, 1980), shows that even the choice to have sex, usually thought of as a mark of a teenager's desire for independence, can occur within the context of a girl puzzling out her relationship with her mother: "I do love her. Why can't I do both, love her and have sex? But still, I get confused." Other adolescent girls often turn to their mothers for advice and support when they become pregnant (Rosen, 1980). While classic teachings about adolescence might regard such mother-daughter ties as pathologic, being-in-relation theory considers adolescence a time of maturation of the relational self. Kaplan and Klein (1991) describe this growth among college-age women as including:

- increased potential for entering mutually empathic relationships, with sharing of one's own empathic states and responsiveness to the affect of others;

- relational flexibility, allowing relationships to evolve and change;
- ability and desire to work out conflicts in relationships while maintaining the emotional connection; and
- feeling empowered through relational connection with others, particularly with their mothers. (p. 131)

Empirical support for a relational model of adolescence comes from a study of teenage girls at Emma Willard School in Troy, New York (Gilligan, Lyons, & Hanmer, 1990). These girls defined their sense of autonomy and independence in terms of their relations with others. While they valued their differentiation from others, they found most meaning in being able to share their experiences. "Although our language implies that independence is the polar opposite of dependence, these women tell us that these are not mutually exclusive experiences. . . . Their discussions of independence involve unusual juxtapositions where separation and connection are linked" (Stern, 1990, p. 81). Similarly, the "connectedness" a girl experiences in her family is reflected in her level of involvement with peers. Disengaged, disconnected girls have few reciprocated friendships; girls strongly connected to their families have more cohesive reciprocated peer relationships (Bell, Cornwell, & Bell, 1988). This vision of adolescence challenges the standard understandings of separation and autonomy as the central tasks of adolescence.

The reinterpretation of adolescence in being-in-relation theory begins with a focus on women's development rather than men's. The choice to look specifically at women does not imply that men do not or cannot develop "in relation"; they do, but the process is deliberately obscured in the standard story of male identity formation with its prescribed trajectory toward autonomy. The focus on women takes as a starting point the assumption of the centrality of relationships to development. Previously, post-Freudian theorists regarded women's connectedness as a manifestation of regression (Kaplan & Klein, 1991); being-in-relation theory allows us to reconsider our assumptions and establish an alternative dynamic in the pathway to adulthood.

If autonomy and separateness are to be replaced by a more complex and less gender-biased vision of development, what would this look like? Being-in-relation theorists offer us a "relationship-differentiation" model of development to replace the "separation-individuation" model so pervasive in medical and psychological teaching. The old model failed to explain the depth of human connection and relatedness; human closeness could be talked about only in terms of mother-infant fusion or heterosexual intimacy (Jordan, 1991a). How would the new model be different? It would enable us to regard relationships as evolving over long periods of time. We could interpret the necessary fluctuations in relationships as the mutual adaptation of those in-relation as they act on their need to move closer and further away from people at different times. Such a theory would provide a more ample understanding of relational networks such as child and adolescent friendships, family ties, teaching and mentoring relationships, and adult friendships. Development would not be seen as unidirectional, because new relational competencies would allow old relationships to be transformed. Finally, women's greater capacity for empathy would no longer be devalued as "more permeable ego boundaries" but rather would merit appreciation as a positive and central feature of development (Surrey, 1991c).

Self-in-relation theory proposes a useful alternative to traditional teachings for primary care clinicians involved in the care of the family. These arguments about the nature of human development are central to a feminist clinical practice. By accepting and promoting an understanding of development based on relatedness rather than on separation, a feminist clinical approach can replace theories based on masculinist ideology with conceptions of development that are more inclusive, more universal, and far more congruent with the values women place on relationships. Such an approach requires that we next examine commonly held views of adult development.

CHAPTER 2

Women's Adult Development

> If one were invested in the reconstruction of social institu-
> tions, what view of human development would most favor
> such reconstruction? . . . Theorists who uncritically set out
> to describe contemporary patterns of development typically
> lend implicit support to the status quo.
>
> Kenneth J. Gergen, "The Emerging Crisis in Life-Span
> Developmental Theory" (1980), p. 57

COMMONLY ACCEPTED VIEWS of adult development are based
on the notion of men's developmental trajectory toward presumed autonomy. Written primarily by men about men, these
accounts define male development in terms of separateness instead of
relationships. Medical discussions of adult development have uncritically incorporated these male constructions of development patterns as
the template for all development. The scant medical literature on
women's development considers women's growth only in terms of
their heterosexual and reproductive roles. In contrast, a relational view
of development would not restrict women to such roles but rather
would allow us to discover the variegated paths women pursue.
Clinicians who work with adults of all ages in networks of relationships
with friends and family should find the assumptions underlying a relational picture of development more compatible with clinical work.[1]

Gilligan's work on women's moral development (1982) supports the
popular belief that women tend to define themselves in terms of relationships and men do not. The code words "caring perspective"
became a shorthand term for defining women's difference. An unintended effect of Gilligan's work was to perpetuate common expectations about women's and men's gender roles: men are achievers,
women are nurturers; men accomplish out in the world, women care
for others in the bosom of their families; men are agentic, women are
communal; men are instrumental, women are relational. No thoughtful
look at development can fail to recognize that these stereotypes limit
the full range of possibilities for both sexes. Racism as well restricts

what people of color can accomplish, both by limiting opportunity in the outside world and by creating individual self-doubt and despair.

A more adequate model would take into account how racism and sexual oppression produce a set of developmental problems not addressed in the standard approach to adulthood. For women, such oppressive experiences include child sexual abuse, date rape, wife battering and marital rape, chronically reduced occupational opportunities, excess household and caregiving responsibilities, and well-documented medical and psychiatric morbidity in adulthood. Racism shapes each of these forms of oppression in a distinct manner; women of color may interpret their experiences of, for example, household chores and child care differently because of the racism they and their male partners encounter outside the family setting. A basic question we can ask of any description of adult development is, does it recognize how racism and gender roles circumscribe developmental options? Does it recognize, for instance, how customary expectations about gender roles play directly into cultural prescriptions of men's violence and women's acquiescence? (Kaplan, 1988). The study of human development should not be a study merely of what is, but of what can be.

Surprisingly, the story of adult development is almost absent from medical texts. This omission is all the more striking since development is central to medical thinking about children and adolescents. Outside of medicine, the failure of the adult development literature to address women's development is well recognized (Evans, 1985; Gilligan, 1979; Josselson, 1991; Kaplan, 1988; McGoldrick, 1988; Wrightsman, 1988). Medical texts, however, continue to rely on a model of development based on men. Psychiatry texts typify this orientation by drawing heavily on the stage models of Erikson (1968), Levinson (Levinson, Darrow, Klein, Levinson, & McKee, 1978), and Vaillant (1977) (Kaplan & Sadock, 1985; Stoudemire, 1990). Family practice sources also rely on these standard studies of men (Leaman, 1980; Medalie, 1984). Otherwise, beyond adolescence, medical sources nest adult development within the theory of the "family life cycle."

Medical authors who initially address male midlife development often lapse into generalizations about all adults. In this passage from an article entitled "New Visions of Adulthood," the implication unfolds that male development *is* adult development:

> Each stage is concerned with a familiar life process: separation/individuation—the process by which people "grow up," which includes giving up one's dependence on others, and as a result of this, developing one's own sense of worth and skill, one's own personality, one's own independence. . . . This process (which begins after birth and continues through adulthood) consists of transition periods which are always concerned with separation, followed by periods of settling

down and using one's abilities and skill. Perhaps it is surprising to some that this is the work of adulthood, yet this is the case, and adults, in going through these processes, become increasingly self-sufficient and independent. (Vanderpool, 1977, p. 95)

The values of self-sufficiency and independence permeate writings about physicians as young adults as well. The assumptions about adult development derived from the male studies are applied to all physicians in training, who are seen to be negotiating the predictable stages of individuation and autonomy (Bauchner, 1988; Bergman, 1988). The fact that such stages do not fit the experience of many residents, particularly women, goes unnoticed.

If adult development is synonymous with men's development, what is women's development? The scant references in the medical literature lead the reader to some pernicious false conclusions: that women's development is inconsequential; that women's development does not differ significantly from men's; that women's development is obvious (that is, the family life cycle says all there is to say about women's development); that all women's development is the same, obscuring differences of race and class; and most insidiously, that women's development is *complementary* to men's development. At times this implication of complementarity is interpreted biologically: "With advancing age, sexual differentiation becomes less pronounced as women become more masculine and dominant while their voices deepen and facial features sharpen. In a complementary way, men become more feminine and less dominant and their faces soften and breasts enlarge" (Medalie, 1984, p. 214). This fantasied symmetry ties adult development to sex-linked hormonal changes, a leap unsupported by empirical evidence. The assumption of a biological complementarity between men and women is most insidious because complementarity confines women's identity to heterosexuality and reproduction: caring for husbands and children and, later, aged parents and ailing spouses; maintaining the family while men appear to become increasingly self-sufficient and independent.

The idea of complementarity is overt in Erikson's writings on adult development, and it is also assumed in the empirical studies of Levinson and Vaillant. All three based their work and their theories on the study of middle-class, predominantly white men. Erikson posited four stages in adulthood: identity, intimacy, generativity, and integrity. Men first discover their identity when they establish themselves as separate from others. After identity comes intimacy, a "counterpointing as well as a fusing of identities." Women pose a difficulty for this orderly sequence which Erikson called the "problem of the identity of female youth" (1968, p. 265). For women, according to Erikson, the stages of identity and intimacy are fused: "The stage of life crucial to the emergence of an integrated female identity is the step from youth to maturity, the state when the young woman, whatever her work career, relinquishes the care received from the parental family in order to commit herself to the love of a stranger and to the care to be given to his and her offspring" (p. 265).

Erikson states that young women wonder whether they can "have an identity" before they know whom they will marry (p. 283). It is Erikson himself, however, who seems to believe that women cannot have a meaningful identity outside of their heterosexuality:

> Granted that something in the young woman's identity must keep itself open for the peculiarities of the man to be joined and of the children to be brought up, I think that much of a young woman's identity is already defined in her kind of attractiveness and in the selective nature of her search for the man (or men) by whom she wishes to be sought. . . . Womanhood arrives when attractiveness and experience have succeeded in selecting what is to be admitted to the welcome of the inner space "for keeps." (p. 283)

Speaking twenty years later, after his model had been criticized for its view of women, Erikson still maintained the notion of the openness of women's identity: "It could be that in women the completion of identity might remain relatively open through the intimacy and even some of the generativity period" (Erikson & Erikson, 1981, p. 267). For Erikson, a woman does not shape her own identity; rather, her identity remains to be defined by husband and children. Not surprisingly, research on women using Erikson's model does find that women form their identity in the context of relationships, but this finding is not used to challenge the relevance of the model for women (Josselson, 1991). Family practice sources accept Erickson's highly sex-stereotyped vision of the formation of identity:

> Because the boy's identity will largely be defined by what he does, he spends a great deal of time and energy thinking, planning, and worrying about his future, particularly vocational future. The girl, on the other hand, while not unconcerned about a future vocation, usually is more concerned about finding a desirable (marriage) partner. (Medalie, 1978, p. 169)

In Erikson's sequence, the next step in adulthood after intimacy is generativity: "the concern for establishing and guiding the next generation" (1968, p. 138). For women, generativity is dominated by the maternal role (procreativity), while for men it includes productivity and creativity. Although Erikson's later views permit women access to these other forms of generativity, he remains preoccupied with women's obligation to fulfill procreative responsibilities. His concept of generativity applied to women is inextricably tied to and constricted by motherhood and child care. Erikson's failure to construct a durable notion of women's development is obvious today, but before we dismiss him as outmoded, it is important to recognize that *every current source* on adult development acknowledges a debt to Erikson's work without disclaiming his portrayal of women. Given the stereotyped vision of gender development that he articulated for women, today's reader must also wonder about the utility of his theories of adult development as they apply to men.

The classic empirical studies of adult development omitted women entirely. In 1937 the frequently cited Grant study, described by George Vaillant in his book *Adaptation to Life* (1977), began a longitudinal investigation of several hundred undergraduate men at Harvard.[2] Although Vaillant stated in 1977 that the omission of women was unacceptable, the study continues today (Vaillant & Vaillant, 1990). Similarly, in 1978 Daniel Levinson and his colleagues published their popular book *Seasons of a Man's Life*, based on a study of another forty men. Again the author lamely comments, in the introduction, on the omission of women. These two works on men's development are invariably cited in medical discussions of adult development. We have no comparable studies of women's lives. What is more, any such study of women's lives is not likely to be essentially comparable.

In *Seasons of a Man's Life*, Levinson and his colleagues attempt to construct a universal schema of men's development from a limited sample. Their book achieved instant popularity in part because it addressed a widely felt need to make sense out of men's adult experiences. The relevance for women's development lies not in proving or disproving Levinson's "seasons" of life for women (or men) but rather in identifying the conception of women and of relationships that prevails in *Seasons of a Man's Life*. In Levinson's analysis, the young man's development is shaped around his construction of "the Dream," his fantasied goal in life. He hopes to find a "Special Woman" to nourish him in the quest for his dream. Thus, women appear as adjuncts to men's development who are chosen to further men's careers and ideals. A man's relationship with a woman is a stepping-stone, not an end in itself. Similarly, the relationship with "the Mentor," a senior figure who supports and promotes the young man in his climb up the ladder, is also valued as a means, not an end. The young man uses relationships to achieve, not to define himself.

Levinson's view of men's development as a process in which women are subsidiary and relationships serve men's needs may fit a masculinist image of men's development, but it sheds little light on women's development. Subsequent attempts to apply such a stage model to middle-class white women have not succeeded in validating either the timing or the sequence of stages for these women (Harris, Ellicott, & Holmes, 1986; Reinke, Holmes, & Harris, 1985; Richardson & Sands,

1985). Not surprisingly, they are even less applicable to a forty-year-old Puerto Rican grandmother, an African-American mother with three children on welfare, or a woman who has left her entire family in Vietnam.

Stage theory is problematic even when it is not explicitly masculinist. Real-life examples reveal how it poses problems for a theoretical understanding of both men's and women's development. First, stage theory is difficult to disprove because the data from any individual's life are so rich that the theory becomes "empirically unfalsifiable" (Dannefer, 1984, p. 103). Second, variations are so common that so-called normal development may not be the pathway for any given individual. For instance, the adult life patterns of gay men neither fit nor disprove the model (Kimmel, 1978). Likewise, the study of a single age group tends to obscure the wide range in ages at which persons go through various life changes. For instance, Levinson and Vaillant studied men of the same age group rather than men of different ages doing similar things. The wide variation in ages at which women enter the workforce, complete their education, or have a first child makes stage theory even less relevant to women's development. A perspective that begins with age constancy diminishes the possibility of seeing variation as normal and in fact makes variation seem deviant.

Stage theories also do not take into consideration social conditions and historical events. The study of a group of people of the same age obscures the influence of events experienced uniquely by the whole group, such as the Depression and World War II by Vaillant's group, or childhood in the conservative 1950s and coming of age during the Vietnam War by Levinson's group. Being a thirty-year-old man in 1950 (the typical age of Vaillant's subjects) had meanings and possibilities different from those available to a thirty-year-old man in 1970 (the typical age of Levinson's subjects). Vaillant reports, for example, that the marital satisfaction of women married to the men in the study deteriorated, compared with that of their husbands, after thirty years of marriage (Vaillant & Vaillant, 1993). This finding appears to be correlated solely to the duration of marriage; the study design does not take into account how these women's marital satisfaction may have related to changes in the status of women, to the media portrayal of women, or to the increased visibility and valuation of older women during the 1980s. Such forces influence men's and women's experiences, shape their roles, and frame their development, yet stage theory minimizes their contribution to adulthood.

Stage theory also ignores the fact that every social and historical context contains prevailing belief systems, or "common knowledge," about adult development. "Such knowledge may operate as self-fulfilling prophecy, producing or reinforcing the patterns it presumes" (Dannefer, 1984, p. 108). Social expectations about "normal" development lead people to judge themselves and others by whether they are proceeding "on time" on the adult timetable (Neugarten et al., 1968). Class and culture construct the interpretation of "on time": a contemporary young Puerto Rican woman may feel delayed if she does not become pregnant within a few months of starting a sexual relationship. Historical time also affects what "on time" means: marriage upon college graduation, a goal for educated white women in 1960, has been replaced by the more biologically driven goal for many similar women in the 1990s of having their first baby before age thirty-five.

Lastly, stage theories are essentially organismic: preordained development unfolds from within. Erikson's stages are analogous to embryology in their sequences and are literally based on anatomy when it comes to women, whose identity depends on "filling up" their inner space. A theory rooted in women's biology posits a claim that is immutable and universal. Environment may be harsh or supportive, but it is not key to the trajectory of development. This view of development ignores the role of girls' and women's real experiences. At a fundamental level, such a theory excludes the possibility that women shape and are shaped by the social reality of their lives (Enders-Dragaesser, 1988). Unfortunately, notions of development based on biology quickly devolve into a version of development limited by biology. At a time when biologically driven theories are gaining ground in every discipline, a biologically determined view of women's development is likely to prevail in medicine. Yet whenever such notions are invoked, as frequently occurs in medicine, whenever women's reproductive function is made central if not essential to her identity, women's potential is circumscribed.

A critical approach to women's development must carefully examine the empirical evidence for a reproductive (biological) explanation for social and psychological events. The heterosexual reproductive definition focuses on "filling up" the inner space; emphasizes marriage, childbearing, and mothering functions; ties caring for children, the aged, and the disabled to reproductive caring; and portrays the empty nest as a catastrophe and menopause as the end of meaningful existence. To satisfy this construction of women's adult development, successful completion of biologically driven tasks should result in measurable well-being for women. Loss of such roles should diminish well-being.

But empirical data do not support these assumptions about women. Instead, we find that becoming a parent causes a decline in marital quality (Belsky, Lang, & Rovine, 1985; Cowan & Cowan, 1992; Ross, Mirowsky, & Goldsteen, 1990). When investigators measure the positive and negative aspects of the mothering role among white middle-class women, pleasure is not a significant feature of their experience (Baruch & Barnett, 1986). Among Hispanic women professionals, who are stereotypically expected to become mothers, having small children is associated with decreased personal and professional satisfaction (Amaro, Russo, & Johnson, 1987).

In contrast to the Eriksonian assumption that women's well-being is tied to our reproductive role, empirical data suggest that for women who are mothers, health, longevity, self-esteem, and life satisfaction are related in complex ways to participation in multiple roles outside the family (Miller, Moen, & Dempster-McClain, 1991; Moen, Dempster-McClain, & Williams, 1989). Moreover, the so-called empty nest has long been known to have positive effects on women's individual as well as marital well-being (Glenn, 1975; Harkins, 1978). Many women actively look forward to the departure of their children. Although some mothers must negotiate loss in some role functions, the gains for women and sometimes for married couples are more diverse and profound (Rubin, 1979). Many college-educated women find that the fifties are the prime of life (Mitchell & Helson, 1990). Nevertheless, adult development theory holds only empty or negative imagery for women during this period, implying an end to meaningful development with the end of the reproductive phase (Gergen, 1990).

Menopause itself requires rethinking (Barnett & Baruch, 1978). Cross-cultural studies suggest that culture frames women's view of the process and their symptoms (Lock, 1991). Western physicians have considered women to be far more troubled by menopausal symptoms than women themselves report (Cowan, Warren, & Young, 1985; DeLorey, 1989; Raymond, 1988). Using early studies of small and unrepresentative samples, physicians have been willing to generalize about menopause for all women (Kaufert, 1988; Wilbush, 1981). Physicians seem to think that middle age starts earlier for women than for men, further linking the end of reproduction with aging (American Board of Family Practice, 1991). Even before the current recommendation for widespread use of estrogen replacement therapy to prevent osteoporosis and coronary artery disease, medicine regarded menopause as a deficiency state, and middle age for women as a problem to medicate. The possibility that middle age might be a time of enhanced well-being for women does not arise within the medical approach, with its reliance on a masculinist view of women's adult development.

Women's caring is not tied to reproductive functions. Caring is a kind of glue that holds women in connection to others. Beyond their own children, women care for parents, spouses, grandchildren, siblings, in-laws, neighbors, coworkers, and friends. Women's activism is an extended form of caring about the communities where they live; such caring cannot be passed off as an extension of biological mothering (Naples, 1992). But in the absence of adequate social support, caring can also become an onerous burden. Women's relational ties and relational self-definitions, not heterosexuality and reproduction, motivate their caring.

Thus, the reproductive and heterosexual construction of women's adulthood does not fit empirical findings about their adult experiences. An acceptable model of women's adult development must be applicable to the vast majority of adult women.[3] Yet the normative picture of the reproductive definition is the white middle-class housewife, a picture that reflects less and less of the population and, by omission, defines alternative family structures and people of color as deviant. Single-parent families and so-called minority families are now more representative of the U.S. population than the white middle-class nuclear family (see chapter 3).

Another damning criticism of the reproductive definition of women's identity lies in its implications for those whom it does not "fit." In the reproductive model of development, single women, childless women, and lesbians without children have no hope of achieving a meaningful identity—or their accomplishments are seen as compensation for what they have "lost" or "missed out on." No model that makes so many out to be deviant is acceptable (Allen & Pickett, 1987).

Finally, the reproductive definition omits the importance of paid work in women's identity. Employment for women is associated with lower mortality and better perceived and measured health (Rosenfeld, 1992). Nevertheless, medicine adheres to the belief that working women who are also wives and mothers experience role strain and role overload. The implication of this belief is that it is paid work that adds the strain or overload; the division of labor at home, which often leaves working women with too much to do, is not questioned. Analyzing the sources of women's stress and satisfaction, the sociologists Baruch, Biener, and Barnett (1987) found that family stress was associated with women's psychological distress and illness more than work stress. They argue that it is the quality of roles, not the quantity, that determines life satisfaction. Their work shows that self-esteem correlates with working status: work is a central feature in women's development.[4]

The fact of middle-class and white women's increasing rate of paid employment pushes theorists to incorporate "productive" as well as reproductive roles into an understanding of women's adulthood, overlooking the fact that working-class women and women of color have always had to take on paid work in order to feed their families. The refusal to recognize the importance of work to women also results in the exclusion of women from research on the impact of unemployment (Baruch et al., 1987). Racism compounds this omission by making the false assumption that women with strong cultural ties do not mind the loss of work and the return to their "natural" role. In fact, despite racial and sexual discrimination, Latinas who lost their jobs because of a factory closure suffered long-term economic and family distress (Romero, Castro, & Cervantes, 1988).

Work, of course, is yet another setting in which women may be devalued. Women's work roles often mimic their position in the traditional nuclear family; their lower pay and status are justified by the assumption that theirs is the supplementary wage and that their work is an extension of their nurturant or supportive roles at home (Chow & Berheide, 1988). Consideration of the importance of work in women's adult development must therefore take into account the idea of the *quality* of roles. Race as well frames how women view their family and work roles. Employment may give women more clout in oppressive family situations, but home may be viewed differently by some black women "who view the family as a refuge from the racism of the larger society and who find family work, in contrast to market work, affirming of their humanity" (Dugger, 1988, p. 440). Supporting this viewpoint is a study of black women employed in low-paying, low-status jobs, such as laundry workers, between 1880 and 1930 in Washington, D.C.; the study found that women's unpaid work in their homes was a source of self-worth and pride, unattainable from their paid jobs (Harley, 1990). Clearly, a vision of women's development must consider the race and class context of women's work and family lives. This context may be best understood through women's own portrayals of their lives.

In summary, men's development studies fail to consider women's development at all and mention women only in the role of being complementary to men, of providing the heterosexual and reproductive setting in which men develop. Based on stage theories or biological views of development, commonly accepted notions of women's development not only exclude women who do not conform to these expectations but fail to integrate employment or career into an understanding of women's life course. The experiences of family and work of women of color play no role in shaping the prevailing view of women's adulthood. Not surprisingly, women's own views are missing.

Most problematically, theories of adult development do not consider relationships (as opposed to roles) to be central: the maturation or unfolding of the person does not depend on the context of relationships. For men, relationships are something to separate from (in infancy and adolescence), to acquire (marriage or intimacy in young adulthood), or to use (the Special Woman and the Mentor). Since the tasks of adult individuation for men involve the development of a separate sense of self, relations are not seen as defining or constitutive of (male) identity. For women, relationships disappear into reproductive and heterosexual roles. Exactly how relationships are important in women's adult development is obscured by theorists' preoccupation with marriage and motherhood. Finally, because women's adulthood is envisioned within family roles, it is difficult to understand the relevance of the concept of autonomy for women.

A FEMINIST PERSPECTIVE

Being-in-relation theory provides a very different way to think about how a person develops. A relational sense of self unfolds from infancy through adulthood and is not associated with reproductive or gender role obligations. "For everyone—men as well as women—individual development proceeds *only* by means of affiliation" (Miller, 1976, p. 83). Men are prevented from recognizing this aspect of their development by their quest for autonomy. Women tend to see their affiliations primarily as responding to others' needs. This self-definition can take many forms, but it is likely to become problematic when a woman comes to accept service for others as her main goal, as if she has no needs of her own. Miller argues that this form of affiliation grows out of "the basic domination-subordination model" of human interaction: men achieve mastery and power through separateness, while women place affiliation at the center of their lives. Although affiliation carries the potential for advancing how human beings relate to each other, "the only forms of affiliation that have been available to women are subservient affiliations" (p. 89).

When women define themselves entirely as caretakers and assume that caretaking comprises a relational self, they fail to take care of themselves and thus accept a subservient definition of their adulthood. Miller states that such sacrifice makes women feel depressed and angry and precludes any clear formulation of why they feel that way. Feminists have argued that the antidote to such oppressed caring is more autonomy for women. By this they may mean women's right to economic security regardless of marital status, their right to occupational and educational advancement, their right not to be solely responsible for household and domestic functions, or their right not to have to put others first in every decision. Enforcing these "rights" is essential if we are to move beyond domination and subordination in male-female relationships, but the implication of these concerns for women's development is unclear. Must women, to escape subordination, define themselves as separate from other persons? What would separateness mean for intimate relationships with men and women or for bearing and raising children? Would it require women to put career achievement ahead of relationships with coworkers? The challenge of being-in-relation theory for women's development is to construct development in terms of affiliations and relations that do not compromise the potential for women's autonomy *as women define it*. To see why women's own understanding of autonomy is important, we need first to examine some common understandings of the word *autonomy*.

Hare-Mustin (a family therapist) and Maracek (a philosopher) (1986) distinguish three senses of the word *autonomy*. First, autonomy is self-sufficiency, the opposite of dependence. This is the commonsense use of the term: implied is a Thoreauvian ability to sustain oneself without the help of others. The meaning of help in this context pertains to material goods and services: young adults leaving home and supporting themselves, or older persons wanting to remain in their own homes, not wanting to become dependent (unable to support or do things for themselves).

A second sense of the word *autonomy* is the freedom to choose: having the power to make decisions or take action implies influence, competency, and mastery. The opposite of such autonomy is being subject to paternalism or coercion. This is the ethical or legal sense of the term that pertains in discussions of patient rights. Material dependence (lack of autonomy in the first sense) may result in subordination (lack of autonomy in the second sense); it is frequently true that the one who controls the material goods in a relationship makes the decisions.

Hare-Mustin and Maracek call the third sense of the word *autonomy* the "transactional sense"; they see autonomy and relationship as two opposite ends of a spectrum. This third sense defines a masculine vision of self-identity: achieved free of relationships, independent, separate. Identity involves being in relation to others only insofar as one is free to succeed and free to leave. (This notion of autonomy is sometimes used to justify sexual infidelity; alternatively, infidelity may be an effort to demonstrate this kind of autonomy.) The transactional sense is the gist of the male rendering of autonomy in popular music: "I am a rock; I am an island."

All three meanings are problematic for women's adult development: setting material and physical self-sufficiency as a goal excludes all but middle- and upper-middle-income women and denigrates the development of women who cannot support themselves and their children alone. "Economic dependence, responsibility for children, and institutionalized lack of power rule out self-determination for most women" (Hare-Mustin & Maracek, 1986, p. 209). Having as a goal the freedom to decide one's fate or make choices over one's life appears to value women's rights, but it also supports the illusion that such decision-making occurs detached from relationships with others. In reality, intimate relationships often form the very context of decision-making (Jecker, 1990). The third sense of autonomy insists that identity is achieved only apart from others and denies that relationships are essential to identity. Autonomy in this sense cannot be accepted as the goal of adult development.

These common understandings of the word *autonomy*, based on men's reality, disenfranchise women.

> [Autonomy] carries the implication—and for women the threat—
> that one should be able to pay the price of giving up affiliations in

order to become a separate and self-directed individual. . . . Women are quite validly seeking something more complete than autonomy as it is defined for men, a fuller not a lesser ability to encompass relationships to others, simultaneous with the fullest development of oneself. (Miller, 1976, pp. 94–95)

On the other hand, to criticize autonomy as an alienating concept for women "because it does not reflect their psychological and emotional world"(Yanay & Birns, 1990, p. 252) poses a problem: it appears to confine women to service to relationships without allowing them a sense of selfhood. "Characterizing the woman as other-directed while emphasizing the caring properties of her motivation provokes, reinforces, and reproduces traditional gender stereotypes and images" (Yanay & Birns, 1990, p. 252). Being-in-relation scholarship identifies this problem and pushes for a redefinition of autonomy that recognizes women as in-relation but does not relegate them to oppressed caring, or caring-while-dependent (Miller, 1976; Stiver, 1991c; Yanay & Birns, 1990).

A feminist understanding of autonomy requires reexamination of the meanings of both *dependency* and *independence*. Academic women in a qualitative study conceived of independence in terms of "authenticity of expression"—the ability to say what they really feel. Dependency resided in finding it difficult to express feelings freely, particularly if they might provoke a confrontation. They saw dependency as "an experience of apprehension and withdrawal from expression" (Yanay & Birns, 1990, p. 258). This group of women repudiated the goal of self-reliance in favor of an involved independence—"A relational concept determined not by how well one can separate oneself from others, but rather by how well one can incorporate others into one's life without conflict or tension" (p. 254). These women also pointed out a more positive sense of the word *dependency*: mutual attachment and emotional involvement.

How does this discussion relate to women who are poor? Increasingly today, the term "dependency" has become shorthand for "welfare dependency," implying a condition that is socially and politically objectionable. Clearly, poverty prevents a kind of freedom that is crucial to women—freedom from injustice and freedom to control their own lives. Yet the opposite, "lonely self-sufficiency," is not the center of a feminist revision of autonomy. Connection to kin and neighbors, connections within a culture, are crucial. Women reject the cruelties and injustices but are not seeking detachment (Griffiths, 1992). Emotional and material reliance on parents and children, neighbors and kin, are meaningful kinds of sustenance (Dula, 1994); we do not want to lose this kind of dependence in our revision of autonomy.

The contribution of self-in-relation theory to adult development is the definition of healthy selves as constituted in relations, and as having some recognition that they are so defined. This recognition is one of the real accomplishments of adult development. According to self-in-relation theory, self-definition in terms of subservient relations or relations in which a person is not free to express herself represents an oppressed or unhealthy condition. Furthermore, once we accept the idea that persons are constituted by relations, then we can recognize that the condition of apparent separateness (the transactional sense of autonomy), even when flaunted, is a pretense and, in fact, not healthy (Hare-Mustin, 1988; Hare-Mustin & Marecek, 1986; Miller, 1976). Untangling the knots of pretense and unhealthiness tied to the notion of separateness will enable us to advance our understanding of adult development in relation to others.

For women, the posture of self-reliance is often a cover-up for feelings of insecurity (Yanay & Birns, 1990). Many men adopt the pretense of separateness. The busy male executive or doctor who sees himself as autonomous because of his successful career—and by implication, his lack of dependence on others—is failing to recognize his dependence on the various women who enable him to function in the world: the secretaries, administrative assistants, and nurses who organize his work life to run smoothly; his wife, who maintains the household, the family relations, and the children. He may rely on them to intuit his moods and relieve his emotional distress even when he cannot articulate it. He may acknowledge that choosing the "right" support staff is a key ingredient to success, but this fact does not challenge his belief that the success belongs to him. His autonomy, however, is a self-delusion.

Autonomy defined as separateness is unhealthy for both the person and those around him or her. First, living in a state of pretense is one form of ill health; the aggressive assertion of independence (considered typical of some coronary-prone people) may disguise an internal war between inner feelings of dependence and an outward refusal to acknowledge them (Radley, 1984). Such conflict may explain the erratic swings between recklessness and helplessness that characterize some men's response to becoming ill. Individuals locked in this struggle have trouble attending to their own bodies' symptoms and caring for their bodies properly.

Second, defining oneself as not-in-relation is psychologically unhealthy. I am not referring to the condition of being single; many single people, especially women, do define themselves in terms of relations—with friends, family, the church, and so on. Rather, I am referring to the person (usually male) who defines himself by not-being-in-relation. Such a person may have sexual relations with someone, even over a long period of time, may even father children, but he does not see himself as defined by those connections. This person lives in a state of deprivation. He cannot admit that he needs relationships, and needs that cannot be admitted cannot be easily filled. Isolation and loneliness are the inevitable result; some would call this alienation.

Third, when a person does not define himself in terms of the real and crucial relationships he does indeed have with other human beings, then whatever connection he does claim with them is the connection of a person to an object. Such a connection results in either a posture of indifference toward others in his life or the illusion of ownership or control over them. The posture of indifference has dire consequences for the future:

> There is every reason to react with alarm to the prospect of a world filled with self-actualizing persons pulling their own strings, capable of guiltlessly saying "no" to anyone about anything, and freely choosing when to begin and end all their relationships. It is hard to see how, in such a world, children could be raised, the sick or disturbed could be cared for, or people could know each other through their lives and grow old together. (Scheman, 1983, p. 240)

The illusion of ownership or control over other human beings is unhealthy because it creates a climate that legitimizes destructive forms of social relations, including the physical and sexual abuse of women and children.

Fully developed and mature human beings recognize that they are not relationally self-sufficient, that they are in fact defined by and in terms of relationships. The fullest and most complete sense of autonomy must include an appreciation of our deep connectedness and interdependence with other human beings, especially those closest to us, and an appreciation of noncoercive, collaborative ways of making decisions that affect ourselves and those we are connected to. Miller uses the term "authenticity" for a woman's growing sense of her own center, "a continuous process of bringing forth a changing vision of oneself, and of oneself in relation to the world" (1976, p. 111).

Now we can ask, what is required for a working model of adult development in clinical practice? A satisfactory model of development must address the previous criticisms: it must incorporate a historical and social context; it must be applicable to women without limiting their development to their biology; it must consider the centrality of work as well as family to women's lives; and it must be broad enough to consider women who make a variety of choices—single, without children, with children, working, in-career, noncareer, lesbian, heterosexual. It must take racism into consideration in looking at the experience of women of color. Moreover, such a model must consider development within the context of relationships rather than separate from them, and it must view critically the idea that development consists in striving toward the goal of male-defined autonomy.

One contribution to thinking about adult development that incorporates the historical variables is life-span development theory. Life-span research examines the influence of historical forces on groups of people across time. For instance, American women who were forty years old in the late 1970s were three times more likely to return to paid employment after child-rearing than women who were forty in the early 1970s (Moen, Downey, & Bolger, 1990). Stepping away from stage theory allows us to see how the sequence and timing of life events influences the many paths of women's development (Brim & Ryff, 1980; Hultsch and Plemons, 1979). With approximately thirty years of potential reproductive time overlapping with fifty years of available time as paid workers, women have a wide range of possible choices, timings, and sequences in their family and work lives. Because the status of women—that is, what women are socially and economically permitted to do over the course of their development—is closely tied to changing historical conditions (Lopata, 1987), studies of life span and timing of events have much to offer the study of women's development. The socially constructed meaning of employment itself undergoes transformation across time, even during an individual's life span (Spenner, 1988). Such variation makes the idea of a "model" of development very difficult; women do not pursue a smooth and unidirectional course. Recognition of the historical setting of life events is particularly useful to clinicians, who already acknowledge the differing impact of, for instance, marriage at eighteen and marriage at thirty-five, for both partners; or career change at thirty and career change at fifty; or the implication of unemployment for someone who grew up during the Depression compared with the attitude of someone who grew up during World War II.

The study of life span and timing of events is useful but incomplete. A historically situated vision of women's development that rejects the notion of complementarity with men must also recognize the importance of crucial ongoing adult relationships with persons other than the sexual or marriage partner: such relationships include a woman's friendships with other women (Fox, Gibbs, & Auerbach, 1985), her relationships with siblings, particularly her sisters (Lee, Mancini, & Maxwell, 1990), and her continuing connection with her own mother (Boyd, 1989). The adult daughter-mother relationship can be viewed as an example of friendship or as a model on which friendships are based. Empirical study shows that daughter-mother relationships are stable and enduring despite the role changes for both members of the dyad (Baruch & Barnett, 1986; Boyd, 1989; Walker, Thompson, & Morgan, 1987). Among college women, many list their mother as their best friend or the most important person in their lives (Fox, Gibbs, & Auerbach, 1985; Gleason, 1991). For black and working-class women, the mother-daughter tie may be even more important than it is for white middle-class women (Barnett, Kibria, Baruch, & Pleck, 1988). Whether marked by conflict or intimacy, a woman's ongoing relationship with her mother plays a central part in her adulthood (Stiver, 1991a).

Finally, a satisfactory vision of adult development must be able to make a place for a woman's own conception of her growth, her self-definition (Peck, 1986). One's self-concept is formed amid a matrix of family and social relationships, over the course of time. Though it responds to social expectation, each person's self-concept is distinct. For instance, a woman who reaches her late thirties without a long-term intimate relationship or children makes decisions that may affect how she views her adult development. She may buy a house in which she plans to live alone, or she may consider job and career changes. Her decisions may also be based on her rich friendships with several other women, her close ties to her parents, her deep attachment to her dog, and her active relationships with her nieces and nephews. Her choices reveal how she shapes her own self-definition.

Teresa Peck designed an image that places a woman's self-definition at the center of development (see figure 2.1). Social and historical time, at times constricting, at times flexible, provides the ongoing context of attitudes toward women in general and toward women of her race and class. This dimension draws on theories of life span and timing of events to place a woman's chronological age within real time. (Peck shows how two unmarried women experienced pregnancy differently in 1947 and 1980, reflecting varying degrees of flexibility in the social setting of the same life event at a different historical moment.) A woman's relationships determine the various "spheres of influence" that both press on and respond to pressure from the central core of her growth. Her relationships have a "bidirectional" quality; she shapes and is shaped by them. These relationships include those with her family of origin, sexual partner, friends, and children, as well as those developed in her work. In Peck's model, relationships are characterized by *flexibility* and *elasticity*. Flexible relationships can expand or contract to include or limit new relationships, but inflexible ones (such as marriage to a battering man) narrowly restrict other connections. Elastic relations stretch to meet changing needs in a woman's self-definition; inelastic relations freeze her into expectations that she has outgrown. Peck portrays the self-definition as a spiraling motion showing the woman monitoring her own growth in terms of her relationships. "Spiraling also captures the importance of the woman's ability to change subtly her degree of involvement in relationships as the prime factor in a clearer self-definition" (1986, p. 281).

Peck's image, illuminated by personal narrative, offers a historical framework for a relational theory of development. Her image is neither a comprehensive theory nor a do-it-yourself manual. It is a visual image we can use to check out theories of adult development. We can enrich Peck's image with biographical techniques that fill in the color and shading of personal narrative (Barry, 1989). We can "collect" a life history, a person's own story, and look at it in the context of her relationships (her "embeddedness") to help us see what is obscured by differences in class, race, and income and to show how she constitutes herself across time (Geiger, 1986; Porter, 1988). The life-history method encourages us to focus on the narrative, the way a person constructs his or her own story; the narrative offers us a rich source for understanding how people view their world. These methods are highly compatible with medical work (Shapiro, 1993).

Being-in-relation theory constructs a vision of adult development based on relations—the mature person situated within the relational context of home, work, family, and community. This vision is missing

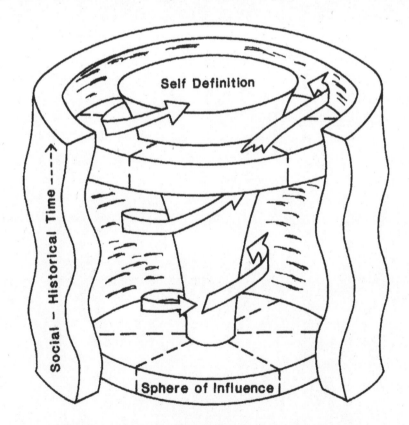

Figure 2.1   A Model of Women's Self-Definition in Adulthood.
Reproduced from Teresa A. Peck, "Women's Self-Definition in Adulthood: From a Different Model?" *Psychology of Women Quarterly* 10 (1986): 278. Reprinted with the permission of Cambridge University Press.

from medical views of adult development. Instead, in the absence of explicit studies of women's development, medical texts have placed women's development within the family life cycle, reducing women's lives to the requirements of heterosexuality and reproduction. In its assumption that the family life cycle *is* women's development, medicine has ignored the meaning of work and relationships outside the home for women. As we see in the next chapter, the assumption that women's development is identical with the family life cycle reinforces stereotypic gender roles and creates a constricted view of women centered on their reproduction.

CHAPTER 3

The Family Life Cycle

> To say that the family, as a social group, has a life cycle in the same sense that single plants and animals may be spoken of as having life cycles, is to tread upon difficult philosophical ground.
>
> Charles Price Loomis,
> *The Study of the Life Cycles of Families* (1936), p. 196

IF MEDICINE ESPOUSES the masculine ideals of separateness and autonomy as the goals of child and adult development, what implications does this approach hold for how medicine views individuals as members of families, and how it views family life itself? Apart from two little-known research studies on families and health conducted in the 1930s (the Peckham Experiment in England) (Ransom, 1983) and the 1940s (the Family Health Project in New York) (Richardson, 1945/1983),[1] the idea that the family is the crucial context of individual life and health went unstated and unrecognized in medicine until the formal recognition of family medicine as a medical specialty in 1969. In a parallel fashion and at the same time, family therapy appeared to spring full-blown into the world of psychotherapy. Though the origins of family medicine and family therapy extended back several decades (Candib & Glenn, 1983), their simultaneous emergence signaled a sudden and widespread recognition among progressive helping professionals of the importance of the family.

Acknowledgment of the family as the context for health and illness made possible the potential recognition of women's concern and feeling of responsibility for family health, the challenges and confinements of the family for women, and their economic, physical, and psychological vulnerabilities in families. Likewise, the rise of the women's movement and the women's health movement led to increased social awareness of women's individual and collective health concerns. One family medicine scholar, G. Gayle Stephens, even directly addressed the potential congruence between the goals of feminism and family medicine (1989). Theoretically, within the deliberately more contextual family approach, a relational view of women—one that acknowledges the complexities of the relationships that shape identity in different ways, in different classes, cultures, and moments in history—might have found expression. Nevertheless, in the early years of family medicine and family therapy, practitioners rarely challenged conventional family roles or admitted women's vulnerability in families.

Instead, both family medicine and family therapy have cleaved to one dominant metaphor—the family life cycle—as an organizing principle.[2] The metaphor has taken on the status of a cherished icon in textbooks of family medicine and family therapy; clinicians nestle child and adult development within its ample arms. In fact, family medicine often uses the family life cycle concept to distinguish itself from the medical specialties that maintain an individual focus on adults or children; typically, family medicine texts open with a chapter on the family life cycle, setting it up as the context for all that follows (Hennen, 1987).

The family life cycle metaphor draws a parallel between species going through specific stages in their development (for example, larva to moth) and families going through various transitions over time. By analogy, families, too, go through metamorphoses in the course of development in a unilinear sequence. Typically the family life cycle describes a set of specific stages in family life: the young couple, the preschool years, the school-age years, the launching phase, the empty nest phase, the retirement years (see table 3.1). Each stage has specific developmental tasks to be accomplished. If these tasks are not "successfully" completed, the family is likely to have problems: symptoms in a member, difficulty with a transition, or trouble at a later stage. These stages are then the subject of study; normative generalizations can be made about the family during each stage. Masking its kernel of truth—the crucial relatedness of human beings—the metaphor itself has come to stand for how human beings form themselves into families.

In family medicine, the family life cycle has traditionally served as the dominant schema to situate the patient in life and to picture what she or he might be going through (Hennen, 1987; Medalie, 1978, 1979, 1992; Rakel, 1990; Taylor, 1983). Although some family therapists have become exquisitely aware of the risks of generalization (for example, McGoldrick, Anderson, & Walsh, 1989), the model imported into family medicine and promulgated in family medicine textbooks is a normative one: women in pregnancy and postpartum experience thus and so; families with young children experience thus and so; the family in the launching years goes through such and such events, and so on. Thus, the family life cycle idea conveys an ageless vision of men and women, their tasks and their needs, their thoughts and their feelings. The metaphor conveys a gendered view of human nature: men *are* this way; women *are* this way. Although these texts concede that individual, social, and cultural experiences make each person and family unique, they maintain an assumption, occasionally explicit, of the universality

Table 3.1. Summary of Family Life Cycle Stages

Stage	Developmental Issues
Stage 1: The new couple	Intimacy and autonomy Freedom and commitment Shared values Family loyalties—old and new
Stage 2: Birth of the first child	Symbiosis Integration of parental roles into family patterns Recommitment to the couple relationship Altered relationship with families of origin Increasing autonomy of growing child
Stage 3: The school age family	Family and society—boundary issues Maintaining couple commitment Styles of mastery
Stage 4: The adolescent family	Identity Independence Sexuality New dependence of grandparental generation
Stage 5: The launching family	Dependence to interdependence Realign family subsystems
Stage 6: The empty nest	Return to couple alone Aging and preparations for old age
Stage 7: The aging family	Ego integrity Dependency Death and loss

From R. B. Taylor, ed., *Family Medicine Principles and Practice*, 2d ed. (New York: Springer-Verlag, 1983), p. 15. Reprinted with the permission of Springer-Verlag New York, Inc.

of experience. It is, of course, from the standpoint of this ideal of the timeless family life cycle that the contemporary family appears to be "in crisis" and undergoing change that breaks radically with the past.

In a hallowed position for many years, this organismic notion (Elder, 1981) of family life cycle received little criticism except from social scientists (Aldous, 1990). Critiques of the concept as "ahistorical, static, culture bound, and unduly focused on the impact of children on the parental relationship" (Featherman, 1983, p. 37) never penetrated clinical thinking. Although early proponents of the family life cycle metaphor were the first to recognize its limits and to discuss variations—particularly of family structure and ethnicity (Carter & McGoldrick, 1988; McGoldrick, Pearce, & Giordano, 1982)—these reservations did not prevent the elevation of the family life cycle metaphor to the level of theory.

When we turn to history to understand the contemporary family, we find not only that the family has existed in very different forms at different times, but that every *vision* of the family has been shaped by its social and historical period (Gergen, 1980). Visions of the family have not necessarily conformed to what families were, for in truth there have always been many different kinds of families in various classes. Rather, the image of the family in every era was the result of how some people, usually upper- and middle-class, looked at or thought about the family. John Demos, a family historian of the early settlers of Plymouth, Massachusetts, points out that "the family" was not a self-conscious construct before the nineteenth century; instead, the family was seen as a microcosm of the wider community. That community—of which the family was a subset—was the grouping that provided for the material, physical, social, educational, and spiritual needs of its members.[3] In the nineteenth century, the family as "refuge" was idealized: the family was the domain of the virtuous woman who provided a tranquil haven where she educated her children in moral values while the man went out into the competitive, vicious, and immoral world of industry to bring back a living.[4] This ideology of "separate spheres" persists today (Lopata, 1993). In the 1950s television fostered the image of the white, middle-class, home-owning American family as an ideal from which the culture has still not recovered (Coontz, 1992). These visions of the family served the needs of the societies from which they emerged, depicting and justifying the historically embedded expectations of men and women in families.

The reigning view of the family shapes the accompanying portrayal of women. As a theory, the family life cycle concept serves an ideological function: it perpetuates a highly gendered vision of the family in which the workings of power are obscured. It enables clinicians to make out certain things plainly while hiding other ways of looking at families. If we were to look back on our own era from a vantage point a century from now, we might recognize the family life cycle as one of these historically determined visions of family life. Let us try now to decipher the central belief underlying the family life cycle metaphor prevalent at the end of the twentieth century:

> The nuclear family composed of a heterosexual, childbearing couple and their children is the primary, enduring, and therefore best organization for human beings. Variations exist, but they may be detrimental and need to prove their viability in the face of the standard.

Although individual human beings may survive and even thrive without conforming to this ideal of the family life cycle, most will conform, and most will do best within its framework.

Although family scholars and practitioners might quibble about the exact wording of these assumptions, most would subscribe to the statement as outlined.

There are a number of presuppositions in and corollaries to the above statement. Let's examine the corollaries first.

COROLLARIES

- Men and women play distinct and complementary roles in families.
- The nuclear family is the best organization for women and children.
- Transitions in the family life cycle cause persons to become symptomatic.
- Paid work for women is peripheral, or if central, problematic.
- Roles, not relationships, constitute family life.
- Central to women's roles throughout the family life cycle is taking care of others.

COMPLEMENTARITY

Complementarity, an idea rooted in Talcott Parsons's structural functionalism, contains the illusion that men and women have separate, distinct roles to play in the family (Glenn, 1987; Goldner, 1988). These roles are based on presumed biological differences between the sexes: each sex supplies what the other lacks, thus complementing each other in a harmonious whole.

Here is an example from a family life cycle text of the distortion of gender relations based on complementarity of roles. In this view, the family structure serves the "needs attainment" of its members; no member gets his or her needs met better than any other. When any family member reaches a new level of maturation, changes occur in the family structure. In the nuclear family in the following description, the youngest child, a girl of five, has just learned to dress herself. The mother no longer needs to do it for her. This change provokes other family members to try new behaviors in adaptation to the new change in structure. "Inevitably, conflict emerges between elements of structure that were previously well-integrated, but now are dyssynchronous" (Terkelsen, 1980, p. 36).

Instead of dressing her child, mother now goes directly to the kitchen, and has more time to attend to her husband and two boys. Husband gets fed faster, but now finds himself criticized for reading at breakfast. The boys have more time for verbal repartee with mother, but simultaneously have acquired an increase in maternal supervision of their play. Father, in turn, may object to mother's supervision, initiating a discordant interaction between husband and wife. (p. 36)

In other words, the mother used to dress the five-year-old and then rush to the kitchen to make breakfast while the father read the paper and the boys played. The example implies that the previous arrangement had been just dandy for all concerned until the five-year old no longer required assistance in dressing. What is missing from this account is the mother's point of view. Was she thinking: "Maybe we can all have breakfast together now; that would be a better way to start the day." Or: "Dammit, I wish he'd get breakfast started instead of just sitting there. No wonder the boys expect to be waited on!" The notion that the "elements of structure" are "well-integrated" in this family in which the mother waits on the husband and children perpetuates the myth that such a structure is the ideal, that a family structure oppressive to women is both acceptable and unchallengeable. Conflict is acceptable when it emerges in the course of developmental change, but the conflict inherent in unequal relations goes unrecognized. Thus, structural views of the family that rest on the notion of complementarity between the mother and father accept the subservient position of women within the patriarchal family structure (Luepnitz, 1988). The notion of complementarity leads directly into the next corollary: ideal organization.

IDEAL ORGANIZATION

Family life cycle theory implies that the nuclear family, composed of a heterosexual couple and their biological children, is the best arrangement for women and children. It overlooks the fact that for many people, heterosexual unions have not proved salubrious (see chapters 4 and 5). Despite the economic and psychological stress of single-parenthood (Landale & Hauan, 1992; McLanahan & Booth, 1989), for some women and children it is a better choice than living with a physically or psychologically abusive or addicted man. Clinicians do, of course, support individual women in pulling themselves out of destructive relationships with men. Cognizant of the difficulties of single-parenting, however, they may also still believe that a "good" relationship with a man should be a woman's goal, in part for the sake of the children.

Complementarity provides a covert argument in support of people forming themselves into heterosexual couples and children needing two parents: men and women complete each other; without the other, each is lacking. But this idea misconstrues what persons in-relation provide for one another. What is apparently lacking for a single parent is the role functions of the other partner, but the real loss may be of adult company and companionship, shared responsibility for child care, and economic support.[5] Adherence to the idealized roles of the nuclear family becomes more important than promoting authentic alternative ways for women to be in-relation.

TRANSITIONS CAUSE SYMPTOMS

Family life cycle thinking portrays the dynamic of the family during any given stage as smooth and unconflicted. It is only when a transition occurs—as when the five-year-old child began to dress herself—that symptoms emerge. A common example is the textbook attribution of women's symptoms at midlife to the departure of children from the home, again linking women's symptoms to motherhood (see, for example, Crouch & Roberts, 1987). Clinicians are advised to help families prevent symptoms by preparing them for transitions beforehand, using what pediatricians call anticipatory guidance. One family medicine textbook offers the following example of how a clinician might anticipate a problem before it happens (see table 3.2):

The man is having a recognizable midlife crisis over his work. He is unhappy but cannot risk a job change; instead, he takes the risk of having an affair. The woman, denoted only as wife, appears preoccupied with her body. By implication, the child's departure from home triggers her pathologic descent into alcohol abuse, depression, and suicidal overdose. The man is understandable, if not admirable; the woman is sick. The author's message is that if the doctor had anticipated the problems of the transition in the anticipatory stage, perhaps the problem could have been averted.

This scenario, clearly somewhat stereotyped in the interests of brevity, reflects a traditional view of women's and men's adulthood and a fundamental acceptance of conventional gender roles. The story fails to acknowledge what is evident to the woman, the bankruptcy of the marital relationship, and any effect of the collapsing family on their child. The disconnection and inauthenticity of each of the relationships go unrecognized. Crises do not emerge from real problems in the ways men and women relate to each other but rather from expectable transitions from one "normal" stage to another in an unremarkable family. The message is that if couples would only prepare better for upcoming transitions, they could avoid crises and continue their presumably harmonious relations.

WOMEN'S WORK

The next corollary of family life cycle theory is that paid work for women is either peripheral or, if central, problematic. The original depiction of the family life cycle (Duvall, 1988) placed women in the

Table 3.2. Stages of Problem Recognition

Anticipatory Stage	Screening Stage	Symptomatic Stage
Things are right for problem to happen, given individual and family development stages.	Problem is happening but is not yet apparent.	Problem is evident.
Man in late forties ponders a late career change; wife is having hot flashes and feels she's lost her figure; oldest child is due to enter university away from home.	Man feels unfulfilled but can't risk job change; happens upon attractive and sympathetic receptionist at work; wife drinks alone in afternoon watching soap operas; child is doing well at university.	Man has affair; wife takes overdose.

From B. K. Hennen, "The Family Life Cycle and Anticipatory Guidance," in D. B. Shires, B. K. Hennen, and D. I. Rice, eds., *Family Medicine: A Guidebook for Practitioners of the Art*, 2d ed. (New York: McGraw-Hill, 1987), p. 30. Reprinted with the permission of McGraw-Hill, Inc.

home as wives and mothers. It is assumed that the married woman with small children remains at home at least until the youngest is in school. Even if employed, the mother is portrayed as focused on the children. Drawing on the standard teachings about male adult development, family life cycle theory portrays (male) young adulthood as the time when the central tasks are selecting a (female) partner and choosing meaningful work. The traditional description of men's adult development emphasizes the importance of work to their self-concepts; women's own work and the complex and varied ways in which those women who marry might support their husbands' careers remain invisible in this stage (Cunningham & Antill, 1984; Pavalko & Elder, 1993). For example, a chapter on the family life cycle in a 1990 family practice textbook offers a 1957 table of "vocational life stages" to describe career development, alongside the example of a young man who chooses to pursue his career dream of becoming a physician. When career development does not follow this linear pattern, "individuals are at risk for difficulties in their family life cycle development, since they may feel unsettled and insecure about their careers, resulting in floundering at a time when they may need to feel settled" (Liese & Price, 1990, p. 47).

The possibility that women's career development may not bear any resemblance to the standard pattern remains unexplored.

More modern conceptions of the family life cycle recognize that many women choose to work or have to work, even during the child-bearing years (Carter & McGoldrick, 1988). But life cycle theory promotes the formulation that paid employment for women is an additional stress in family life. The older notion of separate spheres has been reconfigured as role conflict (Lopata, 1993). Women who work full-time outside the home at their chosen work are portrayed as caught in a double bind between the demands of career and family. To reduce the conflict, women have to suppress their resentment at working the "second shift" at home if they want to remain married (Hochschild, 1989). The finding that, for middle-class women, job roles combined with family roles (parent and partner) protect their mental health is still not reflected in medical thought (Barnett, Brennan, Raudenbush, & Marshall, 1994).

In the textbook description of the family life cycle, maternal employment is depicted as voluntary, despite the reality that 58.6 percent of married white women and 70.9 percent of married black women with children under age six are in the workforce (U.S. Bureau of the Census, 1994). Invisible are working-class and poor women, women who have always worked—in factories, farms, shops, or services—because they have no choice.[6] Family life cycle theory has been unable to squeeze women's work—middle-class, working-class, or poor—into an idealized portrayal of family life.

The omission of women's work from the family life cycle up to this point does not prevent a peculiar reversal when the children enter school or enter adolescence. Suddenly, without any previous groundwork, the family physician may recommend career and personal development for a mother to prevent her from getting bored or to redirect her energies away from the children (see Liese & Price, 1990). The implication is that women who do not work outside the home are liable to become overinvolved with their children. This theme harkens back to the 1950s notion that overprotective mothers are the root cause of children's problems (Coontz, 1992). The recommendation of employment for women with school-age children is usually made with no consideration for the low status and low pay of most jobs available to women who have had no special training (Barrett & Roberts, 1978). And for a poor woman receiving Aid to Families with Dependent Children (AFDC), taking a job may cost her one of her few benefits: health insurance for herself and her children.

Thus, in family life cycle thinking, women who choose to work walk a perpetual tightrope; women who work because they have to are invisible; and women who do not work outside the home are bored, unfulfilled, and potentially pathogenic for their children. With marriage and motherhood primary in family life cycle categories, paid work for women is problematic and peripheral in women's development. (For men as well the emerging contradiction between work and fathering suggests that the standard vision of men's work in the family life cycle is also deeply deficient.)

ROLES

Another corollary of family life cycle theory is that roles, not relationships, constitute family life. Conflict between family members and unequal power relations are obscured (Ferree, 1990). The prescription of certain roles for women renders deviant those who do not conform— for instance, women (and men) who do not marry. Yet at different times in history, marriage was not a foregone conclusion for all of the young adults in a family. Many women in the nineteenth and early twentieth centuries chose not to marry; some became nurses or schoolteachers. Others remained home to care for younger children or aging parents. A study of the households of nineteenth-century Providence, Rhode Island, revealed that over 60 percent of married couples over age seventy had children coresiding with them, and over 70 percent of widows had an adult child at home (Chudacoff & Hareven, 1979). Adult daughters did not, as we have been led to believe, become spinsters or "old maids" because of some inherent marital ineligibility; rather, they made their choices within a context of commitment to family and economic necessity. Here are the words of one such woman:

> I brought the children up, and I used to take care of the house and the kids, make up the beds. See, my mother was never too well. She had very serious operations. I thought we were going to lose her so many times. . . . That is why I stayed home so much. . . . She didn't like to go anywhere because she would say I would be left alone at home. . . . That was her excuse so she didn't have to stay anywhere because she just wanted to stay with me. (Allen & Pickett, 1987, p. 522)

Today a family practitioner might say that this woman "failed to complete her young adult task of separation from her family because of enmeshment with her chronically ill mother." But such an interpretation ignores historical conditions and trivializes the deep commitment involved in caring for the parents and children of one's family of origin instead of starting a new family.

Women who marry but have no children or fewer children than they wish for are also stigmatized by their failure to achieve the idealized role of mother within the family life cycle. In colonial times, infertile women were more likely to be accused of witchcraft (Demos, 1986). Today the quest for biological motherhood leads women to pursue expensive, dehumanizing, and invasive therapies in the effort to conceive and bear a child. Even when it is her husband who is infertile, a woman will still take on a sense of failure at her designated role of mother (Greil, Leitko, & Porter, 1988).[7] Thus, marrying or not marrying, having some children, none, or many, are life cycle activities that are historically situated and historically interpreted. Deviation from the socially prescribed and expected roles can result in a sense of personal failure as well as social stigma. Family life cycle thinking, by highlighting normative role expectations, tends to transform difference into deviance.

The focus on roles, not relationships, as constitutive of family life portrays the woman as separate from others, involved in a function called being a wife, or being a mother. In this way, women's various relationships are constrained within reproductive and caretaking roles and stages. The implication is that once the role is no longer active—small children are in school, adolescents have left the home—the relationship is no longer central. Crucial relationships may be overlooked: relationships with adult children, with siblings, and with parents in adulthood get short shrift in family life cycle thinking. For instance, in the so-called postparental years, our attention returns to the "marital dyad." Yet people do not just stop being parents; relationships with adult children are of great importance. Deep and abiding connections persist and are reinforced by mutual aid in both working-class and middle-class families. Similarly, a woman's relationship with her parents is frequently portrayed in terms of the need to assume increasing responsibility for their physical needs as they get older. This focus on women's caregiving role overlooks the rewards and heartaches of relationships with aging parents; the persisting intensity and complexity of the relationship is lost (Aldous, 1987; Fischer, 1986).

The focus on roles in family life cycle thinking also does not account for the power and duration of sibling bonds across the life span (Connidis, 1992; McGoldrick, 1989a). Yet relationships with siblings, particularly those between sisters, may be the most enduring bonds as marriages become shorter, families get smaller, and people live longer (Goetting, 1986). Strong variations in the importance of this bond exist across cultures; sibling relationships in industrialized countries tend to be more discretionary than obligatory (Cicirelli, 1994). Nevertheless, in a 1975 U.S. study of people over age sixty-five, among the unmarried group with siblings, three-quarters had seen a brother or sister the week before they were interviewed (Shanas, 1980). Thus, the relationships of unmarried women and widows with their adult siblings may be among the most important yet are relatively invisible from the perspective of the family life cycle.

The role orientation of family life cycle theory confines women to reproductive and caretaking roles, obscures certain ongoing relationships within the family, and fails to recognize other central connections.

Women's relational identity—woven into the complex fabric of parents, siblings, partners, children, friends, and coworkers—is compressed into one-dimensional roles that move along through life stages like ducks in the penny arcade. Missing is the vision of each woman involved in a multiplicity of relationships of varying intensity at any given moment, with a rich variation at different times and among women.

THE CENTRALITY OF CAREGIVING

Family life cycle thought recognizes that women do the lion's share of family caregiving.[8] This term usually refers to the work of caring for an aging or disabled parent, spouse, or other elderly family member. About two-thirds to three-quarters of all family caregivers are women: usually the wives or daughters of the one receiving care, but often the daughter-in-law or niece. The same percentage of those receiving care are likely to be women (Stone, Cafferata, & Sangl, 1987). Despite their commitment to caregiving, many women would prefer to share child care or elder care equally with their male partners or brothers. But they are unwilling to abandon the work if male family members limit their contribution (Aronson, 1992). While employed sons limit their hours of caregiving, employed daughters put in as much time as unemployed daughters, probably cutting back on their own leisure (Stoller, 1983). A son becomes a primary caregiver only when no sisters are available: when he is an only child, or the only child living nearby, or he has only brothers. This is untrue for daughters. Over three-quarters of married sons rely on their wives to help care for their parents; fewer than half of married daughters involve their husbands (Horowitz, 1985). These findings suggest that it is not only women's proclivity or willingness to take on family caregiving but also men's relative reluctance that loads caregiving onto women's shoulders.

Widespread social expectations reinforce women's sense of obligation as caregivers. Doctors, nurses, and social workers in acute-care hospitals expect families to care for their sick elders. Government policy—the reduction of the cost of health care—is translated into social policy that affects families and women in particular as the expected family caregivers (Evers, 1985; Finch & Groves, 1983). Hospitals now discharge after shorter stays patients who are frailer and sicker. An army of "discharge planners" pressure families (women) to provide the nursing and supportive care during recuperation that used to be provided in hospitals (Glazer, 1990). This pressure easily slides into a judgmental posture that families ought to do more. The budgetary origin of this moralistic position on family responsibility disappears. As resources become constricted, women are increasingly expected to pick up the slack in supportive and health care services.

Government policy favoring care in the "informal sector" (by the women in families) is consistent with the conservative vision of family life in which women remain the unpaid caretakers of both young and old. In England, where the state pays an "elder care allowance" to care-givers, only men and unmarried women qualify for the stipend. Married women, presumed to be unemployed, are expected to provide the care for free while being supported by their husbands (Finch & Groves, 1983). Policy makers thus take advantage of many women's expectation that they will be the family caregiver. Within families, elderly women expect their daughters to provide necessary personal care, and their middle-aged daughters and young adult granddaugh-ters expect to provide it (Brody, Johnsen, & Fulcomer, 1984). Women believe that caregiving is women's "normal" and "natural" work and that it takes precedence over other kinds of work (Lewis & Meredith, 1988). Accepting the injunction to care, women may then judge them-selves by their caring and feel guilty when they think they fall short or when others imply that they are not fulfilling their obligations.

The interpretation and experience of family caregiving falls differ-ently on women of different classes and incomes. Middle-class women are more likely to be able to arrange and pay for care for their parents; they become managers of care while retaining their own employment. The perspective of the women they employ, who become the direct caregivers, gets lost when only "family" caregiving is studied (Graham, 1993). Working-class or low-income women are more likely to provide care themselves for dependent family members; they relinquish low-paying or part-time jobs to become full-time unpaid providers of care (Stone & Short, 1990). Middle-class women are more likely to feel a sense of benefit and growth as a manager of care; the poorly paid or unpaid provider of care is more likely to feel burdened (Archbold, 1983).[9] The literature on the burden of family caregiving reports two consistent findings: caregivers with lower income report more distress, more depression, and less satisfaction (Chiriboga, Weiler, & Nielsen, 1988; Fengler & Goodrich, 1979), and social support (for example, shar-ing tasks and family visitation) buffers the stress of caregiving (Chiriboga et al., 1988; Pratt, Schmall, Wright, & Cleland, 1985; Walker, Torkelson, Katon, & Koss, 1993; Zarit, Reever, & Bach-Peterson, 1980). Hence, the context of income and social support shapes the experience of caregiving.

Caregiving seen as a role obscures the positive effect of direct care on relationships (Schulz & Visintainer, 1990). Many women see caregiving as making their link in the chain of reciprocity, as a return for what their mother or spouse had given them (Fischer, 1986; Motenko, 1989). Relationships are more intimate and caregiving is more gratifying when caregivers offer aid out of affection or perceive it as reciprocity than when they consider it an obligation or responsibility (Motenko, 1989; Walker, Pratt, Shin, & Jones, 1990). And caregiving even improves some relationships through the extra time spent together (Walker, Shin,

& Bird, 1990). On the other hand, caregivers feel increased strain when they see themselves in conflict with the elderly person they care for (Sheehan & Nuttall, 1988). Negative effects on mother-daughter relationships are associated with longer years of caregiving, lower incomes, and less previous intimacy with their mothers (Walker, Shin et al., 1990). Part of what makes the care of elders with Alzheimer's disease so difficult is the loss of the intimacy in the relationship (Blieszner & Shifflett, 1990). These findings show that family caregiving is a unique personal experience embedded within a social and economic context.[10]

Any interpretation of family caregiving must place it within the context of the lifelong relation between the one cared for and the caretaker (Walker & Pratt, 1991). Family caregiving is more than a role—it is an extension and a complication of a relationship in process, not just a squeeze amid competing responsibilities. To understand it, one must examine the "caring biography," the history of the caregiving over time (Lewis & Meredith, 1988). A being-in-relation understanding of caregiving would make the perspective of the cared-for central. Focusing on the caregiver assumes that the viewpoint of the able-bodied is the most important and makes peripheral yet again the viewpoint of the sick, frail, or disabled (Graham, 1993).

The six corollaries of family life cycle ideology restrict women to culturally circumscribed roles within the family. The focus on roles obscures the power relations between men and women and clouds any understanding that many women construct their lives from the fabric of relationships rather than roles. Further obfuscation emerges from the assumption that crises result from transitions in the life cycle, not from any problem in relationships. These corollaries discourage clinicians from considering whether something is wrong with the institution of the family itself.

PRESUPPOSITIONS

Obscured within family life cycle thinking are also a number of hidden presuppositions. Although any given practitioner might not subscribe to these assumptions, family life cycle theory takes them for granted:

- Homosexuality is deviant.
- White families are the standard by which to compare African-American (or Hispanic, or any other racial grouping) families.
- Middle-class families are the model for the family life cycle.
- The functioning (competent) nuclear family should be economically self-sufficient.

HOMOSEXUALITY IS DEVIANT

It is correct to say at the outset that family life cycle thinking fails to deal with homosexuality or lesbianism at all. Theories of individual development and the family life cycle hypothesize a stage of young adulthood in which the primary tasks for the young person are to separate from his or her family of origin and to choose a heterosexual mate. Hence, McGoldrick notes that therapists may view lesbians as "unlaunched adolescents," since they have "failed" to choose such a partner and presumably have "failed" to separate from their families (1989b, p. 222). (In family life cycle thinking, failure to separate from the family of origin is believed to be the source of a host of problems, for both the young person and his or her parents, in young adulthood as well as in later years.)

Since the theory "looks" only at persons who choose heterosexual mates, it cannot "see" lesbians and gay men. The organizational schema renders them invisible. Although family clinicians may personally eschew homophobia, the original statements of family life cycle theory did not recognize, much less legitimate, homosexuality. Genograms, the visual technique of drawing relationships within biological families on a family tree, have no formal notation for homosexual relationships or sexual orientation, and the only text devoted to genograms contains no entries under the words *gay, lesbian,* or *homosexual* (McGoldrick & Gerson, 1985). Thus, even the signature tool of family clinicians, the genogram, highlights heterosexual and reproductive unions and makes homosexual unions invisible.

In the past five years, family therapists have increasingly recognized the inadequacy of life cycle theory in addressing the issues of lesbians. Newer texts devote sections and even chapters to lesbian issues (see, for instance, Carter & McGoldrick, 1988; Goodrich, 1991; Goodrich et al., 1988; McGoldrick, Anderson, & Walsh, 1989; Mirkin, 1990).[11] Nevertheless, apart from texts that address women's concerns, in mainstream texts lesbians and gay men do not appear to participate in the family life cycle. AIDS has made gay men more visible in medical settings, but it has also encouraged medical providers to focus on "high-risk" sexual behaviors, not to sensitize them to the concerns of gay men and lesbians or to the ways in which homosexual unions resemble or differ from heterosexual relationships. It is as if AIDS provides the only context in which a clinician might encounter a homosexual person, an assumption that chains male homosexuality to pathology and ignores lesbians completely. Of course, lesbians and gay men do constitute themselves in families. Lesbians are not only lovers; they are daughters, sisters, mothers, and grandmothers. Gay men are sons, brothers, fathers, and grandfathers as well as lovers and friends. Regardless of the personal beliefs and practices of individual clinicians, the inability of family life cycle theory to take an open position on sexual orientation suggests that it does not consider homosexuality a serious option for human beings. If family life cycle theory cannot accept and address the specifics of gay family experiences, the unique strengths and commitments of homosexual relationships will remain lost to family clinicians.[12]

WHITE FAMILIES AS THE STANDARD OF COMPARISON

Phrases like "the multiproblem poor family" and the "ethnically diverse" family show that white families are the norm; others are interesting but problematic variations. Embedded in this viewpoint is the assumption that over time, through acculturation, ethnic families come more and more to resemble white middle-class families, retaining perhaps some interesting or exotic vestiges of their ethnic legacy (see, for example, Falicov & Karrer, 1980). The underlying assumption is that whiteness defines what family life is about. The family experiences of people of color—of being marginalized and diminished in the dominant society—are subsumed under "ethnic variations." We lose sight of the pernicious effects of racism and continue to hold up the image of white family life as the standard.[13]

If for a moment we were to take families of color as a model for life cycle study, we might call the centerpiece of family life the link between grandmothers, their children, and their grandchildren. The traditional intergenerational connectedness of black women and the interdependence of Hispanic extended families would emerge as essential family strengths. Adolescent autonomy and the separation of young couples from their families of origin might appear as problematic issues of loneliness and isolation. From a black perspective, white nuclear families might appear impoverished in the relation between daughters and mothers or between children and grandparents. Detached from extended family and cut off from community and religious connections, the white family experience might appear deeply deficient.

I put this alternative forward as bluntly as possible because it will take a strong corrective for white people not to see themselves as the standard (Zinn, 1990). Empirical studies suggest that black women have stronger ties to their mothers than white women do (Barnett et al., 1988); that black families frequently "absorb" additional children (the "extended caring role") (McCray, 1980); and that black families continue a tradition of interdependence within the black community (Stack, 1974). Single-parenting is not the primary issue for African-American families, who have always raised children in a variety of family formations; rather, the main problem for female-headed households is poverty (McAdoo, 1988). Moreover, the debate about the effect of maternal employment on the family appears irrelevant. African-

American women have always had to engage in paid work outside the home to make ends meet (Turner, 1984). Clearly, if one belongs to a group that the (white) mainstream regards as a "variation" or an "alternative," one's way of life possesses less theoretical centrality and ultimately less social legitimacy. From the vantage point of the white family life cycle, black family life disappears from view. Unless family scholars correct their lenses, they run the risk of entering the twenty-first century with a theory that says less and less about more and more of the families in clinical settings.

THE MIDDLE CLASS AS MODEL FOR THE FAMILY LIFE CYCLE

Taking the middle-class family as the standard for the family life cycle assumes an economy in which one salary is adequate to support the average family. This presupposition does not recognize that social and economic forces outside the family have rendered the idealized vision of the single-income middle-class family a fantasy. This presupposition not only puts poor and minority families on the fringes, it marginalizes working-class families as well. For instance, it fails to acknowledge that macroeconomic factors, such as rising unemployment, coupled with falling housing subsidies create higher rents, increased shortages, and more homeless families, through no intrinsic family deficit.

Two further assumptions undergird the fantasy of the single-income middle-class family. First, the idea that meaningful work is what the mature adult chooses is closely related to the Horatio Alger myth that any person can make it, with enough hard work. This assumption in turn rests on the notion that the economy offers fair and equal opportunity to all. While individuals recognize that race, sex, class, and limited education function as barriers to equal opportunity, theory continues to rely on models of individual and family development that pretend that these barriers do not exist or are only rarely operative. For instance, in discussions of young adulthood, life cycle theory emphasizes that a key task is choice of career. That discrimination, sex role ideology, and poverty narrow or even obliterate that choice is rarely acknowledged.

Second, family life cycle theory considers men's and women's economic trajectories identical with that of nuclear family. Men and women are not regarded as separate economic beings. The illusion of economic parity between men and women assumes a world in which marriages are permanent, economic conditions are stable, and divorce, retirement, and spousal death have the same economic impact on women as they do on men. Clearly this is not the world we live in. Nevertheless, the standard use of family income statistics obscures the economic experiences of women and children not living with a male breadwinner (Hondagneu-Sotelo, 1992; Landale & Hauan, 1992;

McLanahan et al., 1989). The income of women and children is severely affected by divorce and widowhood, while men's income actually rises 43 percent after divorce (Weitzman, 1985). One-third to one-fifth of all women will spend some time in poverty, and about one-third of all children will fall below the poverty line at least once before age fifteen (Duncan & Rodgers, 1988). Put another way, compared with women, men have a 23 percent higher standard of living (Duncan, 1988). Thus, the use of "family" income indicators hides the economic vulnerability of women and children and supports an illusion of prosperity. Whose interest is served?

THE ECONOMIC SELF-SUFFICIENCY OF THE NUCLEAR FAMILY

Finally, the most obvious but perhaps the least questioned assumption is that the nuclear family should be economically self-sufficient. This idea flourished in the 1950s despite the reality that federal subsidies for families peaked in that decade through federal loans for housing and education (Coontz, 1992). In other eras, family and community collaboration have been necessary to manage large or expensive activities: barn raising, communal cattle grazing, loss of homes to fire, and so on. Black families both poor and middle-class still collaborate (McAdoo, 1980; Stack, 1974), as do immigrant families, who may pool the AFDC check of a single mother, the disability check of the grandfather, the under-the-table earnings of another member, and the salary of the able-bodied. Family transitions into and out of poverty continue to depend to a large degree on the earnings of "secondary earners" other than parents (Duncan & Rodgers, 1988). Thus, extended family support is essential to the survival of low-income families, even though contemporary ideology still holds that the "adequate" nuclear family should be able to make it alone. This notion of adequacy rests on the illusion that the economic system is fair and just: if people work hard, they will do all right, and if they cannot make it, it is they who failed. Hence, the view of family competency within life cycle theory accepts the U.S. economic system as a reasonable and healthy milieu for family life.

This series of economic assumptions—that individuals who work hard should be able to make it, that a single earner should be able to support a family, that "competent" families should be self-sufficient, and that family economic life takes place in a context that is fair and just—do not now and probably never did reflect economic reality for contemporary American families. Grounding family life cycle theory in these false assumptions serves an ideological function: to obscure the inequality and injustice of the environment in which family life takes place. In the next two chapters, we will see how the climate of inequality and injustice is replicated within the internal environment of family life.

Of course, humans constitute themselves in family groupings, and these groupings serve to protect, nurture, and promote the growth of the members. These groupings change over time as members join and leave, as children are born and grow up, as adults age and die. History, culture, politics, and economics all influence how these groupings that we call families shape themselves. In all classes, among all racial and ethnic groups, in a variety of family constellations, many women bear children, and many women marry. But many do not, and some establish their primary and supportive relationships with other women. Many women work, much of their lives, outside the home, sometimes at work they value and even enjoy. Their diverse experiences call for a theory of family life that recognizes the richness of relations with others at home and at work; that confronts poverty, abuse, racism, and homophobia; and that celebrates the caring connections women forge with each other. Anything less is a distortion of women's identities. In the next two chapters, it will become clear how such distortions work to damage women through physical and sexual abuse.

CHAPTER 4

Violence against Women, Not Family Violence

THE MEDICAL PORTRAYAL of child and adult development and of the family life cycle offers a harmonious picture of gender relations. Despite inevitable transitions, struggles, and crises for individuals and between family members, the lives of girls and boys, women and men, are assumed to evolve in predictable and usually positive ways. Words like *power, domination, assault, brutality*, and *victimization* seem out of place in the medical profession's version of the family drama. Rape, battering, and child physical and sexual abuse are viewed as the obnoxious acts of a deviant few trapped in cycles of violence: physically abused boys grow up to be batterers, sexually abused women allow their daughters to be abused, battered women revolve in the wheel of violence. The unfortunate children are doomed to repeat the sins of their parents. The mythical quality of these cycles resists examination of the connection between gender and power in family life. In this chapter, I show how medicine avoids facing the issue of power in its approach to violence against women.

The explosion of media attention has jolted medicine into awareness of the frequency of violence against women. Reform efforts acknowledge medicine's past failure to recognize or diagnose violence against women (Council on Scientific Affairs, 1992). Current efforts concentrate on the need for medical professionals in all settings to recognize women who have been battered (American Medical Association, 1992; McFarlane, Parker, Soeken, & Bullock, 1992; McLeer & Anwar, 1989). Yet despite the publicity, the sheer frequency of violence against women remains a surprise to some medical care providers.

Because battering typically causes acute traumatic injuries, the medical literature has concentrated on the detection of battered women among women who come into the emergency room setting (McLeer & Anwar, 1992). Advocates recommend paying attention to the specifics of the history of the injury, the injury itself, and the circumstances surrounding the patient's decision about when to seek medical attention.

Despite this attention, training programs and protocols to improve the detection of battered women have no lasting impact without consistent reminders. One emergency room increased the identification of battered women from 5.6 percent of women with a history of trauma to 30 percent after instituting a protocol. However, eight years later the rate of identification had fallen to 7.7 percent (McLeer, Anwar, Herman, & Maquiling, 1989). Emergency rooms with protocols for the care of battered women frequently fail to follow the procedures outlined in the protocol: for instance, filing reports with the police, making psychiatric and social work referrals, and referring women to shelters (Warshaw, 1989).

In primary care and in psychiatry, researchers have concentrated on the detection of battered women through the use of questionnaires or interviews. Of course, many battered women do not openly admit the source of their injuries to medical personnel, partly out of fear of retaliation by the abuser, partly out of shame, and partly because of lack of trust in the medical care system. However, other battered women are quite open about who injured them and will describe their experiences to nurses or physicians who ask. Even so, health care providers often do not identify either group as battered, nor do they refer such women for appropriate services (Warshaw, 1989). Why so many women are battered is not often asked.

Medicine's new awareness about the prevalence of violence against women has not yet informed or changed other areas of medical practice. For instance, medical students are taught the importance of preventive health measures: safer sex, seat belt use, avoidance of tobacco. These appear to be gender-neutral practices that any reasonable person would follow. Unacknowledged is the fact that a woman in a relationship with a controlling, abusive, or violent man is in no position to insist on his using a condom. Invisible are the rape and sexual abuse survivors who, for complex reasons, are less likely to practice good preventive health (Koss & Heslet, 1992; Koss, Koss, & Woodruff, 1991; Springs & Friedrich, 1992). In a similar vein, public health policy advises that HIV-positive women notify their sexual partners of their infection, without considering their vulnerability to physical assault from angry partners (North & Rothenberg, 1993). In medical texts, violence against women stays compartmentalized as a discrete problem located in chapters on rape or adult battery.

Medical sources fall back on several commonplace beliefs to explain violence against women. First, it is a global problem: the whole society is violent. No one, except for the impersonal media, is responsible for such violence; no one perpetrates it; it just happens. It is a cultural norm. Also, it runs in families. Children who witness violence in their families grow up to be violent in their own marriages; it is learned behavior (Smilkstein, Aspy, & Quiggins, 1994). Alternatively, clinicians may invoke psychological theories to explain the sick behavior of violent men: they are impulsive, dependent, lacking in self-esteem, victimized themselves, and so on. Women who live with such men are sick as well: they are helpless, dependent, lacking in self-esteem, and subject to multiple somatic complaints. Such explanations fit easily into the medical model, which can turn any situation into a problem of individual pathology.

Academic medicine, like the social sciences, prefers to view battering within the rubric of "family violence" (Kurz, 1989), as if it were a quality pertaining to a given residential grouping or genetic makeup. In this view, the family itself is violent. Hitting between spouses and hitting of children by parents are direct results of past experiences of witnessing or being hit in the family of origin—it just runs in the family. Gender and power disappear as critical factors in discussions of conjugal violence. For example, medical texts now include the "cycle of violence" first described by Walker (1979): the tension-building phase, the battering incident, and then the "honeymoon" phase (Taylor, 1988). While this sequence is often chronologically accurate, the cyclical imagery suggests that the violence is inevitable, that it is out of the hands of either party. Invisible is the fact that the batterer uses all three phases—the tension, the blows, and the apologies and promises—to control the woman (Jones & Schecter, 1992). The so-called honeymoon phase functions to make her ambivalent about her previous assessment of the batterer and uncertain about her own judgment. Thus, the cycle itself is an instrument of domination, not a feature of "family violence."

Use of the family violence framework obscures recognition of the far more serious injury women experience at the hands of their male partners and of the climate of fear that dominates the lives of such women and their children. Placing the family at the center of analysis allows medicine to dodge the reality that violence against women is about gender domination. If instead we placed gender at the center of the discussion, we could see that violence is a mechanism of domination, a way that men try to control women, and a way that adults try to control children. This approach better explains the data: women's excess of injuries, women's reaction to battering, and women's inequality in the family and in society at large (Warshaw, 1989).

To look at violence against women as a problem of gender domination is foreign to medicine. While the facts themselves are unambiguous—men comprise the vast majority of the perpetrators, and women and children the victims—scholars and practitioners are reluctant or unable to acknowledge how gender shapes violence. Clinicians prefer to maintain a stance of apparent value neutrality toward controversial issues like violence against women. Choosing to focus on violence and not on violence against women, on spouse abuse instead of on wife battering, reflects an understandable desire to be neutral. Practicing physicians and medical educators may not wish to identify violence against women as an issue of domination because they do not wish to be inflammatory. Talking about violence against women as a gender issue makes teachers and learners alike uncomfortable. Pointing out that it is men who perpetrate violence against women makes people squirm—men because they are implicated by other men's abuse (and perhaps by their own potential violence against women), women because they have been taught to protect others' feelings.

Physicians and nurses may also be unable to see the gendered basis of violence against women because they take care of patients within sexist institutions, the same institutions where they trained. Medicine develops as a set of values and practices within these educational and medical institutions. That women patients continue to receive sexist treatment is unarguable. Humiliating conduct toward women students and insulting teaching practices are still commonplace in medical training (Ehrhart & Sandler, 1990; Komaromy, Bindman, Haber, & Sande, 1993; Moscarello, Margittai, & Rossi, 1994; Warshaw, 1993). Within this climate, medicine cannot see that men's violence against women and children is both formative and ubiquitous. From the five-year-old girl whose uncle fondles her genitals to the woman medical student confronted with slides of *Playboy* models during orthopedics lectures to the woman repeatedly raped and battered by her husband to the fear of any woman walking to her car in a dark parking lot—the vulnerability is universal. Yet medicine has not made awareness of this vulnerability central to its approach to women. Given the gender hierarchy in medical settings, medicine is unlikely to scrutinize its own participation in male domination.

Medicine resists the recognition that men's violence against women is a systematic assault on women *as women*. This resistance consists in the denial of two key ideas. First, medicine fails to recognize that the various forms of violence against women are connected. They are neither random events nor isolated behaviors; men who commit one kind of violent act against women are likely to commit other violent acts against women and children. Taking the events one at a time, or the individuals case by case, or the kinds of violence separately, avoids this recognition. Chopping the whole into gender-neutral parts—"spouse" abuse, rape, courtship violence, and child sexual abuse—obscures the fact that women are the primary victims and men the main perpetrators.

Second, medicine resists the recognition that sexism (the systematic devaluing of women) is central to violence against women. Medicine prefers to consider sexism an individual point of view rather than a continuum of attitudes and behaviors that function to keep men in charge and women fearful for themselves and their children. The sexist attitudes held by individuals are supported by powerful social institutions (the media, the legal system, the medical care system, the educational system) that collude in ignoring, maintaining, and even promoting men's violent practices. Institutions and their routine practices, academic disciplines and their ways of looking at the world, all participate in an ideological milieu in which sexism is taken for granted. Even when medicine recognizes "the cultural reality of male dominance in society," the recommendation is for "the suppression of violence and the advancement of rational discourse as the ultimate goals," not for the end of male dominance and female subservience (Smilkstein et al., 1994).

THE CONTINUUM OF VIOLENCE AGAINST WOMEN

Violent acts against women are connected; they are not random acts, and they do not occur in isolation or in a vacuum. The connection is both personal and ideological: personal in that the same individual who perpetrates one kind of violence against a woman is likely to perpetrate other forms of violence against her, her children, or other women; and ideological in that men support their own and other men's violent acts against women (and children) through a belief in men's "right" to dominate women physically and sexually. Support for the ideology of male domination may come from pornography (Jensen, 1995), from male peers who encourage and abet sexual violence against women or, more broadly, from male authorities who have ignored, and at times sanctioned, men's violence toward women.

BATTERING AND RAPE

Men do not just batter. Men who batter their wives also rape them and use force to make them perform other sexual acts. Large surveys of battered women report that between 46 and 75 percent were previously raped by the batterer, and that up to 80 percent were forced to perform sexual acts (Campbell, 1986; Cowan, 1991; Shields & Hanneke, 1988; Walker, 1987; Walker & Browne, 1985). One-third of rape victims have a documented medical history of battering, and 58 percent of rape victims over age thirty have been battered (Stark, Flitcraft, Zuckerman, Grey, Robison, & Frazier, 1981).[1] In a survey of women family practice patients, 15 percent had experienced forced sex; there was a significant association between verbal and physical abuse and forced sex for this group of women (Rath, Jarratt, & Leonardson, 1989). Thus, men who physically abuse their women partners often sexually abuse them as well and vice versa; wife beating and marital rape go together. The linkage between battering and marital rape means that marital violence against women is not a matter of misdirected anger or poor impulse control; sexual domination is central to violence against women in marriage.[2]

The precursor for marital rape and wife beating lies in "courtship violence." Half of battered women report that their male partner began to strike them during the dating period (Roscoe & Benaske, 1985). Among college women, 20.6 percent report being victims of violence on dates. Of these, one-quarter feel that forced sex had been attempted (Makepeace, 1986). These figures are matched by reports that between 10 and 20 percent of college men have used force to have sex with an unwilling woman (Garrett-Gooding & Senter, 1987; Mosher & Anderson, 1986). In large surveys of college women, 15 percent report having been raped, and 12 percent report attempted rape (Koss, Gidycz, & Wisniewski, 1987). Among those who had been raped, only 11 percent had been raped by total strangers. The others had been raped by acquaintances, dates, lovers, husbands, and family members. (After stranger rapes, rapes by spouses and family members were the most violent.) Nevertheless, the stereotypical stranger rape prevails in women's fears. Although 90 percent of college women believe that they need to be cautious in dark and secluded areas of campus, most sexual assaults during the school year take place at parties in dormitories, off-campus housing, and fraternities (Ward, Chapman, Cohn, White, & Williams, 1991). The widespread and institutionally tolerated practice among fraternities of using alcohol to make women more available for sexual relations provides further evidence of the connection between force and date rape: using alcohol to get sex is a form of force that denies a woman consent (Boeringer, Shehan, & Akers, 1991; Martin & Hummer, 1989; Sanday, 1990). That rape and battering are common-place experiences of college-age women suggests that many women's earliest adult relationships with men were abusive.

BATTERING AND INCEST

Male sexual domination over children is established in the setting of force or threat of force. Sexual abuse and incest often occur in a climate permeated by male violence. Among adult survivors of father-daughter incest, 50 percent report that their mothers were physically abused by the incest perpetrator (Browning & Boatman, 1977; Herman & Hirschman, 1981). More than two-thirds of mothers of incest survivors report physical and psychological abuse by the perpetrators (Truesdell, McNeil, & Deschner, 1986). Wife beating typified 44 percent of two-parent families reported to Massachusetts social service agencies for child sexual abuse between 1880 and 1960 (L. Gordon, 1988). Among Iowa social workers experienced in handling cases of child sexual abuse, 44 percent think that the fathers use physical violence and 78 percent consider wife battering "likely" in incest families (Dietz & Craft, 1980). In a group of adolescents who performed self-mutilating acts, prior sexual abuse and family violence were highly correlated (Walsh & Rosen, 1988). Even though most clinical accounts of incest and sexual abuse do not consider battering central to the incest, all sources with adequate detail verify that male violence characterizes about half the settings in which sexual abuse occurs. "He tried to choke me to death when I saw him with my daughter once. He said it wasn't anything and to forgive him. He called me ignorant and alcoholic. I used to beg him to go to bed with me, but all the while he was having something with my daughter. When I reproached him about it, that's when he started beating me" (Russell, 1986, p. 379). In this interview transcript, "family violence" is revealed to mean that a girl child is forced to have sexual contact with her stepfather in an environment where her mother is being beaten.

Incest itself may be initiated by force or threat of force, and it may be maintained through force or threat of force. Approximately one-third of all sexual abuse occurs in a setting of force (Russell, 1986). When violence is not a part of the sexual abuse, the atmosphere of threatened violence may be all that is required. Children may be terrified because they have witnessed their mothers being beaten. The threat of such violence toward the child or others in the family may also serve the same function as the violence: to enforce compliance with the sexual abuse and to guarantee silence. For a child, the implication is clear: if a woman, who is an adult, is powerless at the hands of this man, certainly a child is even more helpless. "He was so much bigger than me, and I was just a child, so he didn't have to hit me" (Russell, 1986, p. 333).

BATTERING AND CHILD ABUSE

Research on child abuse preferentially focuses on characteristics of mothers and omits or ignores attributes of the father (Breines & Gordon, 1983; Martin, 1988). One maternal factor that has been largely ignored is her safety. Among children identified as abused in a Boston hospital emergency room, 59.4 percent of their mothers already had medical documentation of having been battered, compared with 12.5 percent of mothers of control children from the same setting (McKibben, De Vos, & Newberger, 1989). Among children referred to a child abuse team at Yale–New Haven Hospital, 41 percent of the mothers had definite or probable evidence of prior battering on their medical record (Stark & Flitcraft, 1988). A batterer's prior arrests for child abuse correlate with more severe injury to his woman partner (Berk, Berk, Loseke, & Rauma, 1983). The identification of child abuse may actually be one of the most accurate markers for the detection of battering of the child's mother.

Battering of a child's mother is also a major risk factor for child abuse. In one survey, 51 percent of battered women said that the batterer had abused her children; 71 percent of women who finally killed their abuser felt that he had abused her children (Walker & Browne, 1985). In a large self-selected survey of 1,000 battered women, 70 percent of women with children reported that the batterer abused the children as well. And the risk of abuse rose with the number of children in the family, ranging from 51 percent with one child to 92 percent with four or more children. The more severe a man's battering of his wife and the more often he committed marital rape, the more severely he abused their children, including increased use of weapons against the children (Bowker, Arbitell, & McFerron, 1988). Thus, a man who dominates a woman through battering and rape is likely to be a child batterer as well.[3]

The abused mother herself may also beat her children. In fact, women who are severely battered are 150 percent more likely to use severe violence on their children (McKibben et al., 1989). Some survival strategies for getting through the abuse, such as using drugs and alcohol, decrease a woman's ability to care for her children and often predispose her to neglect and abuse them (Jones & Schecter, 1992). A battered woman's abuse of her children appears to depend on whether she is living with the abusive man at the time, suggesting that her violence toward her children is not a characteristic of her personality but rather a response to being beaten (Walker & Browne, 1985). As one battered woman said, "It finally dawned on me that I never acted like this before I started living with him. So I went home to my mama and all of a sudden my 'temper' magically disappeared. I didn't have any 'problem with violence.' My only problem was *him*" (Jones & Schecter, 1992, p. 90).

RAPE AND CHILD SEXUAL ABUSE

Perpetrators of sex crimes are not specialists. In the past, men who committed sex crimes against children were considered pedophiles—men who preferred children, usually of one sex or the other, for sexual relations. Pedophilia was considered distinct from rape, incest, and other sexual problems. However, highly confidential interviews with 561 self-acknowledged male sexual offenders (either court-referred or self-referred) reveal more generalized patterns of sexual crimes. Of 126 men who had raped an adult woman, 44 percent had sexually abused girls outside the family, and 24 percent inside the family; 14 percent had abused boys. Of 224 men who had sexually abused girls outside the family, 35 percent had abused girls in the family, and 25 percent had raped adult women (Abel, Becker, Cunningham-Rathner, Mittleman, & Rouleau, 1988). In the words of one incest survivor: "My father suspected my mother of seeing other men and began parading around the house nude demanding that she make love on the spot. She refused so he grabbed her and raped her right in front of us" (Russell, 1986, p. 363).

The overlapping patterns of sexual abuse against both women and children confirm that violence against women consists of a continuum of offenses against children, family members, and adult women.

Battering and rape in marriage and in dating, child sexual and physical abuse, all take place in a climate of threat. Men use threat to enforce their demands. Surveys of battered women show that batterers use threats of harm to control them—threats to the woman herself, her children, her family, pets, her personal possessions—in short, anything he knows she cares about (Hilberman & Munson, 1977–78). His previous destructive violence is adequate proof that he is capable of carrying out his threat. She complies. "Nonphysical abuse [threat] *in the context of continuing violence* creates an environment filled with fear—fear that acts to impose the man's will upon his partner" (Edelson & Brygger, 1986, p. 382). Even after treatment, battering men continue to use threat as a means of control (Jones & Schecter, 1992). In dating relationships, men acknowledge using violence and threats of violence to intimidate women (Makepeace, 1986; Mosher & Anderson, 1986). The threat of harm is inherent in the secrecy required for child sexual abuse. Summit summarizes this climate of threat bluntly:

> "This is our secret; nobody else will understand." "Don't tell anybody." "Nobody will believe you." "Don't tell your mother; (a) she will hate you, (b) she will hate me, (c) she will kill you, (d) she will kill me, (e) it will kill her, (f) she will send you away, (g) she will send me away, or (h) it will break up the family and you'll all end up in an orphanage." "If you tell anyone (a) I won't love you anymore, (b) I'll spank you, (c) I'll kill your dog, or (d) I'll kill you." (1983, p. 181)

Or he might threaten to kill the child's mother. All forms of violence against women and children are linked together through threat.

ALCOHOL AND VIOLENCE

Violence and the threat of violence are intertwined with alcohol abuse. Although battering men attempt to excuse their actions as a result of alcohol or drug use (Dutton, 1986; Ptacek, 1988), alcohol does not cause battering. Men batter when they are not drinking, and men who stop drinking continue to batter (Hilberman, 1980; Ptacek, 1988; Randall, 1991). Nevertheless, alcohol abuse often accompanies rape and sexual assault, and the intensity of alcohol use is a predictor among male college students of the severity of their sexual aggression (Koss & Gaines, 1993). In a national sample of adult women, 60 percent stated that someone who had been drinking (presumably a man) had became "sexually aggressive" toward them (Klassen & Wilsnack, 1986). Women college students reported that 75 percent of the times they experienced unwanted sexual contact the men had been drinking; the women had been drinking over half the time. In acquaintance rape (largely at parties), 96 percent of men had been using alcohol and 87 percent of women (Ward et al., 1991). Among self-acknowledged undergraduate date rapists, 76 percent admitted to attempting to get a woman drunk in order to have sex; a significant 23 percent of control students also admitted to this tactic (Kanin,

1985). Correspondingly, 66 percent of college men participating in a study on male sexual fantasies admitted to getting a woman drunk in order to have sex with her (Mosher & Anderson, 1986).

Alcohol-accompanied gender violence is not targeted at adult women only. Alcohol abuse is common among the perpetrators of incest and sexual abuse. Loss of inhibition while drinking is frequently accepted as an adequate explanation of men's actions toward women and children: "He was drunk." Attributing the link between alcohol and sexual abuse to loss of inhibition overlooks a crucial fact: men's alcohol use occurs in settings where they have power over women and children and can abuse it. Drinking intertwines with personal and social expectations of sex role behavior: men are expected to be able to "hold their liquor," yet they are allowed, even socially expected, to be both violent and sexual while they are drinking. Men get drunk as *men* and do what *men* do when they get drunk. Sex role expectations coupled with their socially sanctioned loss of responsibility create a situation in which alcohol abuse reinforces men's violence. In contrast, women's alcohol use makes them (and their children) more vulnerable to victimization. Heavier drinking by women puts them at greater risk of victimization (Fillmore, 1985). Alcohol clouds their ability to make realistic assessments of their safety and weakens their ability to resist unwanted advances. Fraternities even use specially sweetened, extra-proof alcohol mixtures to expedite the process (Martin & Hummer, 1989; Sanday, 1990).

In medical discussions of "family violence," substance abuse is a troublesome lifestyle choice that exacerbates conjugal conflict. Missing is any consideration of the fact that alcohol abuse takes place in a gendered context. The setting, the sex role expectations, peer group activity, and even the differential effect of alcohol on men and women, all reinforce men's power to abuse and all render women more vulnerable. Discussions of the connection of alcohol to rape, battering, and sexual abuse require an analysis of the relationship between alcohol and gender. A similar analysis is necessary in examinations of the relationship between gender and other addicting drugs.[4] Alcohol abuse exaggerates the power difference between men and women; it potentiates men's domination and disempowers women in relation to men.

SENSATIONAL CRIMES AND THE NEED FOR PROTECTION

"You're all a bunch of feminists!" shouted the murderer of fourteen women engineering students at the University of Montreal on December 6, 1989. The most publicized crimes against women—gang rapes and murders—are committed explicitly against women as a gender to intimidate, torture, rape, and kill them. Rape is an instrument of war—in Bangladesh, in Bosnia-Herzogovina, in every country ever invaded and conquered, rape has been a tool to demonstrate who is in charge (Guinan, 1993). In this country, when the victims are women of color, police sometimes attempt to discredit their respectability, or they portray the victims of serial murderers as prostitutes, drug addicts, or street women (Caputi, 1989). Dishonoring the victims reduces the public sense of urgency to identify the perpetrators and diminishes the crime by implying that the victims were somehow responsible. Nonetheless, the fact remains that the targets of serial murderers are almost all women. Rape and murder, the sensational crimes against women, serve as a threat: they remind women that they are never safe, not at home, not in the street, not at their school, nowhere.

Nonoffending men benefit from women's vulnerability to rape in at least two ways. First, women are forced to limit their activities while men are not. Most women internalize this awareness of potential danger and circumscribe their daily activities to limit their vulnerability. Men are relatively unaware of the extent to which women constantly monitor their own behavior out of safety concerns (Furby, Fischhoff, & Morgan, 1991). Second, women become dependent on men for protection (May & Strikwerda, 1994). When men do become aware of women's vulnerability, it is usually their role as masculine protector that is activated in response to women's vulnerability to other men, not any sense of shared vulnerability with women. Male protection becomes essential to safeguard a woman against other dangerous men. But those providing this protection may take on the proprietary attitude of safeguarding their property rather than respecting the vulnerability of their partner. Even convicted rapists, those men society has punished for their crimes against women, state that they would take violent revenge toward any man who attempted to assault "their women." They predict that they would also take revenge on the woman "if she was responsible" (Scully, 1988). Such a man protects a woman for his own use, not for her safety.

At a societal level, violence against women is a "good cop–bad cop" routine: women need good men to protect them from bad men. The bad men "out there" enable the men at home to define themselves as protectors of "their women." Both the men out there and the men at home gain from the vulnerability of women and children: both become more powerful in relation to women (May & Strikwerda, 1994). At home or on the street, women as a gender are at risk in a society characterized by male domination. One male researcher and counselor of batterers reports his recognition of his own participation in this system:

> My repulsion [toward batterers] may have arisen in part from a refusal to acknowledge my own potential for violence. While I was clear at the time that psychological labels inhibit the recognition of commonality with a violent client, what I didn't see so clearly was that moral and political judgments can be just as self-serving if I want to

avoid confronting my own sexism (I'm the "good guy," they're the "bad guys"). Such an exaggerated dichotomization can also slide over into chivalry or paternalism—notions that women need my protection from "those men." That attitude is typically masculine: Chivalry and paternalism represent the benevolent face of men's domination. . . . All men are on a continuum of violence and controlling behavior; I have learned that this can be conveniently forgotten. (Ptacek, 1988, p. 139)

Thus, even the identity of nonoffending men is shaped in response to violent practices against women.

ATTITUDES THAT PROMOTE VIOLENCE AGAINST WOMEN

What are the societal and individual attitudes that support and encourage men's violence against women? The answer is: sexism. For example, the frequency of rape varies across cultures. In an analysis of ninety-five societies, Sanday (1981) has shown that the frequency of rape correlates with the prevalence of "macho" ideology. Frequent warfare and interpersonal violence also correlate with the occurrence of rape. Rape is one expression of the social ideology of male dominance. Likewise, male-dominant marriages are the most violent (Straus, 1980). Although researchers have attempted to make parallel the risk of violence in so-called female-dominant marriages (Coleman & Straus, 1986) and in marriages in which women have more status than men (Hornung, McCullough, & Sugimoto, 1981), it is male dominance in decision-making that characterizes marriages in which husbands use violent tactics (Frieze & McHugh, 1992; Straus, 1986).

Racism interacts with male dominance to put women of color particularly at risk in several different ways. Most directly, women of color are and have always been more vulnerable to white male violence. Even today, black women continue to find it impossible to convict a man of raping them (Adisa, 1992). One specific comparison showed that Hispanic women married to white men experienced more brutality from their husbands compared with white women (Berk et al., 1983). Indirectly, racism works to make women of color more vulnerable to violence from men of color. For instance, black women may interpret black men's violence toward them as an effect of racism and therefore be less able to act to end it (Jones & Schecter, 1992). And women of color may be less willing to call in the police when they are beaten because of the racist treatment their batterer might experience.

Violence against women gains its legitimacy from prevailing attitudes. A wide range of studies of attitudes supports the connection between sexist attitudes and violence against women. Men who witnessed violence between their parents are more likely to subscribe to "conservative" attitudes toward women (Alexander, Moore, & Alexander, 1991). College men who believe in the ideology of male domination (and have "calloused sexual attitudes") are more likely to have engaged in sexual aggression against women. Such men have fewer negative reactions to rape imagery (Mosher & Anderson, 1986). College men, more than college women, are likely to uphold rape myths, to blame the rape victim, to hold adversarial sexual beliefs, and to maintain conservative gender role attitudes (Fonow, Richardson, & Wemmerus, 1992). College men who subscribe to a high degree of sex role stereotyping show a sexual arousal pattern similar to that of rapists (Check & Malamuth, 1983). Male peer groups support male-dominant ideology as well. For instance, college fraternities choose their members for power, control, athleticism, ability to drink alcohol, and "sexual prowess" (Martin & Hummer, 1989). In such an environment, it is no surprise that fraternity members are more likely than other college men to use alcohol or drugs to get sex. Fraternity members are also more likely to associate with other men who engage in coercive or violent sexual acts and are more likely to be reinforced by their friends for engaging in sexual coercion and aggression (Boeringer et al., 1991). Likewise, sexually assaultive young men believe that their friends approve of such exploitative tactics (Ageton, 1983; Kanin, 1985).

Many people, both men and women, believe that rape and battering are justified. But men are more likely to believe it than women (Feild, 1978; Finn, 1986). Men's (and women's) beliefs about rape and battering are connected to their beliefs about women in general. College men, male prison inmates, and adolescent boys who hold more sexist attitudes toward women are more likely to agree with rape myths: that she deserved it, that she brought it on herself (Hall, Howard, & Boezio, 1986). College men who hold "traditional" attitudes toward women are more likely than men with nontraditional attitudes to see women's behavior as justifying rape (Muehlenhard, Friedman, & Thomas, 1985). In a random sample of Minnesota households, respondents with a high acceptance of interpersonal violence (for example, "Being roughed up is sexually stimulating to many women") and a high degree of sex role stereotyping (for example, "A woman should never contradict her husband in public") were more likely to uphold rape myths (Burt, 1980). Forty-four percent of college men who support a high degree of sex role stereotyping acknowledge some likelihood that they would rape a woman if they could get away with it, compared with 12 percent of men who support a low degree of sex role stereotyping (Check & Malamuth, 1983). College men with more calloused sexual attitudes were more likely to have engaged in sexual aggression against women, including the use of anger, threat, and force to obtain sex (Koss, Leonard, Beezley, & Oros, 1985; Mosher & Anderson, 1986). Thus, a person's outlook on rape is set within his or her attitudes toward women, including the extent to which he or she accepts a violent approach to women's sexuality.

Similarly, college students who hold more traditional attitudes (and men are more traditional than women) are more likely to maintain attitudes supportive of men's marital violence against women (Finn, 1986). Among male college students, 79 percent acknowledged the possibility of battering a future wife in one or more of five hypothetical situations (for example, if she had sex with another man, or if she told friends he was "sexually pathetic"). Again, the likelihood of such a reaction correlates with conservative attitudes toward women and high acceptance of interpersonal violence (Briere, 1987). Even among health care professionals, attitudes toward battered women correlate with gender and with global attitudes toward women. Across various disciplines, female therapists accept fewer rape myths than do male therapists (Dye & Roth, 1990). Female physicians and nurses hold more favorable attitudes than male physicians and nurses toward battered women; women are less likely to think that beatings are justified or that women are responsible for preventing beatings (Rose & Saunders, 1986). Finally, women physicians, in interviews with "standardized patients," detect abuse earlier in the interview, take more thorough histories, and are more likely to help make a plan or referral (Saunders & Kindy, 1993). Thus, a person's own gender and his or her attitudes about gender shape how he or she will view violence against women.

Men who batter endorse traditional attitudes toward women (Goldstein, 1983). A typical batterer is morbidly jealous: he attempts to control the woman's every move, her friends, her phone conversations (Campbell, 1986; Hilberman & Munson, 1977–78). That batterers presume the right to control a woman shows the connection between battering and sexism, as well as the fallacy of viewing battering as an act of impulsive violence unconnected to gender attitudes. Batterers attempt to justify their behavior by appealing to the notion that "she provoked it" (Dutton, 1986). The idea that the woman provoked the violence implies "that there is a proper way a wife can address her husband that the husband is empowered to maintain. . . . While his retaliatory behavior is acceptable, her verbal excesses are not" (Ptacek, 1988, p. 145). Although batterers try to explain their actions as being temporarily "out of control," analysis of their own statements reveals them to be very much *in control*. They use violence deliberately to intimidate and threaten their partner—"I grabbed her, and said, 'I'm going to fucking kill you if you do this again to me'"—or to punish her for not being a good wife—for not cooking right, for not being sexually responsive, for not being respectful or deferential, for being unfaithful: "I should just smack you for the lousy wife you've been" (Ptacek, 1988, pp. 150,

147). Thus, batterers appeal to male entitlement to justify their behavior: they deny that the violence is wrong because they believe in their rights as men to have their women be "good wives." Battering women is one way to keep them in line.

Interviews with convicted rapists shed light on how these men look at women. Some rapists maintain the illusion that the rape was consensual and that the victim enjoyed it, even though they broke into the victim's house or used a weapon. They fail to recognize that the woman has any rights or reality as a person. Other rapists recognize the rape as a violent sexual act that humiliated and degraded the victim; that is why it was exciting: "I assume she felt degraded, angry and used. The parts of her body that I touched felt dirty and that was just what I wanted." Convicted rapists lack ordinary empathy for women because they do not see them as persons; to them, women are objects. A man who raped his girlfriend's mother commented, "I don't think I had any feelings for her. At the time I think it was something I had wanted to do and was getting around to doing it" (Scully, 1988, pp. 208–9).

Just as men who batter feel that women deserve it and bring it on themselves, rapists believe that women are responsible for preventing rape; if a woman is raped, it is because she precipitated it (Feild, 1978; Koss et al., 1985). Many rapists see their own behavior as "situationally appropriate" (Scully, 1988, p. 203). The underlying sexism of rapists and batterers reveals that these are not crimes of asexual violence but gender crimes. Consistently, batterers minimize the severity, the frequency, and the effects of their acts on women (Dutton, 1986; Edelson & Brygger, 1986; Makepeace, 1986). Rapists also minimize the impact of their deeds: one rapist considered rape "much ado about nothing" (Feild, 1978, p. 175). Another stated, "It just blew past. I played some basketball and then went to my girl's house and had sex with her. I wasn't worried or sorry" (Scully, 1988, p. 206). These self-admitted and convicted perpetrators of rapes and beatings represent only a tiny fraction of the men who uphold the attitudes that accept and condone violence against women. Such attitudes toward women are widespread in every population that has been sampled.

MEDICAL PRACTICE: THE TRANSFORMATION OF ATTITUDES INTO IDEOLOGY

Offering help to the sick and injured is a standard role for providers of health care. And indeed, doctors and nurses do define helping battered women as within their role. Yet the prevailing attitudes described above do not disappear within medical institutions. Rather, personal attitudes are masked by medicine's tendency to frame violence against women either as a medical problem or as a "public health emergency"—an epidemic. Both stances remove the events from any meaningful connection to the individual professional or to the institutions in which medicine is practiced.

The medical model itself is an important tool that enables physicians and nurses to ignore what battering means: a beaten woman's fear and pain are reduced to, "Alleges punched in eye," or, "States hit in mouth by fist." This process transforms violence against women into unmanned blows landing on random body parts; it *decontextualizes* the battering. The physician misses "the animate connection between her injury and how it happened" (Warshaw, 1989, p. 511). Through the systematic removal of human beings from the events, the medical model actively discourages clinicians from facing the reality of battering. No one did the hitting; no one felt the beating; no children crouched in fear in the corner; all is reduced to, "Facial contusion; X rays negative; ice and ibuprofen." Objectification is a standard technique that human beings, particularly professionals, use to protect themselves from the meaning of what they see and do (Schmitt, 1990).

Decontextualization and objectification are pillars that uphold the medical model. They are essential skills in the education and socialization of physicians in training. They enable students to dissect a dead person, pound on the chest of a dying person, put their fingers up the rectum of a living person, and stick needles into the limbs of screaming children. Decontextualization and objectification excise gender from apparent consideration except for diseases specific to the body parts of males or females. Medical students and residents learn from more senior physicians how to take a history, conduct a physical examination, arrive at a diagnosis, and create the medical record. In the emergency room, the process of transforming battering into contusions is taught and learned as part of medical training. Students learn to write, "Alleges rape," as the chief complaint because of concern over legal accountability. They learn not to take a person's account of her experience as real. Only the discrete, observable findings are true. The fact vanishes that objectification itself formulates the problem to be assessed and treated. Decontextualization and objectification detach violence against women from gender.

Besides allowing physicians to wall off the recognition of beatings and rapes as real events inflicted on women by men, the medical model also denies the personal values of the physician. The valorization of objectivity in the medical model presumes that personal attitudes are irrelevant to assessment and treatment. An individual physician's standing on sex role ideology is reduced to a matter of individual preference, like hairstyle, food choices, or political viewpoints. The same ideology of privacy that discourages physicians from inquiring into patients' personal lives (Burge, 1989; Jecker, 1993) also limits examination of physicians' own values. Yet, as discussed above, a person's attitude toward battered and raped women correlates with his or her attitudes toward women in general. The medical educational setting does not challenge those attitudes as incompatible with appropriate care of women patients; rather, sexism is accepted as a private matter of opinion. The presumption of objectivity in medicine allows individual professionals to continue to maintain sexist attitudes toward women who have been beaten or raped. Societal attention to the "epidemic" of violence has forced medicine as a whole, and individual specialties within medicine, to address the issue of violence against women. The field of family medicine provides ample evidence that medicine is more comfortable addressing violence disconnected or decontextualized from a discussion of gender. Ideally, family medicine could be the source of a feminist analysis of violence against women in the family because of its location outside of mainstream medicine. Family medicine has taken a strong ideological position of opposition to the objectification of patients and to the removal of a person's symptoms from context. Nonetheless, family medicine is ill at ease with making gender central to considerations of violence against women. True to its name, family medicine prefers to see violence against women as part of family violence. This position allows family medicine to avoid awareness of the power difference between men and women.

Discomfort with a gendered understanding of violence against women emerges at both individual and academic levels in family medicine. Recognition of violence against women as a gender issue forces the individual physician to take sides in a marital conflict, an admittedly awkward position, and one that may expose the physician to personal risk. In the long run, siding with one member of a couple may result in the departure of one or both partners from the physician's practice. Moreover, identification of the violence as wife battering threatens the physician's relationship with the man of the house, whom the physician may wish to protect. Finally, acknowledgment of battering and rape as gender issues may raise the specter of abuse in the physician's own family of origin or current home life (Lent, 1986; Sugg & Inui, 1992). For the male physician, it means facing his own impulses to hit or previous experiences of hitting or being hit; for the woman physician, it provokes a sense of vulnerability and may remind her of victimization that she or women in her family have experienced.

Family medicine professionals may not identify the gender issues underlying wife beating because doing so would require acknowledgment of the fundamental sexism of our society. This stance is identified with feminists and with political activists. Many people in medicine do not feel comfortable in this company. Facing the gender issue requires men in particular to reexamine their own position on violence, particularly violence against women. It would commit men to openness of inquiry into the painfully common events of child sexual abuse, date rape and "courtship violence," marital rape and wife beating.

These personal dilemmas for the physician are difficult and complex enough to keep family medicine from identifying or exploring a deeper ideological layer of explanation. Violence against women in families poses a contradiction in terms for family medicine. It destroys the illusion of domestic tranquillity and threatens the idealized vision of the nuclear family as the preferred environment in which to live and raise children. Although an individual family physician may encourage a battered woman to leave her partner and to seek shelter, the ideology of family medicine supports the general notion of keeping the family together. Recognition of the sexism underlying wife battering forces the physician to reconsider how the family is constituted and whether it is salubrious for all its members.

FAMILY SYSTEMS THEORY AND ITS FALLACIES

Violence against women challenges family medicine to reexamine root assumptions about the relationship between men and women. Like family therapy, family medicine assumes that the relations between adults in a family are relations between equals, that troublesome relationships can and should be "treated," and that relationships that do not prove to be amenable to treatment can be left. Family medicine textbooks use family systems theory—the application of systems theory to family relations— to locate the problem of battering in the family, not in gender relations, and to protect itself against the recognition of the power discrepancy between men and women (Christie-Seely, 1984; Henao & Grose, 1985; Ramsay, 1989; Taylor, 1988). In a characteristically "systemic" effort to avoid placing blame, the texts fail to deal with the concepts of responsibility and power in the domestic relationship. By attributing violence to society at large in some instances and to systems maintenance in others, such models fail to offer concrete methods to prevent further battering and physical abuse. Furthermore, family systems theory suggests that by participating in the system the woman herself perpetuates the battering; this stance serves in the long run to blame the victim.

The Fallacy of Equivalency
Medical texts preferentially apply the gender-equivalent terms "domestic violence," "spouse abuse," and "conjugal violence," even while acknowledging that most perpetrators are male and most victims are female (Smilkstein et al., 1994; Taylor, 1988). Other texts uncritically cite crude data to support the notion that violence is equivalent between women and men (Arnold & Jeffries, 1983; Paradis, 1984). This fallacy is closely tied to the assumption in systems theory that the partners in the marital pair are equal (Bograd 1984, 1986; Goldner, 1988). For instance,

in a chapter on "spouse abuse," Arnold and Jeffries take pains to neutralize gender, thereby minimizing the effect on women: "Aside from the factors relating size and physical strength, and the legal, ethnic, and cultural endorsements of male dominance, it is reasonable to infer that for men and women there are many similarities of causation, frequency, injury impact, and management of abuse" (1983, p. 1610). Apart from male dominance, abuse might be a symmetrical issue, but these authors do not make it clear that, at least in our society (and in most well-studied societies), family relations have never existed apart from male dominance.

In contrast to family medicine's assumption of the equivalency of violence between spouses, the social scientists who first recognized that women respond violently to men were also quick to acknowledge that the meaning and effect of a woman's blows against a man are not equivalent to his blows against her (Finkelhor, Gelles, Hotaling, & Straus, 1983; Straus, 1977, 1980). Feminist reexamination of the early social science research on the "myth of sexual symmetry in marital violence" suggests that the methodology systematically underestimated the disproportionate impact of the men's violence on the women (Brush, 1990; Dobash, Dobash, Wilson, & Daly, 1992). In a case-by-case analysis of "domestic violence" in Santa Barbara County, California, Berk, Berk, Loseke, and Rauma (1983) demonstrated that in 262 incidents reported by the police, women were injured 94 percent of the time, compared with 14 percent of the time for men. When a measure of severity of injury was included, in incidents in which a man was injured, the woman's injuries were far more severe.[5]

The psychological impact of experiencing violent assault is not equivalent for men and women. Battering is far more destructive to women's self-esteem than to men's (Mills, 1984). This is consistent with the finding that school-age girls have more problems with self-esteem as a result of parental conflict compared with boys the same age (Amato, 1986). In courtship and marital relationships, men are more likely to use violence to intimidate and threaten, whereas women are more likely to use violence in self-defense (Edelson & Brygger, 1986; Makepeace, 1986). Far from being a mutual arrangement in which two people symmetrically have a fight and come to blows, the repeated battering of women often occurs in a climate of terror in which a trivial dissatisfaction can provoke a random beating.

The battering of a woman by her physically and socially more powerful male partner is an overt display of his power over her. Family systems theory does not recognize this power imbalance but rather views the parents in a family as symmetrical counterparts engaged in mutual combat. The fallacy of equivalency enables the family physician to avoid facing the complex and troublesome issue of responsibility. The problem of responsibility for battering surfaces again when we examine two other connected fallacies: family homeostasis and neutrality toward the system.

The Fallacy of Homeostasis

Family systems theory uses the notion of family homeostasis to explain violence against women. Paradis provides an example of this fallacy at work: "When the tension gets too high, one spouse may trigger the other one to act violently. The nonviolent spouse *remains in control* and can convey the negative message afterwards: 'I didn't lose my temper, you're a beast,' etc." (1984, p. 417, my emphasis). Here the homeostatic metaphor barely conceals an analysis that blames the victim: it portrays the woman who is physically overpowered *and beaten* as, miraculously, having remained *in control*. This bizarre interpretation serves the perpetrator of the physical abuse, not the victim. The illusion of family homeostasis functions to make the woman as responsible as the battering man for the violence.

Belief in family homeostasis clouds the issue of responsibility. Bograd (1986) points out that common to homeostatic explanations is the assumption that the violence plays a role in the maintenance of the family system. Violence is part of the "system"; lost in this analysis is any consideration of who hits and who gets hit. Battering as a pattern of control over one person by another disappears. For example, Arnold and Jeffries consider it "undesirable to assume that wife battering is simply a pathologic condition of the husband which, by analogy with disease, must be cured or eradicated" (1983, p. 1611). Rather, they see violence as a "failure of adaptation" in the marital system. Likewise, Smilkstein, Aspy, and Quiggins see violence as "a non-normative conflict resolution tactic" (1994, p. 113). This approach reveals a desire to be "fair" to the men; it also appeals to the physician's desire to be impartial.

The Fallacy of Neutrality

Systems theory provides family medicine with the illusion of avoiding blame and maintaining a neutral stance. Pittman claims, "Anyone, even the family doctor, who crosses family boundaries to champion one party of a domestic dispute" is destructive:

> It is characteristic of families in crisis to loosen their boundaries and cry for outside help. The police officer, the divorce lawyer, the mother-in-law, the hairdresser, and the family physician may all cross the boundary at the same time and all may be equally destructive if they see their function as protecting one family member from another one. ... The function of the intruder in the family crisis—the physi-

cian—is *to respect and protect power alignments sufficiently to help stabilize the family.* (1985, p. 352, my emphasis)

Taking sides is destructive; neutrality is the ideal. This stance ignores the woman's need for safety in favor of "stabilizing" the family. Here systems theory clearly champions existing power arrangements and fails to confront the power discrepancy between men and women. While purporting to be value-neutral, such an approach actually endorses existing power relations.

Systems neutrality poses a particular dilemma for the family physician, who usually relates to patients as an advocate. The advocacy role conflicts with the tendency in systems thinking to regard all helpers as overly involved with families and as therefore contributing to the problem rather than the solution. Family systems analysis promotes disidentification with helpers by portraying them as misguided perpetuators of the problem. By corrupting the idea of advocacy, this version of family systems theory consigns the family physician to the disinterested posture most compatible with rational distancing and detached objectivity—the hallmarks of a traditionally male value orientation.

Michele Bograd, in her critique of family therapy's approach to wife abuse, shows that family systems theory provides not to the battered woman but to the *clinician* a protected and remote vantage point from which the real physical events, the beatings, are lost from view. In contrast to the decontextualization provided by the medical model, systems theory "overcontextualizes" violence. Battering becomes a sign of systemic dysfunction—"diffuse boundaries, structural rigidity, or runaway positive feedback loops" (Bograd, 1984, p. 560). The reality of bloody faces and broken bones disappears in this linguistic sleight of hand.

These three fallacies disguise the relevance of gender to violence against women. The fallacy of equivalency denies the social and psychological context of male dominance. The fallacy of family homeostasis attributes violence against women entirely to the family system and thus implicates women as partners in the violence. Family homeostasis also implicates caretakers and helpers in the abuse ("enmeshment") and thus disallows the protection and support a woman may receive from caring relationships outside the family. The maintenance of systems neutrality discredits women's subjective experience of violence. Taking these family systems fallacies as truth leads family medicine away from being able to recognize violence against women as gender violence, as part of the system of men's domination of women.

FEMINIST APPROACHES

In conventional medical interactions, physicians take a prescriptive role: the doctor tells the patient what to do and considers the patient noncompliant if she does not do it. This directive approach can recapitulate in the medical setting a woman's experience of not being in charge of her own life. In contrast, feminist clinical work with battered women is based on respect for a woman's ability to make the necessary choices in her life and confidence in the healing potential of a nonabusive clinical relationship. Physicians and nurses might do well to borrow the methods from feminist family therapists that acknowledge and confront the power difference between men and women (Bograd, 1984, 1986; Goldner, 1988; Hare-Mustin, 1987; Luepnitz, 1988; Swift, 1987). Feminist treatment of families in which men batter women insists on making safety a prerequisite of treatment. Physicians could adopt this requirement.

Battering takes place in an atmosphere marked by fear and social isolation. The women have fewer and fewer contacts with adults outside the family and find it increasingly difficult to assess whether their view of reality is accurate. Mills describes this as "loss of the observing self"; it is difficult for a woman to get any outside perspective on the violence. "Without this outside validation, the woman is caught in a closed system, weighing her perceptions and her husband's judgments, and getting confused in the process" (1985, p. 114). Even in dating violence, the young woman becomes cut off from family and friends, who may know about but not take a stand on the violence. She becomes trapped in a kind of tunnel vision that does not allow her to put the violence in perspective (Rosen & Stith, 1993).

Outside influences—such as a physician, nurse, or social worker—can provide the crucial function of outside validation. The battered woman is uncertain of her own reality—did she do something to get hit? Did she deserve it? Is she just supposed to put up with it? The clinician can take a clear stand about the abuse: it is not tolerable. The woman has a right to safety. Nothing she does causes her to deserve being beaten up. This position can be made perfectly clear to the woman and can thus serve the function for her of reality testing. In the process of reinterpreting her relationship with the battering man, she can draw on this clear position statement to make choices in her life. Swift argues that "leaving the batterer is often preceded by a transformative experience in which another person, one who stands outside of the battering relationship, reflects the woman's reality in a way that enables her to acknowledge and assess her risk more objectively" (1986, p. 12). How important such a statement from a professional can be is demonstrated by these quotes:

> One weekend I took an overdose of pills and had to go to the hospital. So, they said since I took an overdose I had to see a psychiatrist. And the funny thing about it, he said the problem was my husband

and not me. He said that if I got away from him, I'd be a lot better off. I thought that was pretty good because I thought maybe I was the one that was crazy. (Mills, 1985, p. 115)

Once I went to the emergency room, and when the nurse checked me over, I had bruises everywhere. I wasn't seeing them. I knew my shoulder hurt, but I didn't realize that my entire back was black-and-blue. I said, "I don't have bruises." And this nurse said, "Honey, either you've got bruises, or you're out of your mind. Now which one is it?" It took that experience to open my eyes. (Jones & Schecter, 1992, p. 33)

To extricate herself from a violent relationship, a woman goes through a process of reevaluating the relationship and then restructuring her sense of self (Mills, 1985; Jones & Schecter, 1992). Clinicians can help initiate this process by asking the woman future-oriented "as if" questions:

- "How will you know when his sincere apology and his good intentions are not enough?"
- "Five years from now, will it still be OK for him to hit you as long as he still loves you?"
- "How will you know when it's time to move on?"
- "What would be a last straw?" (Rosen & Stith, 1993, p. 431)

Without telling a battered woman what to do, such questions allow her to imagine what she might do in the future. They give her the possibility of imagining herself to be different.

One useful restructuring tactic is to use the concept of survivor instead of victim. Survivors can be responsible actors who take responsibility for their future (Wendell, 1990). Survivors seek to establish new social networks that support their new vision of themselves. A supportive relationship outside the battering relationship can provide the setting where a woman begins to make sense of her experience and consider other life possibilities. Swift calls this "the restorative and healing function of connection" (1986, p. 16). The beginnings of such a network can form in the powerful bonds women make with other women in the safety of a battered women's shelter. Another connection that strengthens a woman's conception of herself as a survivor can occur within the healing relationship with a medical practitioner. A clinician willing to make a long-term connection with a battered woman can offer a consistent, caring, nonabusive, and nonsexual relationship at a time when no other relationships have these qualities. Offering a relationship rather than neutrality stands in sharp distinction to the distance and noninvolvement of the systems approach.[6] Clinicians committed to the concept of relationships as the medium through which healing and growth occur will find their work compatible with this feminist vision.

IMPLICATIONS

Medicine is reluctant to make the connection between all the forms of violence against women because doing so would require acknowledgment of how power is aligned in society. Medicine itself participates in this power alignment: men dominate the institutions of medicine, structure the organization of medical knowledge, and dominate the majority of interactions among medical personnel as well as between doctors and patients. The recognition of this power dynamic threatens individual men with loss of power. Their respectability is also threatened by being associated with abuse of power by other men. That male physicians themselves abuse the power entrusted in them is well documented in recent studies of sexual abuse of patients by physicians (Bates & Brodsky, 1989; Gabbard, 1989; Rutter, 1989). Recognizing the power to abuse and rejecting it, refusing to accept that power as legitimate—this is the challenge that medicine faces.

If medicine does not recognize gender violence as the systematic abuse of men's power, physicians run the risk of recapitulating the abuse. To address only the physical sequelae of abuse is to reinforce "whatever feelings of helplessness, isolation, and futility at not being seen or responded to that the woman may have already felt" (Warshaw, 1989, p. 511). Interactions with health care professionals result in further "disconfirmation" of a woman's abuse, compounding the distortion of her experience and the minimization of her injuries by the batterer (Rieker & Carmen, 1986; Warshaw, 1989).

> By reducing the battered woman's lived experience into medical facts and not acknowledging the feelings they avoid by doing so, medical staff inadvertently recreate the abusive dynamic between themselves and their patients. . . . Together, the doctor, nurse, and patient construct a "medical history" that is, in fact, ahistorical—one that extracts an event from its context, even from its status as an event, something that has happened in time and space. The dynamics of an abusive relationship are recreated in an encounter in which the subjectivity and needs of the woman are reduced to categories that meet the needs of another, not her own, a relationship in which she as a person is neither seen nor heard. (Warshaw, 1989, pp. 512–13)

"Seeing" and "hearing" patients requires recognition of the gender violence that women experience. Failure to do so replicates the disempowerment and abuse of women by denying their reality. But women's experience of gender violence begins long before adulthood. Just as the family often proves to be the setting in which men dominate women, we will see that the family is also the place where children, particularly girls, have their first experiences of gender violence. The next chapter examines medicine's way of looking at the incest and sexual abuse that women experience as children.

CHAPTER 5

Incest and Sexual Abuse

Someone trusted has used force to enter this space.
Margaret Randall, *This Is About Incest* (1987), p. 48

INCEST AND SEXUAL ABUSE are acts of domination—domination of an adult or an older person over a younger, weaker, and more vulnerable child, and usually domination of a man over a girl. Scrutiny of the medical construction of sexual abuse is important because it reveals medicine's ideology around issues of gender and power. Girls constitute the majority of identified sexual abuse victims.[1] The increasingly recognized sexual abuse of boys by men reveals that during childhood boys share sexual vulnerability with girls (Lew, 1988). For women, however, sexual abuse continues into adulthood as date rape and as rape and sexual abuse inside and outside of marriage. That girls and women are the primary target for sexual abuse by men both inside and outside families underscores that sexual abuse is an exercise in the practice of male domination.[2]

The women's movement of the 1960s and 1970s legitimated disclosure and political action about the rape and battering of adult women. That process of public consciousness-raising laid the groundwork for raising professional consciousness about incest and sexual abuse. Physicians are now aware that sexual abuse is prevalent in the community as well as among their patients. Two kinds of research studies have examined the history of incest and sexual abuse among adults: studies of unselected women, and studies of "special" (selected) clinical populations. To determine the prevalence of past sexual abuse among women in general, epidemiologic surveys study unselected populations of women in community and college settings and registered patients or patients attending annual exams. Because patients seeking medical care have health concerns that might relate to a past history of sexual abuse, community and college surveys are generally thought to be more accurate measures of the prevalence of sexual abuse. Nevertheless, since by definition clinicians see women who have already defined themselves as patients, samples of random medical patients do reflect the prevalence of past sexual abuse potentially detectable in clinical work.

UNSELECTED POPULATIONS

Women as Community Members

Comprehensive community surveys of randomly chosen women in San Francisco (Russell, 1986), Los Angeles (Wyatt, 1985), New Zealand (Mullen, Romans-Clarkson, Walton, & Herbison, 1988), and Canada (Bagley & Ramsay, 1986) have demonstrated the widespread prevalence of past incest and sexual abuse and the burden of symptoms among survivors. These studies come up with strikingly similar results: sexual abuse of girl children is commonplace. About 10 percent of girls experience genital sexual abuse before age twelve on one or a series of occasions; up to half of the respondents report less severe sexual abuse, still involving physical contact, by that age. A survey of professional women revealed a history of sexual abuse of 26.9 percent, with abuse defined as sexual contact (from fondling to intercourse) before age sixteen with someone more than five years older (Elliott & Briere, 1992).

Community surveys demonstrate a significant burden of excess symptoms among adult women who experienced childhood sexual abuse. One-third of sexually abused women reported having suffered extreme trauma, with long-lasting negative attitudes toward men, toward the perpetrator, and toward themselves dominating their reports. Women reported more trauma when the abuse was more severe and persisted over time, when the perpetrator used force, and when the father or stepfather was the perpetrator (Elliott & Briere, 1992; Herman, Russell, & Trocki, 1986; Russell, 1986). On clinical measures, abused women acknowledged more symptoms of physical and emotional morbidity: greater symptoms of depression, anxiety, and phobic worry, more dissociation, more suicidal ideas or behavior, more drug and alcohol abuse, more sleep problems and sexual problems, recent psychiatric treatment, and much poorer self-esteem compared with nonabused women (Bagley & Ramsay, 1986; Burnam et al., 1988; Elliott & Briere, 1992; Mullen et al., 1988). Because these women were randomly selected community members, these studies confirm the burden of symptoms carried by unrecognized incest and sexual abuse survivors.

College Students

Surveys of North American college students find frequencies of reported abuse ranging from 8 to 22 percent of women (Peters, Wyatt, & Finkelhor, 1986).[3] Again, unselected students who are sexual abuse survivors carry an excess symptom burden of depression, anxiety, phobic anxiety, dissociation, somatization, and thoughts of suicide and self-harm

(Briere & Runtz, 1988; Fromuth, 1986; Gidycz, Coble, Latham, & Layman, 1993; Sedney & Brooks, 1984). These symptoms are more intense and more distressing than symptoms among unabused students. Previously abused college women have a greater likelihood of being hospitalized for anxiety and depression and are more than twice as likely to consult physicians for relief of symptoms (Sedney & Brooks, 1984). Sexually abused women have damaged self-esteem: they consider themselves more "promiscuous" than other women despite a lack of difference in their actual sexual behavior compared with that of nonabused women (Fromuth, 1986). Again, the level of symptoms correlates with violent or prolonged abuse, the age of the abuser, the total number of abusers, parental incest, and completed intercourse (Briere & Runtz, 1988).[4]

Thus, surveys of sexual abuse in community and college populations find an excess of symptoms among respondents who were able to acknowledge a history of sexual abuse to an interviewer or on a questionnaire. Their symptoms serve as evidence that even women who are not identified as medical or psychiatric patients undergo distress related to their history of abuse. Such symptoms provide common reasons to seek medical care, yet often neither the women nor their health care providers recognize the connection between their history of abuse and their symptoms.

WOMEN MEDICAL PATIENTS

Between 17 and 37 percent of women seeking routine medical care give a history of childhood sexual abuse, depending on how the question is asked and how sexual abuse is defined. These unselected patients report more medical problems, more psychological distress, more total symptoms, more office visits, more morbid obesity (more than fifty pounds overweight), and more negative "health risk behaviors" than nonabused women from the same settings (Felitti, 1991; Friedman, Samet, Roberts, Hudlin, & Hans, 1992; Greenwood, Tangalos, & Maruta, 1990; Lechner, Vogel, Garcia-Shelton, Leichter, & Steibel, 1993; Springs & Friedrich, 1992; E. A. Walker et al., 1993). Measures of negative health risk behaviors include age at onset of smoking, amount of cigarettes, alcohol and drug use, age at first intercourse, total number of sexual partners, and frequency of pap smears. Only 2 to 6 percent of abused women have ever disclosed their history of abuse to a physician (Friedman et al., 1992; Lechner et al., 1993; Springs & Friedrich, 1992; E. A. Walker et al., 1993).

SELECTED POPULATIONS

The second kind of study examines specially defined clinical populations for a past history of sexual abuse, sometimes comparing members of the selected population with controls. Ample research documents that specific clinical populations contain a high proportion of sexual abuse survivors: pregnant teenagers, psychiatric patients, women with somatoform or somatization disorders, women with particular kinds of pain (chronic pelvic pain or gastrointestinal symptoms), teen and adult women with drug and alcohol problems, and women at risk for HIV infection.

PREGNANT ADOLESCENTS

Depending on the vantage point, teen pregnancy is considered a societal problem, a problem of welfare "dependency," a high-risk obstetrical problem, or a pediatric problem ("babies having babies"). It has been variously attributed to promiscuity, poor self-esteem, inadequate sex education, and poor compliance with contraception. Only recently have clinicians made the connection between teen pregnancy and prior sexual abuse. Among a racially diverse population of 535 pregnant or parenting teen women in Washington State, 51 percent gave a history of sexual molestation beginning at an average age of 9.7 years; 54 percent were molested by a family member; 77 percent were molested more than once; and 24 percent said that their abuse began at age five or younger. About 44 percent of the women gave a history of rape at an average age of 13.3 years; half were raped more than once; and 17 percent reported rape by someone in their family. Sixty percent experienced some kind of physical abuse in childhood, and 50 percent had been beaten by a sexual partner (Boyer & Fine, 1992). Pregnant teenagers, it emerges, may be one of the more visible yet medically unrecognized groups of sexual abuse survivors.

PSYCHIATRIC PATIENTS

Women psychiatric patients consistently report a high rate (up to 50 percent) of childhood sexual abuse when asked, but focused questioning and careful documentation are necessary to demonstrate this finding (Bryer, Nelson, Miller, & Krol, 1987; Goodwin, Attias, McCarty, Chandler, & Romanik, 1988; Jacobson & Richardson, 1987). When the childhood sexual abuse was inflicted by a family member, hospitalized women are likely to show more trouble with trust and more self-blame and shame manifested in more serious self-destructive acts, resulting in longer hospital stays (Mills, Rieker, & Carmen, 1984). Likewise, women seeking outpatient psychotherapy report a history of incest or sexual abuse at rates ranging from 33 percent in private practice (Rosenfeld, 1979) to 70 percent in the emergency room setting (Briere & Zaidi, 1989). Those seeking outpatient psychiatric help specifically for incest are likely to have experienced more violent, repeated, and prolonged abuse and severe physical abuse from older men, fathers, or stepfathers compared with sexual abuse survivors identified outside of psychiatric settings (Herman et al., 1986). In other words, survivors who become identified as psychiatric patients probably experienced worse trauma.

Psychiatric patients diagnosed with borderline personality disorder report a past sexual abuse rate of 67 to 86 percent. Women with this diagnosis experienced a significantly higher rate of childhood sexual trauma than men with the same condition (Herman, Perry, & van der Kolk, 1989). Self-mutilation among adolescents in psychiatric treatment, often considered a hallmark of borderline personality, correlates highly with a past history of sexual abuse, as well as with a history of witnessing family violence or family alcoholism (Walsh & Rosen, 1988). In fact, self-mutilation may be a very specific marker for previous experiences of violent sexual trauma (Shapiro, 1987). Similarly high percentages of patients with the diagnosis of multiple personality disorder have a history of incest or child sexual abuse (Morrison, 1989; Putnam, Guroff, Silberman, Barban, & Post, 1986; Stern, 1984). This almost universal finding of severe trauma in the background of such patients has provoked a reconsideration of the diagnosis of "borderline personality" as a childhood adaptation to severe abuse, a kind of trauma response (Herman, 1992; Saunders & Arnold, 1991).

PATIENTS WITH SOMATOFORM DISORDERS

In contrast to identified psychiatric patients, patients who manifest body distress primarily attend medical providers, making many visits to specialists as well as generalists and emergency rooms in search of relief from their relentless symptoms. Their chronic and acute symptoms result in multiple medical workups involving innumerable diagnostic tests, invasive procedures, and surgery. Moreover, these patients' uncoordinated use of many medical care sites guarantees further cycles of referrals as well as polypharmacy. Such patients, often classified with a disorder of somatization or a somatoform disorder, are legion on the lists of physicians.[5]

People with somatoform disorder are perhaps the most misunderstood of all medical patients. Sad, depressed, and miserable, yet demanding and insatiable, they are dreaded and even despised by the physicians charged with their care. No visit is long enough, no medicines are effective, and all the care and attention possible do not make the patient feel better. Few clinicians want to provide comprehensive care for patients with so many complaints, and those who try find that it is nearly impossible to prevent them from "breaking through" to make visits elsewhere. Sadly, despite their persistence in seeking medical care, these patients get little relief and even less satisfaction from any given provider or encounter; often they become angry at a system that continues to give them the runaround.

The medical literature is replete with accounts of the difficulty such patients pose for clinicians. Somatoform symptoms are the hydra of medical practice: for each logical attempt to diagnose and treat a symptom, a new one springs up. Practitioners become frustrated, depleted, powerless, and finally angry. Frustration with the relentlessness of the symptoms ultimately leads most clinicians to seek personal relief from the perceived demands of these patients by making psychiatric referrals. Patients then find themselves literally divided into categories—physical or mental, body or mind, medical or psychiatric—for a set of symptoms that, above all, requires an approach that integrates rather than bifurcates the treatment pathway. In the last few years, clinicians have begun to recognize that many patients with diffuse somatic symptoms are sexual abuse survivors (Bachman, Moeller, & Benett, 1988; Koss & Heslet, 1992; Shearer & Herbert, 1987). In research among primary care medical patients, two thirds of women who met the criteria for the diagnosis of somatization disorder gave a history, when interviewed by a female researcher, of prior sexual abuse (deGruy, Dickinson, Dickinson, Candib, Hobson, & McIntyre, 1994).

Patients diagnosed with somatization disorder by psychiatrists are highly likely to have been sexually abused during childhood (Loewenstein, 1990; Morrison, 1989).[6] This finding is not surprising considering that incest and sexual abuse cause many somatic symptoms in children, that girls are more likely to be sexually abused, and that women comprise the vast majority of patients classified as having somatization disorder. Most of these women do not, however, primarily attend psychiatrists. Rather, they visit the offices of innumerable subspecialists in search of relief. Studies emerging from the subspecialty setting show that gastrointestinal pain and pelvic pain—common symptoms among patients with a somatoform disorder—are strongly associated with a history of childhood sexual abuse (Caldirola, Gemperle, Guzinski, Gross, & Doerr, 1983; Drossman et al., 1990; Walker, Katon, Harrop-Griffiths, Holm, Russo, & Hickok, 1988). Women with normal findings at laparoscopy for chronic pelvic pain had a strong likelihood of a history of childhood sexual abuse (64 percent before age fourteen, and 48 percent after age fourteen) compared with the control group (23 percent abused before age fourteen and 13 percent after age fourteen) who underwent laparoscopy for sterilization or for infertility (Walker et al., 1988). Such a finding in the control group also reconfirms the very high rate of sexual abuse among nonclinical samples.[7]

WOMEN WITH ALCOHOL AND DRUG ABUSE PROBLEMS

Women alcoholics and incest survivors have many commonalities: stigma, denial, secrecy, family alcoholism, abusive relationships with men who are often alcoholic as well, family disruption and loss, defiance, distrust, poor self-esteem, depression, and sexual dysfunction (Hurley, 1991). Adolescent and adult women with drug and alcohol problems also have frequently suffered childhood sexual abuse (Edwall

& Hoffmann, 1988; Hurley, 1991; Loftus, Polonsky, & Fullilove, 1994). Sexually abused adolescent girls in treatment for substance abuse used more alcohol and stimulant drugs, had a higher frequency of suicidal ideation and attempts, and a significantly higher rate of psychiatric hospitalization than girls who had not experienced incest (Edwall & Hoffmann, 1988). Like teen pregnancy, self-mutilation, borderline personality, and somatoform disorders, substance abuse by women may actually serve as a marker to clinicians of a history of sexual abuse.

WOMEN AND HIV

Women (and men) at risk for acquiring HIV infection have a high likelihood of being sexual abuse survivors (Allers, Benjack, White, & Rousey, 1993; Klein & Chao, 1995; Zierler, Feingold, Laufer, Velentgas, Kantrowitz-Gordon, & Mayer, 1991). High-risk behaviors associated with HIV infection—drug and alcohol use, early intercourse and early pregnancy, and multiple sexual partners—are also associated with a history of childhood sexual abuse. Sexual abuse survivors may be less able to protect themselves from subsequent abusers and less able to enforce safer sex practices with their male partners. Long before the HIV epidemic, incest and childhood sexual abuse were understood to be precursors to later activity as a sex worker (James & Meyerding, 1977; Kluft, 1990b, 1990c; Russell, 1995; Simons & Whitbeck, 1991). Both women sex workers and intravenous drug users (often overlapping groups) are at particular risk of acquiring sexually transmitted infections, and both are particularly disempowered from protecting themselves from infection.

All sources emphasize the burden of symptoms carried by survivors, whether or not they make a connection between their symptoms and their history of abuse. While retrospective studies cannot prove causality, the brunt of the evidence supports an etiological connection between abuse and later symptoms. In the last ten years, feminist therapists treating sexual abuse survivors have recognized the connection between past abuse and current symptoms. Medical care providers, although increasingly aware of the frequency of past sexual abuse, are just beginning to learn how to tailor medical treatment to sexual abuse survivors (McKegney, 1993). Clinicians' first step in shaping treatment is to recognize survivors' accounts of their abuse experiences. One woman who was well known to a group practice for her dramatic suicide attempts finally confided in her physician of five years that she had been raped at age thirteen. She was unable to talk about this event in person and chose to write to the doctor:

> Dear Dr. Huliot:
> No one on this earth is going to tell me this pain I have is in my head. You didn't believe that my ankle was in such terrible pain when I was working, now you don't believe that I have this pain in my back-

side, right. Well, you're wrong. It's there. You have just made me realize that I don't ever need to go to a doctor for myself. I have suffered
pains that doctors claim there's no reason for for 19 years. No you
aren't the only one. But I will never go to any other doctor again. I
have suffered 19 years but believe me I am not going to wait to suffer
another 19 years. I was raped when I was 13 and a half and got gonorrhea. I was never treated until 18 years of age. Nobody nor no book
will never make me convince anyone that Gonorrhea is not a painful
disease. From 18 to 21 I was treated for gonorrhea and no one can tell
me that they cured it. Those pains have never gone away nor the signs.
When I am dead, you people have me cut open and you all see that I
am infested with that damn disease. Then you all will see that the
abdominal pains weren't in my head that they were real.

When her doctor told her that she had given the letter a lot of thought,
the patient sent another:

Please Dr. Huliot don't take that other letter personally. Because
even if you did believe I was in pain, even if the other doctors believed
I was in pain, none of you could have done anything about it. I was
raped in July of 1961 and I have been suffering since then oh not in the
same way. I know now how to stop getting the rash and burning feeling but not way back then. But that's 19 years of it. Coming and hiding, now it's got no where to hide. I've had it too long nobody can get
rid of it now, they tried in 1966–68. So believe me Dr. Huliot, I am not
angry at Dr. Huliot, only medicine.

Love Always, Good by,
Bianca d'Angelo.

For this survivor, medicine's failure to identify and treat her deep sense
of contamination echoed the earlier failure of responsible adults to protect her from harm and to recognize when harm had been done. The
result for her was a lifetime of stigma. Enabling her to reinterpret her
experience would require that both clinician and survivor ground their
understanding of the abuse within the context of male domination.

MEDICINE'S RESPONSE: PSYCHIATRY

Historically, medicine has been slow to acknowledge sexual abuse and
unwilling to admit that it results from male abuse of power.
Ambivalence about incest and sexual abuse pervades the history of
psychiatry. Freud, of course, made the original connection between
childhood sexual abuse and adult somatic symptoms when he attributed so-called hysterical disorders among thirteen women patients in

1896 to childhood sexual trauma. He later recanted this assertion, and his followers, friends, and family attempted to obliterate the remnants of his insight from his published writings and letters. Thirty-five years later, his friend and disciple Sandor Ferenczi came to the same conclusion and met with the same cold response from psychoanalysts, including Freud himself (Masson, 1984).

It was anathema in psychoanalytic thought to dwell on the actual sexual abuse; what was important was the fantasied sexual life of childhood. An emphasis on real sexual traumas, the psychoanalysts held, would undermine the theories of infant sexuality and the Oedipus complex and thus weaken the entire psychoanalytic method (Masson, 1984). Recognizing the sexual abuse as real would also implicate the fathers, uncles, and grandfathers in the respectable European families whose children were the first psychoanalytic patients. As Masson argues, Freud was unwilling to risk his entire professional career on a concept that would alienate not only his professional colleagues but also the very patrons who provided his livelihood.[8] The brief awareness that Freud instigated of the prevalence and destructiveness of past sexual trauma disappeared from clinical consciousness for almost a century (Herman, 1992).

In later accounts of childhood sexual abuse, when overt sexual contact could not be denied, the girl herself was held responsible for being at least willing, if not seductive. In 1937 Bender and Blau described the "conspicuously charming and attractive personalities" (p. 516) of fourteen multiply sexually abused children who were hospitalized on a children's psychiatric ward for prolonged evaluation. The authors of this frequently cited study concluded that the children were active participants in the sexual relations and that sometimes they initiated it. For decades, these and other psychiatric authors argued that incest and sexual abuse did not necessarily damage the child (Bender & Grugett, 1952; Yorukoglu & Kemph, 1966).

The psychiatric view of children as willing participants fit with the social service reports from the same era that dwelt on how girls from poor neighborhoods would allow sexual contacts for money, candy, or oranges. Social workers considered a girl morally defective once sexual abuse had occurred (Gordon, 1988). Any bad outcome for the child was not a result of the sexual abuse but rather a problem intrinsic to the child herself. Those children who did develop psychiatric problems as teenagers and adults were thought to have been manifesting the beginnings of their psychiatric illness in their early sexual activity: "Their sexual behavior in childhood, rather than predisposing to a psychotic adjustment, had more likely been but one aspect of their generally confused reaction to the beginnings of a fundamentally disrupting process" (Bender & Grugett, 1952, p. 829). Such accounts, which denied or minimized the effect of sexual abuse or ascribed its occurrence to moral depravity or childhood psychopathology, formed the backdrop of the contemporary psychiatric understanding of incest and sexual abuse.

The incest literature up until the 1970s consisted of a scattering of articles confounded by methodological weaknesses: unrepresentative and tiny samples, lack of control groups, preoccupation with father-daughter incest, and author bias about incest (Carlson, 1977). In overt expressions of misogyny, the theme of maternal collusion or maternal responsibility for incest became central. For instance, Lustig et al.'s "Incest: A Family Group Survival Pattern," invariably cited in later discussions, concluded that incest depends on five factors: (1) role reversal between mother and daughter; (2) "impaired" sexual relations between the parents; (3) "unwillingness by the father to act out sexually outside the family related to a need to maintain the public facade of a stable and competent patriarch"; (4) fear by all family members of family disintegration; and (5) "the conscious or unconscious sanction of the nonparticipant mother" (Lustig, Dresser, Spellman, & Murray, 1966, p. 39).

Of these five characteristics, only one (and a dubious one)—that the father is unwilling to go outside the family to meet his sexual needs—is an attribute that belongs directly to the father. Underlying this assertion are two unexpressed assumptions: that a man has a *right* to get his sexual needs met in "his" family, and that any sexual problems in the marriage result from the wife's "frigidity." The focus on individual pathology portrayed mothers as frigid, dependent, inadequate; fathers, although they behaved like patriarchs in the family, felt inadequate and unsure of their masculinity. When the wife refuses sex with the husband and, what is more, reverses roles with the daughter, the man appears entitled to have sexual access to his daughter. Apart from personality shortcomings, the incestuous or sexually abusive father in the early incest literature appears to be acting in a completely rational and understandable manner.

The daughters depicted in these case studies were "pseudomature" yet afraid of family disintegration. Their attempts to avoid, run away, disclose, or stop the incest were either invisible or appeared dysfunctional. Incest became a pre-Oedipal wish-come-true of the daughter, who was enmeshed in a family system in which the mother was centrally at fault (Gutheil & Avery, 1977; Lustig et al., 1966; Machotka, Pittman, & Flomenhaft, 1967). The notion proliferated that incest was caused by the family's response to the fear of separation. "The daughter's sexual gratification of the father clearly served to reduce family tension and the danger of family dissolution" (Lustig et al., 1966, p. 36). The incest was transformed into a service "to protect and maintain the family . . . serving to reduce family tension by preventing confrontation with the sources of tension. The preservation of the family group is the central function of incest to the group" (p. 39). Nowhere does this version of the incest family make the father an active agent who uses his daughter in sexual ways for his own gratification.

Belief in the seductive child and in the maternal role in incest were prerequisites to the evolving family systems interpretations that portrayed incest as the response of the entire family. The family systems approach centers on the appreciation of the "interpersonal triangle" created by the incest. The role of nonparticipant (usually the mother) appears more "interesting" than that of the participants; it is her denial that creates the "secret," not the perpetrator's insistence on silence. In the reformulation of incest as a family problem, the father appears "passive" despite his "overt culpability," and the mother emerges as "the cornerstone in the pathological family system" (Lustig et al., 1966, p. 30). In a still cited family therapy case report from 1977, Gutheil and Avery (1977) persist in the view that the role of the incest in the Jones family was to defend against separation anxiety. This case warrants detailed description because it shows how family systems thinking refuses to recognize that incest is sexual abuse, that responsibility for the abuse is deflected onto the mother, and that missing or misinterpreted in the report are the mother's and girls' experiences of abuse.

Their pediatrician referred the Jones family for therapy because of the revelation of incest by two teenage daughters. The family consisted of the father, the mother, and seven daughters, ages nineteen, seventeen, sixteen, fifteen, fourteen, and twins of nine. The mother's pregnancies were complicated by "sickness, discomfort, and renal disease." After the birth of the twins, Mrs. Jones "insisted" that her husband have a vasectomy. At about this time, the father began incestuous relations with the oldest daughter (then age ten), then with the fifth daughter (age five or so), then with the second, third, and fourth. The twins were not identified as sexually abused. The oldest daughter married and moved out when she turned eighteen, and the second daughter "ran away" early in treatment. The text does not clarify whether the incest continued with any of the younger daughters during the course of the treatment.

As the case unfolds, we learn that in the early years of the marriage the father had repeatedly enlisted voluntarily for duty in the Antarctic, causing prolonged absence from the family when the children were small. On one later occasion, the mother left precipitously with all seven children but returned a few weeks later. Mr. Jones's reaction to "this shattering experience was to bury himself in work and bowling to deny the loss" (Gutheil & Avery, 1977, p. 110). The authors' interpretation was that the family had never "integrated" the trauma of these separations. They attempted to get the family to agree that the incest was a way for the family to prevent separation, pointing out the parents' problem with the eldest daughter's marriage. They located the onset of the incest as having occurred after the birth of the twins, the vasectomy, the mother's departure and return, and the hospitalization of one of the twins when the father accidentally backed the car over her foot.

The viewpoint of the mother during these years is totally missing. We can infer, nonetheless, that she must have recovered from a complicated and possibly dangerous twin pregnancy, looked after two infants as well as five children between the ages of five and ten with little help, and then dealt with the hospitalization of an infant whom her husband had injured. There is no mention of how desperate those times must have been for her, only "the shock and pain" of the father at the mother's temporary departure. Instead, the authors describe the mother as sexually rejecting. They offer little explanation for why she might not have wished to have intercourse with her husband, only that "both partners accused the other of being insatiable and bound to rigidly prescribed foreplay." Also, she saw him "as too demanding, selfish, and perverse in his interest in such variations as dorsal intercourse."

Openly contemptuous of the mother's low self-esteem, the authors consider her worries about the children being taken away because of the incest as "quasi-paranoid" (p. 112). Their inability to accept the mother's anger is overt:

> Mother's anger flared as she described her husband as dictatorial. She compared him to a king and the rest of the family to his subjects. The salient differences in the power allotment reduced to mother's perception that father was free to kick her out of bed or to leave himself, whereas she could do neither. . . . Her theme was that men were privileged to have their sex wherever they wanted it, but women were uniquely vulnerable to abandonment. Furious at her own notion of the entitled male, she began to ridicule father's sexual interest in her. "What have I got down there that's so damn precious?" she blurted out through tears, and fled the room with father in pursuit. Our interpretation of this outburst was that mother could not contain her sense of being cheated because she was a woman. Rather than bear her envy of the idealized male genital, she sought to reverse roles through ridicule and abandonment of father. (p. 112)

This interpretation demonstrates the authors' inability to tolerate the appropriateness of the mother's rage. Finding her position incomprehensible, they fall back on penis envy as the only explanation for why she would be so outraged. They could not recognize as "salient differences in the power allotment" the humiliation and powerlessness this woman experienced at the hand of her husband, who had abused five of their seven children.

After six months of treatment, mother and daughters were both furious at the father. The authors find this perplexing and contradictory:

Rather than face the issues of *mother's* failure in the nurturant role, the women resorted to a "sexist" defense of deploring *father's* failure to provide the care. . . . Father was made to appear the only entitled one, who had hurt everyone. Having made father the culprit, mother angrily revenged herself both on him and the male therapist by summarily deciding to take the children and flee after the 22nd session. We felt this flight represented an acting out of long-deferred anger against her own mother's failure to nurture, and subsequently separate from, her own growing daughters. (p. 112, emphasis in original)

Today the authors' incredulity is comical. They could not acknowledge that the final result constituted both a failure of their explanation of incest and yet a clinical success in terms of preventing further incest or abuse. Today we might view the "flight" of the mother and daughters as evidence that they had been adequately empowered to depart from male-dominated family and therapeutic systems and to reinstate the mother's authority and confidence in managing her family. What is paradoxical is that this kind of therapy could have yielded this result!

Gutheil and Avery's interpretation of the Jones family incest demonstrates how diffusing responsibility to the whole family system absolves the father from responsibility for his actions while actively holding mother and daughter(s) responsible. Published almost twenty years ago, this case is still cited as a respected source. For instance, in a recent family therapy text, Combrinck-Graham (1988) nests incest within a chapter on adolescent sexuality. Citing the case of the Jones family, she repeats the familiar generalizations. The mother is sexually unavailable through illness, absence, or, "often, her preoccupation with her own mother." The father's "strong morality" prevents him from seeking sexual relationships outside of the marriage. (This peculiar vision of morality makes sense only if one accepts the notion that a married man's sexual relations with his daughters somehow fall within his morally acceptable sexual options.) When the daughter reaches adolescence, the family "pulls together to resist strong developmental centrifugal forces" that are normally expressed through the adolescent's sexual exploring outside the family. "If the forces holding the family together are so strong, then it may be equally difficult for the maturing daughter in the family to seek sexual relationships outside of the family" (p. 122).

Thus, modern psychiatric and family therapy approaches to incest have failed to define incest as sexual domination over a child and often over her mother; rather, they identify the mother as collusive and pathological. As with physical violence against women (chapter 4), the reigning orthodoxy diffuses responsibility onto the family, distracting attention away from male responsibility for sexual abuse. Neither men's abuse of power in families nor men's domination of women in the larger society are subject to question. Moreover, strikingly absent from clinical incest reports is any awareness of the perspective of the women and girls who survived the abuse (Johnson, 1992). By failing to recognize that incest survivors and their mothers have a voice, the psychiatric approach to incest, until the 1980s, denied the reality of the incest experience for the girls and women to whom it happened.

MEDICINE'S RESPONSE: PEDIATRICS

Pediatrics has a split consciousness about incest and sexual abuse. On the one hand, the typical description of the incest family has been uncritically imported into pediatric teachings: the *Nelson Textbook of Pediatrics* again portrays the father as "rigid, patriarchal, and emotionally immature," unlikely to seek sex outside the marriage; the mother is depressed, unavailable, and often a childhood sexual abuse victim herself; the "pseudomature" daughter has taken on the household tasks in the "closely knit," socially isolated family (Behrman et al., 1992, p. 81). Hoekelman et al.'s *Primary Pediatric Care* (1992) repeats these stereotypes and then quotes the hackneyed words of Lustig et al. (1966), that incest is a symptom of defective family functioning that serves to preserve the family system (Rosenfeld & Sarles, 1992).

On the other hand, when the problem is defined as "child sexual abuse," the pediatric literature places an urgent focus on detection of the abhorrent violation of the vulnerable young. All clinicians, as well as teachers and social workers, are schooled in the recognition of the physical signs and behavioral symptoms of child sexual abuse. Pediatricians in particular have concentrated on the identification of the often subtle signs of sexual abuse in small children. Pediatric consideration of the sexually abused child focuses on emergency evaluation, the legally mandated reporting of the abuse to state authorities, immediate protection of the child, and referrals to social service agencies and to mental health services for the individuals in the family.[9]

A sexually abused child may come to medical attention when sexual abuse is obvious on physical examination because of acute or chronic anogenital trauma or venereal disease. Since these cases are almost indisputable from a medical point of view, they tend to generate strong reactions and immediate social service and legal involvements. More often, however, clinical examination of possibly abused children reveals few or no physical findings of abuse: exposure, pornographic involvement, nonpenetrating touch, and oral-genital sex leave no tangible findings. Or the findings themselves may be subtle. Pediatricians disagree about the standards for defining redness, chafing, and vaginal and rectal dilation associated with sexual abuse (McCann, 1990). Even definite findings may resolve within a few days, necessitating immediate medical examination following disclosure. Later exams may neither confirm nor refute charges of sexual abuse, although in some cases the resolution of subtle anogenital findings after the child has been separated from the perpetrator may serve as verification that abuse occurred and has stopped.

Since the Victorian era, the physician's role in child sexual abuse cases has pivoted on documenting physical evidence of molestation (Gordon, 1988, p. 216). In the debate about the subtle findings of otherwise undisclosed abuse, physicians are divided about which is worse: undiscovered sexual abuse or unwarranted aspersions of abuse. Some pediatricians detail and photograph subtle anogenital findings in sexually abused children and call for careful inspection of children's genitalia during evaluations (Emans, Woods, Flagg, & Freeman, 1987; Hobbs & Wynne, 1987; McCann, 1990; Muram, 1989; Paradise, 1990). Others dispute these findings as within the range of normal and decry the potential damage to children and families from the increased suspicion of sexual abuse and from the exams and interviews themselves (*Lancet*, 1986, 1987a, 1987b; Zeitlin, 1987). Even though medical and legal definitions of sexual abuse do not require trauma or penetration, the current debate about genital findings in sexual abuse continues to direct physician attention to the condition of the hymen and rectum in an effort to obtain physical proof of sexual abuse.[10]

Because of the frequent absence of physical findings, clinicians trying to detect childhood sexual abuse have also focused on the interview with the child. Particularly with young children, experts in child sexual abuse advocate for interviews with children using "anatomically correct" dolls—that is, with penises, vaginas, mouths, and rectums—to enable the child to show what happened. Experienced interviewers are preferred so as to avoid the trauma of repeated interviews (Paradise, 1990). When physical evidence is ambiguous or absent, the evidence of child sexual abuse may be constituted in verbal or behavioral disclosures to a professional in these interviews.

Despite this pediatric focus on detection, clinicians remain unfamiliar with those forces that virtually guarantee that sexually abused children will carry their secret into adulthood.[11] Fear of punishment by the perpetrator or someone else, fear of abandonment or rejection, fear of hurting someone or breaking up the family, or fear of being blamed or not being believed all render children mute. These fears are entirely appropriate considering the climate of threat, force, or violence in which sexual abuse takes place. Even when the abuse itself is not forceful, the threats of harm to the victim, her mother, her siblings, or her pets or possessions may guarantee silence (Lister, 1982). Here is a sample of this climate of threat from Sylvia Fraser's *My Father's House*:

> Desperation makes me bold. At last I say the won't-love-me words:
> "I'm going to tell my mommy on you!"

My father replaces bribes with threats. "If you do, you'll have to give me back all your toys."

I tot up my losses: my Blondie and Dagwood cutouts, my fairy tale coloring book, my crayons. "My mommy gave those things to me. They're mine."

"I paid for them. Everything in this house belongs to me. If you don't behave, I've a good mind to throw them into the furnace." I think of my beloved Teddy Umcline, his one good eye melting in the flames. "I don't care! I don't care! I don't care!"

"Shut up! What will the neighbors think? If you don't shut up I'll . . . I'll . . . send you to the place where all bad children go. An orphanage where they lock up bad children whose parents don't want them any more."

"My mother won't let you!"

"Your mother will do what I say. Then you'll be spanked every night and get only bread and water."

That shuts me up for quite a while, but eventually I dare to see this, too, as a game for which there is an answer: "I don't care. I'll run away!"

My father needs a permanent seal for my lips, one that will murder all defiance. "If you say once more that you're going to tell, I'm sending that cat of yours to the pound for gassing!"

"I'll . . . I'll . . . I'll. . . ."

The air swooshes out of me as if I have been punched. My heart is broken. My resistance is broken. Smokey's life is in my hands. This is no longer a game, however desperate. Our bargain is sealed in blood. (Fraser, 1987, pp. 11–12)

It is remarkable, considering this atmosphere of threat, how many children do try to disclose (Gordon, 1988).[12] Yet medicine, however offended by the practice of child sexual abuse, cannot maintain an awareness of the usual context of domination in which it occurs and the trauma that it inflicts (Herman, 1992). Clinical awareness remains focused on detection.

With physical evidence often absent or debatable and children's disclosures variable or contradictory, physicians lack an organizing schema from which to view childhood sexual abuse. Instead, they have become preoccupied with the question of proof; concerns about the veracity of children's allegations have led to published caveats about children's reports,[13] especially in instances of divorce and custody conflict. For example, the *Nelson Textbook of Pediatrics* states that false accusations of incest are rare "except in cases involving psychotic patients or in some custody disputes" (Behrman et al., 1992, p. 82). Highly publicized custody disputes have hinged on the allegation of sexual abuse, making the physician yet again the final arbiter.[14]

It is at this point of arbitration, when child sexual abuse comes up in the context of a fight over control of children between a man and a woman, that we see how women's ability to protect their children may be invalidated and men's power to abuse strengthened. While common wisdom holds that a mother should protect her child from sexual abuse and do everything possible to protect her child from an abuser, including divorcing him if he is her husband, when she tries to do so, the abuse may be portrayed as an allegation that emerges as part of the vituperative struggle between embittered adults. In this scenario, the child appears to be a pawn in a battle between a man and a woman; women's and children's shared need for safety disappears. Furthermore, concern about protection of the child gets lost because adults outside the family construe the abuse as just another one-sided accusation in a setting where doctors and judges do not believe in taking sides.

Clinicians are more likely to suspect the possibility of sexual abuse and believe in its likelihood in marginally functioning families than in apparently asymptomatic families because of the common assumption that sexual abuse is a deranged act. Only in such "chaotic" families do clinicians imagine that children would be exposed to (or left unprotected with) men so disturbed that they would abuse their own family members. Historically, protective services have focused their efforts on children from such families (Gordon, 1988). However, clinical reports and surveys of adult women and the recollections of women survivors of sexual abuse concur that most sexual abuse occurs in otherwise unremarkable, *ordinary* families that never come to the attention of any medical, social service, or legal authority. Discovery of childhood sexual abuse is unlikely during routine well-child care in such families since clinicians hesitate to raise the subject of sexual abuse with apparently well-functioning families. Both patients and clinicians may equate questions about sexual abuse with insinuation. The fact that ordinary men in ordinary families molest the girls in those families has not altered the clinical work of practitioners who have not been previously sensitized to the issue of incest. Schooled in a system of medical knowledge that idealizes conventional sex roles (see chapter 3), clinicians do not anticipate that the heterosexual nuclear family is a hazardous setting for some female children.

Thus, most sexually abused girls from undistinguished families do not come to medical attention in childhood or adolescence. Despite increased public discussion of sexual abuse, medical providers are unlikely to detect the high frequency of sexual abuse during childhood that adult women later report. Although the symptoms of children known to have been sexually abused are well documented, pediatric knowledge is limited about the medical and psychological development of undetected child sexual abuse survivors. Those children who were not recognized as sexually abused during childhood often come to clinical attention during adolescence and adulthood.

A FEMINIST RE-VISION

Eloquent personal accounts of the discovery of and recovery from incest and child sexual abuse immeasurably enrich our understanding of what it means to have been sexual abused and what it means to survive it.[15] A shared understanding among survivors is that their body symptoms are a reflection of their experiences of victimization (Bass & Davis, 1988). Many survivor accounts detail the years they spent going from one doctor to another, trying to cure the problem with no name, often before they became aware of their previous history of sexual abuse or before they were able to link it to their bodily symptoms.

Personal accounts by survivors convey the unique pain or terror or horror of each child's experience. In line with contemporary feminist thinking, the particularity of each experience is central and must not be blotted out in a dogmatic search for a single version of reality. Particularity requires the acknowledgment that some perpetrators are physically violent and some are not; that some mothers are collusive or actively abusive and some are not; that some girls respond sexually and others retreat from their bodies to other levels of consciousness. The details differ in distinct ways. A cohesive understanding of abuse and its aftermath not only accepts the particularity of individual experience, it is grounded in it. Survivor accounts are not peripheral to a central theory; they are the essential core of our understanding (Barringer, 1992). Survivor accounts contradict the falsehoods that appear when case reports merge biased portrayals of mothers, fathers, and daughters to obliterate each girl's own description of how unwanted was the incest.

"Lie down there, you bitch."

He's not shouting but his voice is hard like steel. I am afraid to look at his face. I don't think that I can move, but I do. He pulls my pants to my ankles.

He lies on top of me after unzipping his pants. He pushes up and down, wrapping his arms around my ribs. I can't breathe. My pubic bone feels sore.

"You cunt," he says. His anger comes out on his breath. I try not to breathe his words into my body but they come in anyway.

My body is confused. Thick, strange feelings come from between my legs. But Kevin feels horrible. He feels hating. He feels old. This is dying. It seems like he will crush my body underneath his weight. I cannot breathe. I cannot move. Every time he bears down on me he calls me a name. No one has ever called me these names before.

But I know what they mean. They mean I'm bad.

"Bitch. Cunt. Whore." My body stops feeling. I become vacant. He is sneering.

"You're liking this aren't you?" he whispers. (Wisechild, 1988, pp. 101–2)

Survivor accounts force us to recognize that male domination—within the family, in the extended family and outside the family, and across generations—lies at the core of incest and sexual abuse.

PATRIARCHY

Male domination works at many levels. At its broadest and most abstract, it generates and promotes an ideology of admiration and respect for what is male and a derogation and disrespect for what is female. This ideology requires an absolute distinction between male and female, and it perpetuates this distinction in every arena of thought, from the classification of garden hose couplers to the color of newborn infant sleepsuits. The ideology of male domination permeates social institutions and perpetuates itself by ensuring that men, who have historically run these institutions, will continue to do so. At the family level, the ideology of male domination ensures that each man feels he is entitled to run his castle and each woman feels it is her job to keep her man happy. From infancy to adulthood, human beings receive a barrage of messages about who is in charge. From the Supreme Court to the magazines at the grocery checkout counter, patriarchy reigns unchecked.

The term "patriarchy" subsumes the protean manifestations of male domination. At a national level, the principle that political sovereignty requires military power depends on acceptance of the legitimacy of physical force to overpower. Physical power determines who is in charge. The fusion of physical force with the act of sex makes rape more than an isolated sexual act: the rape of Jewish women in Russian pogroms, of women in Bangladeshi religious wars, of Catholic nuns in El Salvador, of a white woman runner in Central Park, all show men defining their power through defiling and debasing women. At an ideological level, most clearly seen in pornography, the imagery of male sexual arousal merges with the imagery of physical domination to proliferate the image of sex as an act between the powerful and the vulnerable. Child sexual abuse by family members (as well as by acquaintances and strangers) is not simply a matter of an individual man molesting an individual girl, though this is the final result; his abuse is supported, indeed encouraged, by a network of social, cultural, and historical forces that coalesce to ensure that men will try to molest girls. Within a specific family, patriarchy ensures that age, generational privilege, physical strength, and male gender will enable an adult man to abuse the disempowered children, usually girls, in his world. Patriarchy overdetermines sexual abuse. Hence:

- Incest and sexual abuse occur in settings where male dominance is established by force or threat of force, often accompanied by abuse of alcohol.
- These settings are further characterized by maternal powerlessness. Maternal empowerment is essential to protect children from abuse; in its absence, girls are particularly at risk.
- Within any given incest family, all the children, particularly girls, are at risk. Abusers often molest daughters in sequence. The individual victim is the exception, not the rule.
- Any situation in families in which an older male has unlimited and unsupervised access to a much younger female provides an opportunity for abuse.
- The workings of male domination over time perpetuate sexual abuse across generations.

Let us look at each of these points in detail.

MALE DOMINATION ESTABLISHED BY FORCE

Male violence or the threat of male violence characterizes many of the family settings in which incest and sexual abuse take place (see chapter 4). Although pediatrics texts take pains to distinguish physical abuse, so obviously violent, from sexual abuse (Jason, Williams, Burton, & Rochat, 1982) and even acknowledge that sexual abuse is "a power problem" (Sgroi, 1982), the same texts do not clarify that domination sets the context.

Alcohol use and sexual abuse of children are often associated. Herman reports that fifteen out of forty fathers of daughters reporting incest had been alcoholics (Herman & Hirschman, 1981); Gordon reports that drunkenness was associated with incest in 28 percent of her case records (1988, p. 357); other studies mention alcohol abuse anecdotally in relation to incest (Browning & Boatman, 1977; Goodwin, 1982; Renvoize, 1982). As with physical violence, medicine acknowledges the use of alcohol by sexual abuse perpetrators but fails to interpret how alcohol potentiates men's ability to abuse with impunity and to disown responsibility for their actions. Most studies offer no interpretation of this association but imply or allow the reader to assume that alcohol abuse makes men lose control. Alcohol use may be used to explain so-called accidental incest or to explain an "unhealthy pattern of expressing intimacy" (Coleman, 1982), or incest and alcoholism together may fade out of focus amid the many problems in a "multi-problem" family. Like the connection between alcohol and battering, alcoholism appears to explain if not excuse sexual abuse. The *choice* to use alcohol and the decision to use a child sexually disappear in discussions of sexual abuse that ignore the gendered context of the perpetrator's drinking.

Men's alcohol abuse is only one element, and a variable one, in the structure of male domination. Some form of physical abuse and psychological abuse of mothers is present in more than three-quarters of incest families (Truesdell et al., 1986). Sometimes the father spares the incestuously abused daughter the physical abuse that thunders down on the mother and other children, setting up a situation in which that daughter appears special and may later feel particularly guilty. Just as battering reflects male domination over women, incest and child sexual abuse represent male domination over children, especially girls, in the sexual arena. Traditional psychiatric theories cannot explain why sexual abuse and incest take place in the environment of threatened if not overt violence against women because these explanatory systems avoid examining the power differential between men and women. For instance, one incest perpetrator described as "dependent" inserted a Q-tip, a pen cap, and then a .22 caliber bullet into the vagina of his eight-year-old daughter, making her promise not to tell. The text notes, without comment, that his daughter "was becoming increasingly afraid of him" (Groth, 1982, p. 221). If we are to make sense of incest, we must redefine it as a sexual assault (even when it is not overtly violent) by the more powerful against the most vulnerable in the family. It is not the incest that "functions to hold the family together" (Swanson & Biaggio, 1985) but rather male violence and continued threat of violence that prevent women's and children's escape (Gordon, 1988). With this recognition, we can rediscover with women who experienced sexual abuse that gender is central to why they were abused. *Incest and sexual abuse are the violent practices of male sexual prerogative in patriarchal families.*

Clinicians are not unaware of the violence of perpetrators, but this awareness has not been made central in discussions of incest. For instance, a 1984 case conference in the *Journal of Family Practice* described a family in which the father had committed incest with the older daughter, then with the younger daughter, from ages eight to seventeen. The mother, who was disabled by rheumatoid arthritis, stated, "I am not going back. He was violent these last two years, and it was awful. I was scared to turn around" (Realini, Ortiz, Turnbull, &

Couchman, 1984, p. 537). The younger daughter and her three brothers knew about the previous incest with the older sister. "My brothers and everybody are scared of my father. They have reason to be: he is the monster of all monsters. I have always thought of him that way" (p. 537).

MATERNAL POWERLESSNESS

Deborah Luepnitz (1988) has argued cogently that the modern American family is patriarchal and father-absent, even though the father may be physically present. Analysis of the setting of incest, particularly father-daughter incest, reveals that these families are *patriarchal and mother-absent or mother-disempowered*, though the mother may be physically present. By highlighting maternal powerlessness, I am not attempting to find yet another way to hold mothers responsible for incest and sexual abuse. On the contrary, when mothers of incest survivors receive active support and explicitly feminist therapy, they usually discover their ability to act on behalf of their daughters (Johnson, 1992; Myer, 1984–85). Nevertheless, these women are disempowered in relation to the perpetrators in their families.

Paternal alcoholism and battering exaggerate the power discrepancy even more—together they fuel men's power to abuse and further disable women. When present, maternal alcoholism, like physical or psychiatric disability, disempowers women in relation to men, prevents them from carrying out the socially expected tasks of motherhood, and ensures their powerlessness and their children's vulnerability. Deprived of their mother's ability to attend to her essential functions, including her ability to protect, girl children are at risk of abuse from men in the family, particularly but not exclusively their father.

Absolute authority characterized the fathers, and dependency and powerlessness the mothers, in Herman's study of forty incest survivors (Herman & Hirschman, 1981). She found that 55 percent of the mothers suffered chronic illnesses during their daughters' childhoods, and 38 percent of the daughters experienced separation from their mothers because of their illnesses or inability to look after their children. (Depression, alcoholism, and psychosis were the most common disabilities.) Similarly, in Gordon's eighty-year survey, no mother was present in 22 percent of the incest families; most often she had died and the father was the head of household. When the mother was present, more than three-fourths had one or more characteristics of weakening in maternal authority or disempowerment in relation to the father: 44 percent were beaten; 36 percent were ill or disabled; 34 percent suffered other disabling conditions, such as alcoholism, rejection by their own relatives, recent migration to the United States, inability to speak English, and social isolation (evidenced by rare trips out of the household) (Gordon, 1988, p. 212). In other words, when the mother was not present in her fullest capacity, daughters faced increased risk of incest.

Further historical evidence of maternal disempowerment in incest families is the fact that these mothers gave birth to more children than other women (Herman, 1981, pp. 77–78). Women who bear larger numbers of children are more likely to remain in traditional women's roles and less likely to seek education or employment, which might offer them a separate basis of authority. Thus, an overburdened mother worn down by excessive childbearing and disabled in some way in relation to her husband has been typical of incest families. In the future, however, traditional sex role activities may not typify mothers in incest families as more women enter the workforce and bear fewer children. Rather, a patriarchal father may allow his wife to work for his own reasons, not because he has abdicated any of his authority (Johnson, 1992). Gender domination will structure incest families even if mothers no longer play traditional roles. Each woman's disempowerment is unique; we must listen to each mother's own story to understand how male power has operated in her situation (Johnson, 1992).

Gordon concludes from her historical survey that "mothers' powerlessness prevented girls from internalizing the self-esteem they needed to resist sexual exploitation themselves" (1988, pp. 212–13). Although both parents should be able to foster such self-esteem in their children, when mothers could not do it, fathers did not usually take on the role. Typologies of incest offenders that divide them into dominant or dependent types (Groth, 1982) imply that, whichever type her husband is, a woman is expected to look after the needs of both husband and children. In the cases above, when the mothers were sick, weak, and overwhelmed, the fathers did not assume any obligation to care for the children or to protect them. Instead, both fathers and therapists adhered to a belief in paternal entitlement: fathers can expect to be taken care of in families; if mothers cannot do it, then daughters should. In their view, it is never the father's responsibility to care for children when the mother is disabled. The therapeutic practice that results from this belief system further disempowers and blames the mother for the catastrophes that befall her children when she cannot protect them.

The mother in the case above spoke about her powerlessness:

> My ex-husband was never able to cope with my being handicapped, especially during the time when I couldn't take care of myself or the children. It was a barrier between us. . . . Before I was stricken so badly, I was the one who took them to school, attended PTA meetings, baked them things, all of that. When I was stricken with the arthritis, I was in so much pain, I could hardly move. I wasn't able to watch the children, especially if they would run away from me. Sometimes they even went hungry because I couldn't cook or wash. Jenny sometimes helped after she was 10 years old or so. Occasionally, my husband or

my mother-in-law would help out. My church wanted to send somebody over to help, but my husband would not allow any church people in our house. (Realini et al., 1984, p. 533)

When we interpret sexual abuse as the violent practice of male sexual power in male-dominant families, the predominance of male perpetrators and female victims in child sexual abuse and incest makes sense. The high frequency of wife beating and marital rape fits in the picture as well. The absence, sickness, or helplessness of the mother is also congruent; mothers of incest survivors have functioned in the most traditional women's roles exactly because these are patriarchal families.

Contrary to common belief, about half of sexually abused boys are molested by family members (Spencer & Dunklee, 1986). Careful examination of these families once again reveals patriarchal power operating, often coercively and sometimes across several generations, to cripple the women and children (see Cooper & Cormier, 1982, for case reports). For instance, Humphries, Barclay, & Mohler (1986) describe a family in which the father had serially abused at least two sons and a daughter, and the older brothers had abused the sister and younger brother, who at sixteen disclosed the multiple incest during his third psychiatric hospitalization for a suicide attempt. The authors contemptuously describe the mother as having "dull normal intelligence" and being "overwhelmed by the situation . . . a passive, dependent woman who made extensive use of repression, denial, and somatization to deal with internal and external distress. . . . She was obese and often appeared on the ward with somatic complaints; she was hospitalized twice during her son's [six-month] psychiatric evaluation for nonspecific somatic problems" (p. 47). The authors invoke the traditional explanations of role reversal, parental sexual difficulties, family fear of separation, and maternal collusion to excuse the father's systematic sexual abuse of both male and female children. Here, in the setting of maternal powerlessness, sexual domination cascaded downhill, while professionals reinforced the mother's powerlessness by making her appear despicable. Thus, sexual abuse of boys in families, less frequently disclosed and less often clinically described, operates under the same patriarchal dynamic as sexual abuse of girls and is subject to the same clinical distortions.

IN INCEST FAMILIES, ALL GIRLS ARE AT RISK

Authoritative studies of child sexual abuse warn that when one child in a family has been identified as sexually abused, the siblings are at high risk (Tilelli, Durek, & Jaffe, 1980). New cases of sexually abused children are frequently the siblings of other children already identified as abused. Many of the incest case reports in the medical and psychiatric literature mention that fathers sequentially molest their daughters (and sometimes their sons), beginning with the oldest and working downward (Gutheil & Avery, 1977; Humphries et al., 1986; McCann, Voris, & Simon, 1988; Realini et al., 1984; Weeks, 1976; Wilson, Clements, Cadoret, Pease, & Lammer, 1978; Zdanuk, Harris, & Wisian, 1987). Russell's random sampling of women documents this reality: 31 percent of perpetrators had molested one or more other relatives; stepfathers had the highest frequency of abusing others (50 percent), followed by grandfathers (44 percent) and fathers (32 percent) (1986, p. 277). Clearly in these families no girl child was safe. Perhaps the same grandfathers had also molested the mothers and aunts during their childhoods. Herman found a comparable rate of 28 percent repetition of incest with younger sisters, and suspicion of molestation in another 25 percent (Herman & Hirschman, 1981). When pregnancy results from incest, the incestuous father may regard the offspring as yet another child at his disposal (Courtois, 1988). Additionally, among self-acknowledged incest offenders, half had engaged in abusing girls outside the family as well (Abel et al., 1988).

Nevertheless, despite the fact that clinicians "know" about the documented downward cascade of incestuous abuse, professional descriptions illogically continue to locate the problem in the family dynamics, the role of the mother, or the behavior of the daughter. These reports ignore the evidence against "role reversal" presented by the fact that many perpetrators molest multiple children within a family. Sexual abuse cannot be about roles, since the multiple abused children no doubt occupy a variety of roles. A man without scruples about sexually abusing one child will have a lower threshold for initiating abuse with a subsequent victim. Such a man will try it with any vulnerable female (and sometimes male) in his purview, regardless of his wife. No particular role or dynamic is necessary other than the perpetrator's desire to behave sexually toward a child and his ability to override his inhibitions, including the fear of getting caught (Russell, 1986).

> I then went to see my stepsister, Sarah, who had lived with my father when we were both between the ages of ten and twelve. . . . I handed her the booklet [that the speaker had written about incest] and said, "There's something I want to tell you about, but it's hard. . . ." She read a few lines, then put it down. "I don't need to read it," she said. "The same thing was happening to me." Later Sarah talked to her sister and we found out that all three of us were being molested by my father in the same period of time, and none of us had known about the others. (Bass & Thornton, 1983, p. 63)

Since abusers often molest more than one girl in their family and sometimes girls outside the family as well, it is both unsatisfactory and inappropriate to make the "incest triangle" the centerpiece in the study of sexual abuse. Moreover, the fact that perpetrators initiate the incestuous activity when girls are an *average* of eight years of age means that many of the girls are younger. Clinical reviews that attempt to reframe "multiple" incest as a "defense against separation" (Gutheil & Avery, 1977; Swanson & Biaggio, 1985) fail to recognize that the majority of the girls are *prepubertal children* who are not about to leave home. Efforts to construe incestuous relations between a man and a girl as anything other than sexual abuse serve to defend the rights of men to continue their invasions of girls' bodies.

Men who sexually abuse girls in their families are not pedophiles (adults whose sexual preference is for children) but rather men who claim a right to sex with these specific girls because of patriarchal control. Perpetrators continue the abuse into the time when the girl is sexually mature. Only when the survivor herself leaves the household or in some other way extricates herself from the perpetrator's grasp does the abuse stop (Herman & Hirschman, 1981). Many adult survivors are unable to return home or to see the perpetrator because they know that they will have to repel yet another assault. Many feel at risk as long as their perpetrator is alive. This clarification about pedophiles is important to prevent the marginalization of child sexual abuse to the realm of a few "perverted" men who are sexually attracted to children. The experience of child sexual abuse by one-quarter of all women shows that sexual abuse is common practice among ordinary "family" men who appear in all other respects to have unremarkable sexual preferences.

UNLIMITED AND UNSUPERVISED ACCESS AS THE SETUP FOR ABUSE

Any situation in a family in which an older man or boy has unlimited and unsupervised access to a younger girl sets up the possibility of abuse. Most clinical studies focus on father-daughter incest, even though father-daughter incest represents, for instance, only 24 percent of the reported intrafamilial child sexual abuse reported by Russell (1986). This focus can provide helpful understandings about the specific context of such abuse (Herman & Hirschman, 1981). Survivors of father-daughter incest are likely to have experienced longer and more severe abuse and are also likely to be more symptomatic as adults. On the other hand, the psychiatric focus on "classic" father-daughter incest, by locating the explanation within either individual psychopathology or nuclear family interaction, addresses neither the disseminated sexual abuse that girls face from other male relatives nor the fact that any older male may claim a right to any vulnerable and accessible female in the family.

The largest group of perpetrators in intrafamilial sexual abuse are uncles (25 percent), followed closely by father figures—fathers, stepfathers, and mothers' boyfriends (24 percent)—male cousins (16 percent), brothers and stepbrothers (13 percent), and grandfather figures (6 percent) (Russell, 1986). Taken together, these data suggest that it is men's use of their generational authority, not nuclear family dynamics, that fosters abuse. Any general interpretation of the cause of incest must look beyond the nuclear family to explain why a variety of men in the extended family feel that it is their right to attempt or to force sexual contact with any related girl children.

As with father-daughter incest, abuse by uncles and brothers-in-law may also be accompanied by threats of abuse or harm to the mother, sisters, or other women in the family, reinforcing the context of violence and threat in which incestuous victimization takes place.

> I was staying with my uncle and aunt at that time [age ten]. Every day he used to give me extra money to spend. One day when my aunt was gone, he called me in and tried to get me to play with his penis. (*Did he use force?*) Yes, he tried to force me to jerk him off. He forced me to touch his penis, but I wouldn't jerk him off. At other times when my aunt was not at home he used to reach out and feel my breast. I was afraid to tell my aunt because he might beat her up if I did. (Russell, 1986, p. 328)

Sexual abuse by grandfathers, uncles, and father figures has a higher likelihood of lasting over a year when compared with abuse by brothers and cousins; abuse by these adult figures is also more likely to take place without explicit force. Grandfathers, who have the most cross-generational authority, abuse girls the longest and are the least likely to use force. In contrast, older brothers, at a mean age of 17.9 abusing their sisters at a mean age of 10.7, are more likely to use force, perhaps because they lack generational privilege over their sisters (Russell, 1986). The fact that cross-generational abuse is the longest lasting and least violent reinforces the understanding that, within families, patriarchy grants power on the basis of gender and age to adult men; this authority permits and maintains the abuse with or without the use of force.

INCEST FROM ONE GENERATION TO THE NEXT

Incest tends to replicate itself: as many as 65 percent of mothers in father-daughter incest families may have experienced incest or sexual abuse during their own childhoods (Myer, 1984–85). Why is this true? Incest and sexual abuse force daughters to leave home younger and to marry earlier; like their mothers, they then have more children than average and find themselves in traditional female roles. The incest survivor recapitulates in her own marriage the power imbalance between men and women in her family of origin. She becomes "the exploited, overresponsible caretaker with no rights to reciprocity and no self separate from her caretaking functions" (Gelinas, 1983, p. 325). She goes from being the daughter to the mother in an incest family. Gelinas suggests that the role reversal between the incestuously abused daughter and her mother will recur in the next generation.

> The now-adult parentified incest victim will tend to choose a man for whom caretaking is important. As with her parents, the birth of children may be the beginning of marital estrangement, and out of exhaustion she will begin to parentify her daughter. With increasing marital estrangement and parentification of the daughter, the high-risk family constellation develops and incest often begins in this generation as well. Like her mother, the former victim is unlikely to notice what is happening, as she too has become a depleted avoidant mother. (p. 325)

Thus, survivors' daughters become the third generation of girls and women to live in homes where women are chronically disempowered.

Although this description of the "transmission" of incest again focuses primarily on the mother's role in father-daughter incest, Gelinas does recognize that "untreated relational imbalances" pass along a certain pattern of power relations between the genders from one generation to the next. She describes a case in which four generations of women were incestuously abused by their fathers or stepfathers. The repetition of incest across generations is clearly a matter of more than any one woman's individual responsibility for picking the wrong spouse, someone who would abuse their daughter. Social and family expectations of gender relations contribute to a cascade of powerlessness that flows from grandmothers to mothers to daughters: devalued women enter marriages with authoritarian men who regard it as their right to control and abuse the women and children in their families. Viewing the transmission as the mother's responsibility ignores the constellation of historical, cultural, class, and family specifics that perpetuate patriarchal marital relationships between authoritarian men and disempowered women.

In each generation in which battering and abuse damage children's self-esteem, the boys learn from their own physical (and sometimes sexual) abuse and the abuse of their mothers and sisters that a man's power is defined by his right to abuse physically and sexually the girls and women in his world. The extravasation of male violence from one generation to the next may be a root cause of sexual abuse: when the father sexually assaults the mothers and daughters, his adolescent sons, aware of their father's sexual violence, may feel entitled to take advantage of their younger sisters and, in adulthood, of their wives and daughters. Case reports of intergenerational incest describe fathers having sex with their sons and daughters, the sons having sex with their sisters and later with their own daughters, and the sons encouraging their sons to do the same (Cooper & Cormier, 1982). Concomitant brother-sister incest in settings of father-daughter incest is commonly reported by survivors. Russell's (1986) finding that the sexually abusive brother was an average of 7.2 years older than the sister he abused invalidates the notion of consensual sibling sex and verifies the brother's ability to overpower his sister by force.

The transmission of sexual abuse also takes the direct route from men to boys. Physically and sexually abused boys have greater potential than nonabused boys to become physically and sexually abusive adults (Courtois, 1988). (It is important to recognize that not all abused boys become abusers, only that, among abusers, most have a background of abuse.) Boys more than girls are likely to attempt to resolve their own abuse by perpetrating it on someone else. They may equate the ability to abuse with power and masculinity (Lew, 1988). To boys, the right to overpower and abuse may appear as a right of males within the patriarchy; they only need to get old enough and strong enough to exercise this right.

These five interlocking factors make incest and sexual abuse the predictable outcomes of patriarchal beliefs and practices rather than aberrant deviations. A feminist construction of incest and sexual abuse holds the ideology and family structures of male domination responsible for creating the settings in which individual men exercise their privilege over women and children.[16] Feminist therapy with sexual abuse survivors recognizes the climate of threat and force that surrounded the abuse and holds the perpetrator responsible for the abuse. The role of mothers in families where girls are sexually abused can be reinterpreted with an understanding of women's vulnerability in patriarchal settings (Johnson, 1992; Luepnitz, 1988; McIntyre, 1981; Wattenberg, 1985). Those providing medical care to survivors, however, have not acknowledged the centrality of patriarchy to incest and sexual abuse.

The discovery and treatment of sexual abuse occurs in a specific historical and social context. The climate in which sexual abuse survivors now acknowledge and disclose their past experiences is markedly different from the therapeutic climate even ten years ago, as evidenced by the books on the treatment of sexually abused children and adolescents (Everstine & Everstine, 1989; MacFarlane & Waterman, 1986; Sgroi, 1982; Walker, 1988), the treatment of the adult survivor of incest (Briere, 1989; Courtois, 1988; Davies & Frawley, 1994; Kluft, 1990a), and the family treatment of incest (Renvoize, 1982; Trepper & Barrett, 1989). Explicitly feminist approaches to individual and family therapy have recognized the centrality of sexual violence in work with women (Goodrich, 1991; Herman, 1992; Mirkin, 1990; Walters, Carter, Papp, & Silverstein, 1988). Therapists are familiar with the anxiety and depression that accompany the disclosure and resolution of past sexual abuse and with the connection between past abuses and current symptoms. However, with the recognition of the widespread prevalence of past sexual abuse has also come the popularization of "recovery."

Sexual abuse is now the buzzword to sell workshops, programs, books, tapes, and groups in the "incest-survivor machine" (Tavris, 1993). Widespread consciousness-raising about incest and sexual abuse can free many women of guilt, shame, and a host of symptoms; it can also challenge the legitimacy of male domination in the families and institutions in which girls and women have been abused. However, confronting the patriarchy is not the key to successful marketing. Instead, the recovery movement focuses on individualized personal problems. Media attention to survivors carefully brackets their tearful disclosures with professional assessments of the diagnosis and treatment of their conditions (Alcoff & Gray, 1993). No one—not the television talk-show host, not the sexual abuse survivor, not the professional commentator—names male domination or the patriarchy as the problem.

The commercialization of sexual abuse victimization (not survivorhood) has been accompanied by attempts to invalidate and discredit survivors' accounts. Prominent among such efforts is the work of the False Memory Syndrome Foundation, an organization founded by parents whose adult children had accused them of childhood sexual abuse (Calof, 1993; Fried, 1994). Seeking to proclaim their own innocence, this group has tried to prove the existence of a "false memory syndrome." Less visible but potentially more dangerous is a trend among academics toward discounting retrieved memories. Just as Freud came to discount his own observation about the frequency of sexual abuse among his clients and replaced it with the idea that their accounts represented their fantasies, contemporary psychology is moving toward distrust of retrieved memories of sexual abuse (Olafson, Corwin, & Summit, 1993).

A prominent example is a 1993 article in the *American Psychologist* that questions the reality of repressed memories, Loftus's "The Reality of Repressed Memories." Pointing to the "malleable nature of memory," Loftus argues that false memories can be "planted" or "injected" into memory. She offers detailed descriptions of therapies in which women had finally recalled episodes of sexual abuse. Despite recognizing the widespread prevalence of sexual abuse, Loftus worries more about the effects of therapists who "suggest" the possibility of childhood abuse, "probe relentlessly for recalcitrant memories, and then . . . uncritically accept them as fact" (p. 534). While some therapists, at best overzealous and at worst unscrupulous, may indeed be manipulating patients' memories, such skepticism about survivors' accounts coming from a prestigious source is likely to introduce doubt and confusion into therapeutic work with all survivors. Loftus counsels therapists to maintain an open mind and to be circumspect about "uncorroborated repressed memories that return" (p. 534). Her observations, while apparently wise and balanced, will surely be used to buttress the activities of the False Memory Syndrome Foundation and to further discredit the accounts of many survivors.

Just as Freud's change in stance protected the patriarchs of Vienna, the preoccupation once again has shifted from the experience of the client in therapy to the possibility of "irreparable damage to the reputations of potentially innocent people" (Loftus, 1993, p. 534). As Judith Herman points out in *Trauma and Recovery* (1992), professionals and society allow themselves to acknowledge hideous trauma only for brief periods before shutting it out of consciousness, either by rendering the victim invisible or by discrediting her. She catalogs the disputes "over whether patients with post-traumatic conditions are entitled to care and respect or deserving of contempt, whether they are genuinely suffering or malingering, whether their histories are true or false and, if false, whether imagined or maliciously fabricated" (p. 8).

Because an attack on sexual abuse is inevitably an attack on patriarchy, at the societal level survivors who reveal experiences of sexual abuse are likely to be discredited, just as Anita Hill's allegations of sexual harassment were used to discredit her. (Physicians and social workers may also be discredited; see, for instance, the scandal that arose when a British physician and social worker diagnosed widespread sexual abuse [Nava, 1988].) Discrediting has two parts: disbelief and devaluing. Disbelief takes on the survivor's account at the level of veracity—it didn't happen, it's a false memory, she's making it up to get back at him, to get money, to get custody of the children, and so on. Disbelief operates at the observable, legal, arguable courtroom level: either it happened or it did not. Disbelief is at the heart of what is likely to be an issue in the courts for generations: how can a girl or woman prove that a man sexually abused her when it was done in private, indeed, in isolation? The fallibility and inaccuracy of memory has become a legal argument.

Devaluing is more insidious; it affects the attitude and openness of the listener to the survivor herself, regardless of the content of her account. Devaluing undermines the listener's willingness to believe the survivor based on *who the survivor is*. Medicine now recognizes the reality of incest and sexual abuse and violence against women. Clinicians are eager to latch onto an explanation for the diffuse and complex symptomatology that survivors present in clinical settings. But survivors are also labeled, marginalized, and discredited as bearers of enormous symptoms that refuse to go away. Medical recognition that a woman is a sexual abuse survivor does not heal her pain; it lets doctors feel better about not looking further for multiple causes to explain her symptoms. She can be discounted as a "frequent caller," "fat chart," or "somatoform disorder" or dismissed by a host of other labels that fundamentally devalue her and discredit her pain. Thus, medicine may accept the accuracy of her account but discount her acceptability as a patient.

Discrediting of survivors is already in evidence in medical settings. The recognition that a highly symptomatic woman has been sexually abused can lead to her isolation through labeling. Once labeled a survivor, she carries the stigma of a victim—she, not the perpetrator, becomes devalued for what happened to her. Medicine, like society at large, cannot bear to be reminded of what she experienced and how damaging it was. Some child therapists work closely with a child to gain trust before the incest material is approached, but clinicians treating distrustful, polysymptomatic adults are unlikely to do the same. Too often they hold the bearer of the symptoms responsible for her own pain.

The reality of "revictimization" also makes it likely that clinicians will hold childhood sexual abuse survivors responsible for what happened to them. Because many survivors do not take good care of themselves and are incapable of protecting themselves adequately, they are more likely to be revictimized in a variety of ways. Sexual abuse survivors are more likely to have unintended pregnancies and abortions, multiple partnerships, and brief relationships (Wyatt, Guthrie, & Notgrass, 1992). The persistence into adulthood of the dynamics of childhood sexual abuse—stigma, powerlessness, sexualization, and betrayal—sets up adult survivors of child sexual abuse for later physical and sexual abuse (Finkelhor & Browne, 1985). As adults, sexual abuse survivors are more likely than other women to experience rape, battering abuse and marital rape, and unwanted sexual advances from authority figures and to be asked either to pose for pornography or to enact things seen in pornography (Russell, 1986). In one study, college women who had been victimized in childhood were more likely to have repeat victimization experiences in adolescence and again in college (Gidycz et al., 1993). Incest survivors may marry spouses who not only abuse them but also sexually abuse their children. They may also be more likely than other women to be victimized by therapists and physicians (Kluft, 1990b).

The current understanding of revictimization is inadequate. While characteristics of perpetrators may account for the high frequency of revictimization of child sexual abuse survivors, most discussions of revictimization focus on the victim rather than on the perpetrator, implying that her own characteristics predispose her to being hurt and raped (Russell, 1986). Although most interpreters have moved away from explanations of revictimization based on masochism, the phrase "she was asking for it" continues to drone on in popular explanatory thought. Any woman might conclude that if sexual abuse or rape happens to her more than once, it is her fault.[17]

Explaining how past child sexual abuse predisposes a woman to later abuse without blaming her for the revictimization poses a problem for medicine. The contemporary medical model holds individual patients responsible for maintaining their health through a wise diet, exercise, regular checkups, and avoidance of tobacco, drugs, and too much alcohol; they are expected to recognize and report worrisome symptoms promptly, reduce stress, keep appointments, undergo evaluations, follow instructions, and take medicines as directed. Even though fulfillment of these tasks may not maintain health and prevent illness, doctors are likely to view sickness as a product of the patient's shortcomings. Medicine's attempts to increase "compliance" with guidelines for health promotion and disease prevention fail to acknowledge the likelihood that women who do not comply are likely to be survivors of some kind of victimization (Koss & Heslet, 1992; Koss et al., 1991). The professional and popular notion of personal responsibility for health locates in the individual not only the obligation to maintain health but also blame for the loss of it. This stance holds a woman individually responsible for what happens to her, for her choice of partner, for the risk she runs by going out alone, and for subsequent events. Physicians subscribe to this sense of personal responsibility for themselves as well as for their patients.[18]

On the other hand, adherence to unidirectional or staged notions of development (chapters 1 and 2) leads the practitioner to view the damage of child sexual abuse as permanently crippling and the adult woman as irremediably sick. The enumeration of her myriad symptoms makes her appear pathological. She is the one who acts out, runs away, threatens suicide, uses drugs, gets picked up by the police. She appears out of control and in need of long, difficult treatment. Her problems with depression and low self-esteem make it difficult for her to form lasting positive relationships. She is inadequate as an adult, hopeless as a parent. She appears to have the problem. The label of child sexual abuse victim, like other psychiatric labels, carries the negative prognostication of an unchanging and unimprovable picture.

Physicians now recognize that children who are sexually abused often have mothers who were sexually abused as children. This finding is used to demonstrate that the mother is incompetent and unable to protect her child. Medicine allows women's past experience of sexual abuse to stamp a label of damage on them—not in the sexual sense as damaged goods, but as defective mothers who fail to be responsible for their children. Rather than seeing the repetition of sexual abuse in families as proof of the vulnerability of all women and children in male-dominant settings, medicine uses the fact to invalidate and discredit mothers and to label the sexual abuse survivor as either responsible and guilty or hopeless and sick.

Each of these choices is flawed. Blaming the mother and holding her responsible removes her from her own developmental and relational context; it ignores what is understood about how harmful sexual trauma is to children. Stigma, powerlessness, betrayal, and inappropriate sexualization are the destructive dynamics that shaped the mother's childhood. Blaming the survivor fails to integrate who she is now with who she was as a child, and with the ongoing relationships from her family of origin and the ones she has made as an adult. It also maintains that she brings crises upon herself, and indeed she may think so. Many physicians will agree with her and be unlikely to help her sort out her vulnerability as part of her past.

Viewing the survivor as hopeless and sick is an explanation that assumes her condition to be static. This stance does not recognize the healing and empowerment that survivors are claiming, as well as their right to safety. Both explanatory frameworks—blaming the survivor and holding her responsible, or viewing her as sick—focus on the woman and neglect the larger social setting in which perpetrators take advantage of anyone who is vulnerable and available.

A feminist reinterpretation of revictimization recognizes a woman's childhood and family experiences of abuse as well as the abuse history of her mother and sisters. The purpose of making explicit this genealogy of abuse is to show that her personality and behavior were not causal: she was not responsible for the offenses of her grandfather or father or uncle or brother. The climate of fear that she experienced in relation to her first abuser may be replicated by men in her adult relationships.[19] Whether she enters these relationships with the expectation of closeness, company, nurturance, or escape, she carries her vulnerability with her. Russell holds that incest strips away survivors' ability to protect themselves: "Their self-esteem may be so damaged that they don't feel they deserve their own loving self-protection" (1986, p. 190). Not unlike abused children, some survivors try to block out recollection of how their perpetrators were abusive and attempt to idealize men (Briere, 1989). A survivor's feelings of worthlessness, linked with her desire to please, her feeling of responsibility for the relationship, her loyalty or even fealty to her abuser, and her disbelief in her ability to effect any change, all work together to limit her ability to protect herself in adulthood.

Patriarchy creates a world where a woman cannot afford to relax her vigilance and become vulnerable. Those who revictimize a sexual abuse survivor by abusing her later in childhood or in adulthood are taking advantage of her vulnerability, but they do not depend on it. Just as "men batter because they can," men sexually abuse because they can. Revictimization depends on the systematic construction of heterosexual relationships, both inside and outside of families, that guarantee men power over women and children. Medicine, embedded within the larger social system, is reluctant to acknowledge sexual abuse as a *gendered* abuse of power. The mother blaming that is ubiquitous throughout the clinical disciplines draws attention away from the power relations in a man's abuse of a girl. Families, therapists, police, and courts have not historically behaved as if survivors of physical or sexual abuse deserved protection. Whether inaction that allows the abuse to continue or actions that sometimes lead to further abuse—separation from nonabusing family, foster placement, psychiatric treatment, institution-alization—both condemn the abused survivor to further abuse. Within a patriarchal system, revictimization is the outcome of the usual oper-ating procedures, not an aberrant pattern.

In a world that allows men to hit women or rape women, any woman can be battered or raped and any child can be sexually abused. In fam-ilies in which women are stripped of their power to protect themselves and their children, they and their children are at risk. The intergenera-tional transmission of domination and vulnerability sets up the context in which revictimization of women and children is only a more pre-dictable outcome. Patriarchy takes advantage of the effects of victim-ization to propagate itself; this is the central explanation of the revic-timization of survivors of incest and sexual abuse, not psychological vulnerability, even though abuse certainly creates such vulnerability.

PART II

CHAPTER 6

The Doctor-Patient Relationship as Contract

> The more we ignore dependency relations between those grossly unequal in power and ignore what cannot be spelled out in an explicit acknowledgement, the more readily will we assume that everything that needs to be understood about trust and trustworthiness can be grasped by looking at the morality of contract.
>
> Annette Baier, *Trust and Antitrust* (1986), p. 241

> Contemporary society is in the grip of contractual thinking.
>
> Virginia Held, *Non-Contractual Society: A Feminist View* (1987a), p. 11

THE FIRST PART of this book shows how medicine views all patients through the lens of developmental and family systems based on the idealized notion of the autonomous male. Medicine defines women's identity by their relationships with men, with children, and with any others for whom they provide care. Women are seen not as separate persons but as figures complementary to men; reproduction is upheld as the centerpiece of women's lives. Because women are not defined as separate or autonomous, they do not achieve medicine's vision of full adulthood. Women whom men have battered or sexually abused are perceived as less than persons because they have been victimized. Their difficulty in protecting themselves and disengaging from abusive relations further supports the impression that they are not full adults, that they are pathologic or defective and therefore unable to achieve autonomy.

The idealization of autonomy likewise suffuses writings on the doctor-patient relationship. Patient autonomy has emerged as the antidote to medicine's domination of patients. Although the problem of domination is now widely recognized as an ethical problem, patient autonomy as a solution has received relatively little criticism. Because the ideal of autonomy arises from a primarily male vision of personhood, it poses a variety of problems for women as patients and as clinicians. It also confines male patients and clinicians to self-definitions they may be ready to shed.

The first part of this chapter reviews the mass of incontrovertible evidence of "power-over" as the kind of power active in the doctor-patient relationship and shows how language serves as the vehicle through which power-over is exercised. All ways of looking at the doctor-patient interaction—from outcome studies based on diagnoses or procedures to linguistic microanalysis of conversation—demonstrate that medicine is a practice of domination, particularly but not exclusively over women. Both feminists and Marxists have been particularly critical of the inequality of the doctor-patient relationship: feminists primarily because of the role the relationship plays in maintaining gender stereotypes and its potential for abuse; Marxists because of the role medicine plays in supporting the ideology of class and gender divisions and in maintaining current social and economic conditions.

Although medicine does not accept the assumptions underpinning these criticisms, it does reject the legitimacy of openly wielding its power to dominate in either malevolent (abusive) or benevolent (paternalistic) ways. With the advent of medical ethics as a field of concern in the last twenty years, medicine has accepted the criticism of paternalism and addressed it by adopting the model of patient autonomy. Medicine now depicts the adult person as autonomous and separate. Relations between autonomous persons (doctors and patients) are construed as relations between equals; contract is the ideal form of this relationship. Differences between the parties in a contract relationship are resolved through negotiation. The second part of this chapter shows how the assumptions underlying the concepts of autonomy, contract, and negotiation pose internal problems for the doctor-patient relationship. Moreover, these concepts reflect a gendered approach to the problem of unequal relations: that is, they address the problem of power-over with assumptions and language that derive from historically male-biased or masculinist viewpoints.

POWER-OVER: AN OLD STORY

We are all familiar with the long history of the domination of doctors over patients and the accompanying pattern of abuses; particularly well documented is the abuse of women patients by male doctors. At times this pattern has been so pervasive and oppressive that it has led us all, even women clinicians, to wonder whether we should just pack up and leave and tell patients to go to the herbalist, the masseuse, the chiropractor, the lay midwife, and chuck the rest of it. (Of course, there are no guarantees that these relationships will not also become abusive; the untested assumption is that clients of such practitioners are less likely to be victimized, especially if the practitioners are women). The indignities of hospitals, the fearsome technologies, the damaging and derailing potentials of drugs, are all real, but perhaps none is so damaging and destructive of trust in medicine as the abuses of power by doctors themselves. The pattern of domination and abuse is so ubiquitous that it raises a serious question: Is there any hope for the doctor-patient relationship?

Many people with means have, of course, already abandoned allopathic medicine for a variety of alternative therapies, but for most poor and working-class people, both in this country and around the world, the doctor is still considered a resource in times of sickness. As long as patients need to go to doctors and doctors see it as their job to attend to the people who come to them, the doctor-patient relationship will persist. The question then becomes: Is there any hope to make it less abusive? Or phrased more positively, what is its potential for healing?

The understanding of power manifested in medicine as power-over is largely derived from the definition of power in political theory: the ability to influence or change another's thinking or behavior (French & Raven, 1959). Feminist critics of doctors' domination have documented the personal, social, and structural elements in the maintenance of power-over. For instance, they have documented how physicians wrested control over childbirth from midwives (Ehrenreich & English, 1972). Even in the latter half of the twentieth century, doctors have decided when they would sterilize women (Mass, 1976) and when they would remove their uteri (Scully, 1980). Doctors decide what information women receive about their bodies and are threatened when women show any authority or self-knowledge about their own bodies (Fisher, 1990; Singer, 1987). Doctors define women in terms of their reproductive roles and claim the right to manage their reproduction (Todd, 1983). Menopause, long ignored by doctors or regarded as a source of neurotic symptoms, has now become the newest terrain for control, through estrogen replacement therapy.

The underlying ideology of medical control, largely outside of the awareness of physicians, permeates medical writings. Reviews of seventeen editions of *Williams's Textbook of Obstetrics* (Hahn, 1987), of dozens of gynecology textbooks (Scully & Bart, 1973), and of the history of obstetrical practice itself (Arney, 1982) reveal medicine's absolute commitment to control over women patients. At the level of ideology, doctors expand their control by redefining social problems into medical phenomena to be managed and controlled—for example, unwed motherhood becomes adolescent pregnancy (Arney & Bergen, 1984). In short, the history of physician domination over women's bodies reveals a long tradition of unquestioned control and repeated abuse.

Doctors do not exert their domination over women only. Any form of status difference compounds doctors' power over patients by virtue of at least one but usually more of the following: gender, class, race, education, social acceptability, and technical expertise. Patients from lower socioeconomic classes get less information, less talk, and less reinforcement from doctors than patients of higher social class (Hall, Roter, & Katz, 1988; Roter, Hall, & Katz, 1988; Waitzkin, 1984a). Doctors volunteer fewer explanations to patients of lower socioeconomic class (Pendleton & Bochner, 1980). Doctors use verbal structures that offer more freedom and respect to patients who are older, white, more educated, and of higher social status (Stiles, Putnam, & Jacob, 1982). These findings show not only that doctors operate within a social class structure but also that their conduct reinforces the disparities of that structure. For patients of limited education, doctors regularly underestimate their desire for information; when such a patient does not ask questions (and less educated patients are less likely to ask questions), doctors conclude that the patient is even more limited (Ventres & Gordon, 1990).

Similarly, racist experimentation in medicine, largely ignored or forgotten by mainstream sources, has included federally conducted experiments from the 1930s to the 1970s on black men with syphilis in the infamous Tuskegee trials (Jones, 1981; Thomas & Quinn, 1991) and experiments on Puerto Rican women with high-dose estrogen and progesterone in the late 1950s and early 1960s (Ramirez de Arellano & Seipp, 1983). Contemporary evidence of differential treatment of patients from communities of color is reflected in inadequate treatment of pain (Cleeland et al., 1994; Todd et al., 1993), suboptimal treatment for HIV infection (Moore et al., 1994), and lower rates of coronary artery bypass surgery (Ford, Cooper, Castaner, Simmons, & Mar, 1989; Hannan, Kilburn, O'Donnell, Lukacik, & Shields, 1991; Maynard, Fisher, Passamani, & Pullum, 1986; Wenneker & Epstein, 1989). Analyses of case presentations reveal that when residents in training mention a patient's race, they are more likely to include a pejorative descriptor of the patient (Finucane & Carrese, 1990). Doctors treat patients differently based on how the patient uses language: when patients use vernacular forms, doctors are likely to devalue them. Dialect speakers wait longer, receive worse service, are thought to be ignorant, and are told what to do rather than asked for their input (Shuy, 1983).

By definition, doctors have more technical expertise than their patients. The power of this expertise is exemplified by doctors' control over decision-making—about drugs, procedures, decisions to treat, and so on. The use of this expertise to exert control is universal but has perhaps been best demonstrated in the treatment of obstetrical patients. Every interaction of the doctor with the obstetrical patient serves to maintain and strengthen his or her control over her (Danziger, 1979; Shapiro, Najman, Chang, Keeping, Morrison, & Western, 1983). Doctors do not explain why they do what they do except in the simplest or broadest fashion. They learn to be reticent as part of their professionalization, itself a process that sets the doctor above the patient through expertise. Doctors also use their expertise to control the information available to patients as they try to make decisions about treatment options—for instance, making the choice between cone biopsy and hysterectomy for treatment of an abnormal pap smear (Fisher, 1990). Many doctors see their role as determining exactly what information patients ought to have (Comaroff, 1976). Even in the relatively less common instance of a physician putting himself or herself in the position of being a patient of another practitioner of presumably equal or greater knowledge, she or he accepts a less powerful role in relation to that physician. But such a physician becomes a patient only temporarily; temporary inequality with doctors does not characterize other people's relations to physicians. Most patients remain socially less powerful after their encounter with the physician has ended.

The difference in power between doctor and patient is not just a matter of structural constraints or disparity in knowledge; it is a central feature of their relationship. The doctor maintains power through the choice of location (Gibson & Kramer, 1965); through participation in the organization of the clinical setting, which is most often arranged for the convenience of doctors, not patients (Lazarus, 1988); through control over the physical position of the patient; through direct control over the length of the interaction; and through the asymmetry of dress and the privilege of touching the patient. But perhaps most telling yet least obvious of all is the doctor's control over the interaction through language.

Linguistic analysis of doctor-patient encounters reveals that doctors use spoken language to maintain and perpetuate their position of dominance. They confine the "discourse" to medical matters and systematically exclude material from the "lifeworld" (Mishler, 1984; Todd, 1983); moreover, the voice of medicine "reinforces the reasonableness and acceptability of the lifeworld in its present form" (Waitzkin, 1989, p. 232). Doctors support the dominant ideology by giving advice that limits patients to their socially expected class, gender, and reproductive roles (Todd, 1983; Waitzkin, 1984b, 1989). For instance, the doctor directs a depressed unemployed man to return to work in order to feel better, or he expects that it is reasonable for a woman incapacitated by heart disease to keep up her housework (Waitzkin, 1984b, 1989). Doctors do not tie patients' personal troubles to larger societal problems—racism, battering, militarism, reductions in social programs—but rather interpret symptoms as evidence of individual pathology (Waitzkin, 1989). Far from challenging social context, doctors consider it marginal to a patient's condition; they do not suggest to patients that they engage in collective struggle against oppressive conditions.

Doctors control conversations with patients to shape their diagnosis and to give their own meaning to patients' voiced concerns (Paget, 1983). Doctors want to hear "words that are consistent with previously defined diagnostic categories. Parts of patients' stories that do not fit neatly into these categories function as unwanted strangers in medical discourse and tend to be shown to the door" (Waitzkin, 1989, p. 230). Doctors believe in giving only as much information as they think patients need (Comaroff, 1976; Waitzkin, 1984a) and actually spend far less time giving information than they think they do. They exclude patients' underlying concerns from discussion, including their preoccupations with causation, side effects of medication and treatment, and mortality (see, for example, Paget, 1983).

Doctors' control over conversation extends beyond content: they shape the length, sequence, and flow of words between themselves and patients. Painstaking scrutiny of transcriptions between doctors and patients show that at every level of analysis doctors use language to exert and maintain power. Doctors control the topics by asking most of the questions, changing the subject of discussion, answering fewer questions than patients ask, shaping the form and length of answers patients can give by using closed or multiple-choice questions, and interrupting patients (Fisher, 1983; Frankel, 1990; Waitzkin, 1984a; West, 1983). Typically, a physician interrupts a patient's initial statement after an average of eighteen seconds (Beckman & Frankel, 1984). This first statement is usually the patient's main (and sometimes only) opportunity to present his or her viewpoint. Thus, language is not just a medium of exchange; not only what is said but also the very structure of language exemplifies the ideology of medical control.[1]

Through closed questions and chains of questions, doctors shape the kinds of answers that patients can offer (Frankel, 1990). Drass's (1982) study of nurse-practitioners and physician's assistants shows that clinicians control the conversation with restrictive questions during history-taking, with commands during the examination, and with information and instruction during the closing phase. Patients challenge the way that clinicians posed the questions in only 6 percent of their replies and challenged the fit of the medical formulation to their situations in only 8 percent of the discussions. In other words, examples of patients' noncooperation with doctors' strategies of interrogation are uncommon. Samples of such interactions are remarkable for making the patient appear to be the problem:

Provider: The diarrhea is gone away and the cramping is still there.
Patient: Well, it's not like a cramp, it's more just like a pain, cramp, you know I mean I know the difference. (Drass, 1982, p. 330)

When patients bring up their ideas about the cause of their symptom at the "wrong" time (that is, during the history-taking or the examination), the clinicians in Drass's study either interrupted them or ignored them. In another study, only 27 percent of medical residents' interviews explored patients' views of their illness. Thus, despite admonishments to ask for patients' views of their illness (Barsky, 1981; Lipkin, Quill, & Napodano, 1984), clinicians do not take this advice seriously. Often doctors view a patient's concerns about causation as evidence that she herself is the problem—that is, that she is neurotic or controlling. For instance, a former cancer patient tries to get her doctor to attend to her concern that her symptoms represent a recurrence. He keeps refusing to take up the subject and instead labels her with psychiatric diagnoses. He maintains control of the subject, the questions, and the diagnosis (Paget, 1983). In another example, a middle-class woman had an ectopic pregnancy rupture at six weeks of pregnancy. When she became pregnant again, she insisted on being evaluated before six weeks to make sure that she did not have another tubal pregnancy. Her demand to be seen very early in pregnancy conflicted with the routine of her "health maintenance" organization. The doctor who saw her dismissed her concerns explicitly and pejoratively with the question, "What's your traumatic story?" (Singer, 1987). These examples of doctors disallowing patients' concerns about their illness provide further evidence that the typical medical conversation does not represent "negotiation," and that patients' participation can hardly be described as mutual collaboration.

Doctors also use nonverbal behavior to manage their interactions with patients. Writing a prescription, washing his or her hands, and standing up are self-evident signals that the clinician considers the transaction to be over. Usually unrecorded, such nonverbal acts can be subtly abusive to patients. One observational study of fifteen family practice residents (nine men and six women) performing pelvic exams in the course of routine care found two instances of inappropriate sexual behaviors: one male resident "rested his hand on the patient's buttock area" while giving an explanation after the exam; another male resident explained his findings "with his hand on the patient's thigh" while she was still undressed (Lang, 1990). Doctors also control the interview through the act of writing; despite appearances, what they are writing down at any given moment may have nothing to do with what the patient is saying at that precise time (Treichler, Frankel, Kramarae, Zoppi, & Beckman,

1984). Richard Frankel (1983) makes an elegant linkage between language and nonverbal behavior when he shows that during a physical exam of a child the doctor attempts to distract the child away from the physical activities through the use of speech. The boy persists in returning his attention to what the doctor is doing to his body. This strategy of touching someone while verbally acting as if nothing is happening is a way of using language for deception. (It parallels some children's experience of sexual abuse and points to the importance of making the connection between speech and behaviors if children are to be encouraged to make sense out of what is happening to them.) The enormous potential of nonverbal behavior for subtle abuse and sexual exploitation in medicine remains almost entirely unexamined.

All of medicine's forms of control—verbal, nonverbal, ideological—assume the legitimacy of existing power relations both inside and outside the medical setting. Failure to criticize social conditions or to challenge gender stereotypes rests on assumptions about the doctor-patient relationship that derive from liberal political ideas: everyone has a right to his or her private viewpoint. The doctor and patient are separate individuals each of whom, as citizens, must work out his or her ideas about the world. Political issues do not belong in the examining room. The doctor-patient relationship is a private transaction that is unrelated to politics. This interpretation of politics implies that the world of elected government officials and electoral party affiliation constitutes the entirety of what is political. The fact that medicine as an institution supports existing social relations, fails to challenge economic conditions, and facilitates gender stereotypes does not, in the medical world, make a political statement. The idea that any power relation has political implications is foreign to medicine, and to contemporary thought in general.

AUTONOMY TO THE RESCUE

Because of the seemingly apolitical nature of medicine, the nonrecognition of power inequities in patients' lives and in the doctor-patient relationship is not identified as the mark of an inherently political position. What medicine did recognize was its own paternalism—it accepted the criticism that doctors act as if they know what is right for patients. Medicine's answer to this criticism was to proclaim that patient autonomy was to be the centerpiece of medical ethics. Patients are separate and autonomous actors with legal rights. In one stroke, paternalism was challenged and autonomy was championed. The outmoded condescending relationship was replaced by the ideal of a contract relationship between autonomous equals. Differences of power were not even open for discussion because of the assumption under liberalism that people are equal. As we shall see, however, the language of autonomy and contract is problematic because it becomes a force in the preservation of power differences.

Without question, no defense remains for the paternalistic authoritarianism that traditionally characterized medical relationships. Its defects are multiple, and its critics myriad. Abuse of power, deciding what is right for the patient and acting on it, deprivation of personhood—all are unacceptable. At bottom, the paternalistic model of the doctor-patient relationship failed to treat people with respect. Because of the subjugation of women by men in society at large as well as in medicine, women have been vociferous critics of the paternalistic model and ardent proponents of patient autonomy and patient rights (Ketchum & Pierce, 1981). Many contemporary victories for patient rights (the patient bill of rights, required informed consent before sterilization, legally required explanation of all available options before breast cancer surgery, and so on) are a direct result of women's efforts to challenge the abuses against women of medical paternalism. This focus on rights was essential to draw attention to the problems of domination.

Widespread abuse of the paternalistic relationship required that any revision of the doctor-patient relationship include a way to protect the less powerful from the more powerful. The solution most often proposed was to privilege the contractual relations between autonomous adults as the ideal. Szasz and Hollender's (1956) relationship of "mutual participation" is the commonly cited exemplar of the ideal relation.

> Realities are interpreted in contractual terms, and goals are formulated in terms of rational contracts. The leading current conceptions of rationality begin with assumptions that human beings are independent, self-interested or mutually disinterested, individuals; they typically argue that it is often rational for human beings to enter into contractual relationships with each other. (Held, 1987a, p. 111)

Advocates of contract in medicine hold that it ensures mutual participation (Gillick, 1992). For instance: "The *autonomous patient*—capable of and inclined toward self-direction by way of rational deliberation— is engaged in a cooperative partnership with the autonomous health care professional" (Meyer, 1992, p. 545, emphasis in original). Patients emerge from the cradle of paternalism as autonomous adults and free agents who contract for what they want and disengage from interactions when they choose. This understanding of the relationship between doctor and patient assumes a relation between two presumed equals, an idea that, in turn, derives from traditional liberal theory (for example, Locke's *Second Treatise on Government*), which regarded adult male property owners as independent bearers of equal rights. Women, however, were not considered equal in the same sense. In its original formulation, this view of persons was clearly determined by both culture and gender.

In the modern era, autonomous adults are thought of as persons essentially motivated to pursue their own life plans. Although they may either choose to be altruistic or prefer that others make decisions for them, autonomous persons usually act in what appears to them to be their self-interest.[2] The weaker must be protected against the stronger, who in the absence of constraints will operate to maximize their own advantage in their own self-interest. Arrangements between persons guided by self-interest require contracts to prevent abuse of one party by the other, in particular, the less powerful by the more powerful. The presumption of each person's autonomy serves as a structural constraint to guarantee rights. Thus, the ethical basis of the contractual understanding between doctor and patient revolves around a central set of patients' rights: autonomy, informed consent, and the choice or refusal of treatment. The doctor's responsibilities include—in addition to specific medical tasks—guarantee of the patient's rights and protection against abuse of power.

Outside of medicine, autonomy has an array of meanings: freedom from influence (she made her decision autonomously), emotional detachment (he preferred the autonomous life of a bachelor), and economic independence (he moved out, got a job, and achieved autonomy). In real life, however, people do not live their lives as autonomous agents, and defining patients as autonomous does not make them so. They are emotionally and financially tied to their families; they also develop strong emotional ties to their doctors. While patients desire as much information as possible, they are not always eager to make many, if not most, of their own health care decisions, particularly the serious or life-threatening decisions (Ende, Kazis, Ash, & Moskowitz, 1989). Declaring patients to be autonomous recasts them as fictitiously independent actors rather than as the emotional and social beings we all are. Moreover, those persons intimately bound to a patient participate in central ways in medical decision-making (Hardwig, 1990). Our intimate relations, in fact, define who we are—a reality that should, but has not yet, transformed our understanding of autonomy (Jecker, 1990). Thus, patients (and persons in general) are autonomous in neither the emotional nor the decision-making sense, even if they are economically independent. Sickness itself is particularly destructive of a person's autonomy (Cassell, 1977). Yet medicine maintains its idealized image of a person as an autonomous being.[3] As I show at the end of this chapter, this central preoccupation with autonomy reveals medicine's deep obeisance to masculinist values.

The concept of patient autonomy narrows our understanding of persons. It is poorly suited to the patient with chronic illness or the patient who requires long-term care; it fails to consider the fluctuations in an illness, the changes in relationships with doctors and nurses, or the family and clinical networks in which patients live (Brody, 1992b; Caplan, 1988; Clements & Sider, 1983; Jennings, Callahan, & Caplan, 1988; Moros, Rhodes, Baumrin, & Strain, 1991; Roth & Harrison, 1991). In other words, the reality of life with chronic illness—with its ties and connections to important others—reveals that autonomy as separateness and independence is a fabrication. Valorization of autonomy makes dependency the enemy but does not acknowledge that integrity, worth, and participation in social issues may be more important to a person than avoiding dependency per se. Agich (1990) offers the example of a wheelchair-bound woman who needs help with the activities of daily living. She is involved in the organization Food for Peace (FFP), for which she stuffs envelopes. She has visitors from FFP and eagerly follows its doings on television. She does not care what time she takes her bath: "Not all choices matter to her, just those that are meaningful in terms of her participatory identification in a larger social context" (p. 16). The medical view of autonomy would look at this woman in terms of her physical dependency, not her personal choice to engage in or support specific political actions.

As with autonomy, the ideology of contract poses a set of problems for medicine. First, unlike a business arrangement or legal settlement, contract does not fit the reality of the doctor-patient relationship. Contract denies the moral and relational grounding of what happens between doctor and patient. Second, it serves a rhetorical function that obscures the power arrangements and hides the physician domination. Third, contract can be coercive in the doctor-patient context.

HOW CONTRACT DOES NOT FIT

THE REJECTION OF PHYSICIAN OPENNESS

The contractual view of the doctor-patient relationship contradicts a fundamental assumption in the classic understanding of the doctor's stance toward the patient: the attitude of what Rogers (1961) called "unconditional positive regard" or what Gayle Stephens, in a 1981 interview, called "grace." "It goes far beyond acceptance as a psychological construct. . . . Grace in its ultimate form says that there is nothing you can do to keep me from feeling a certain way about you. . . . The patient can bring anything to the doctor; nothing's too terrible, nothing's too shameful" (Candib, 1981, p. 4). Joined with such regard is the doctor's implicit promise to the patient: *No matter what happens to you, I will be your doctor.* Contracts fail to deal with the unpredictable, the contingent, the unexplicit in human sickness and human relationships (May, 1975, 1983). A contractual relation cannot provide the basis for the unknown; yet it is just such a journey into the unknown that patients undertake when they bring symptoms of unknown significance to the doctor. This open commitment, or fidelity, derives from a view of the relationship as promised, or to use a religious term, "covenanted" (May, 1975, 1983). This covenanted relationship, in which the doctor promises unconditional positive regard and fidelity, cannot be contracted because it is not up for bargain.

DISCARDING BENEFICENCE

Beneficence—acting for the benefit of others—is an essential feature of medicine. Care of the patient and avoidance of harm are elements of beneficence (Thomasma, 1983). One of the side effects of rejecting paternalism was that beneficence was discarded as well. The idea of contract leaves no room for what May calls the "donative element" in the doctor-patient relationship. All is negotiated; nothing can be given. Fundamental human relatedness is not a consideration. Without beneficence, contract has no role for the caring, human qualities that patients need from the people who take care of them. In contractual relations between parties guided primarily by self-interest, the appearance of caring is useful to enhance satisfaction, but caring is not integral to the relation. Caring becomes a matter of communication.

THE TRANSMOGRIFICATION OF CARING INTO COMMUNICATION

Warmth, empathy, and genuineness—the physician attributes that Carl Rogers (1961) deemed crucial to success in psychotherapy—do not loom large in the contractual understanding of clinical relationships. In fact, the contractual model has no way of thinking about caring. Descriptions of caring are reduced either to issues of style and personal characteristics or to the observation and measurement of behaviors, usually verbal and nonverbal communication, that doctors use in their interactions with patients. Empathy includes congruence (between doctor and patient) and attentiveness. Permitting patients to tell their story without interrupting them and using specific questions, statements, and postures convey attentiveness (Havens, 1978; Mishler, Clark, Ingelfinger, & Simon, 1989). Posture and gaze may convey warmth. In medicine, the interview has become the vehicle for the teaching of such behaviors, and primary care internists now lead the way in teaching how to ask questions, what types of questions to ask, and how to recognize problems in the interview (Lipkin et al., 1984). Proponents of improved interview technique argue for the need to recognize the patient as a person, to explore the experience of illness, and to show empathy. Advocates of the contractual relationship hold that the contract is a way to guarantee that this communication takes place (Gillick, 1992).

The understandable focus on skills has highlighted the importance of communication but dodged the issue of how or whether the doctor cares for the patient. While caring behaviors seem to make a difference in terms of patient outcomes and patient satisfaction (Ben-Sira, 1976; Hall et al., 1988; Hall, Epstein, DeCiantis, & McNeil, 1993; Inui & Frankel, 1992; Wasserman, Inui, Barriatua, Carter, & Lippincott, 1984), caring itself seems to vanish in the process of dissecting the doctor-patient relationship. We have not discovered any way to assess or teach genuineness—a characteristic that may best be manifested by the extent to which the doctor or therapist uses himself or herself as an instrument of treatment and allows the patient to see himself or herself as a person (Candib, 1987; Gilbert, 1980). Instead, we have accepted the aphorism that "you can't teach people to care," and we find ourselves, as a result, trying to teach the proper behaviors to clinicians in training as a substitute for caring itself. Thus, the preoccupation in teaching clinicians how to conduct medical interviews is with the acquisition and application of communication skills, but it is unclear whether improved communication skills actually result in greater caring by the clinician. We teach verbal and nonverbal behaviors as a way to approach "the interaction" from the outside, but we remain removed from the relationship itself.[4] Efforts to describe what happens in the relationship take on a quasi-mystical quality when physicians entrenched in the view of persons as autonomous attempt to describe the "connexional dimension" (Suchman & Matthews, 1988).

The impoverished language of contract restricts caring to a matter of technique. Since caring can be considered only as a form of communication, the discussion of communication serves as a shorthand for talk about the relationship. In effect, communication has become a stand-in for the relationship. Physician behaviors, patient behaviors, illness behaviors, nonverbal behavior—all measuring sticks to describe the interaction at any point in time—have come to signify the relation itself. The healing relationship—that vision of two people, sometimes more, engaged in a mutual project going forward in time, with complex feelings on either side—rarely appears in discussions of the doctor-patient relationship as contract. Even more rare is the consideration of what happens between the two people: love, fear, respect, commitment, sadness, anger, denial, and loss.

THE DENIAL OF TRANSFERENCE AND COUNTERTRANSFERENCE

Transference—the patient's projection onto the doctor of feelings from other important relationships—and countertransference—the doctor's feelings and responses toward the patient—are concepts from psychoanalysis that are germane to the conduct of medical relationships. Like therapists, doctors, often without knowing it, are often the focus of patients' powerful feelings. Likewise, a doctor's intense reaction to a patient can derive from other experiences in the doctor's past. The contractual view of the relationship cannot account for the enormous hidden energy and the resultant power for commitment and healing that suffuse many if not all clinical encounters. Instead, patient recovery or improvement, including the placebo response, can be understood only as evidence of the patient's dependence (where "dependence" carries a pejorative meaning). Perhaps the notion of contract allows doctors to opt out of the healer's heavy burden of responsibility (Cassell, 1985) by denying the importance of the transference. A transformed understanding of dependence is essential to a view of recovery as empowering (see chapter 10).

THE DENIAL OF THE IMPORTANCE OF THE RELATIONSHIP FOR THE DOCTOR

In this era of litigation, we rarely hear of the sustenance physicians receive from ongoing relations with patients. The idea of contract obscures the lifetime indebtedness of the doctor to his or her patients for the privilege of learning from their sicknesses (May, 1975, 1983). It is only when the relationship is blatantly absent that doctors become aware that something is missing. One impact of consumerism on medicine has been the loss of relationship; in the proliferation of medical marketplace jargon, doctoring is now a product to be packaged, marketed, and provided. Contracts between doctor and patient situate the transaction in commercial terms (Stoeckle, 1992). Patients, buying into this mentality, seek to obtain some small measure of control over their medical care by shopping for a service. Services (but not payments) can be negotiated. Although clinicians have been quick to hail negotiation as the panacea for struggles with patients, the commercial origins of the term frequently surface to pose a problem for the "provider." Consumerism is particularly uncomfortable for the clinician, not because the patient is educated and empowered to request, even demand, services but because the long list of requests does not include a relationship. The patient-as-consumer does not seek a person at the other end—she or he is looking for a product. Even physicians who are unsophisticated about the doctor-patient relationship do not relish being treated like a discount department store.

The closure of the relationship between patient and doctor highlights the ways in which contract is an inappropriate construct. Unlike the termination of contractual arrangements, termination of the doctor-patient relationship is a difficult matter. A doctor may legally terminate a relationship with a patient, but in actuality it is hard to do. Doctors who change practices and residents at the end of their training often use denial and avoidance to protect themselves from their feelings of guilt, sadness, or loss about ending relationships with patients (Lichstein, 1982; Macaulay, 1992). Doctor-prompted termination is also fraught with legal risk: patients may sue for abandonment or even libel (Curran, 1982). Likewise, patients may choose to leave a relationship with a clinician but feel great conflict, guilt, or ambivalence in doing so.

These conflicts support the idea that the doctor-patient relationship shares some of the qualities of "permanence and non-replaceability" that characterize relations between a mothering person and child (Held, 1987a) but not contractual relations. In a contractual relationship, each party is replaceable and the interaction itself becomes a commodity to be bought and sold.[5]

THE DENIAL OF THE MORAL BASIS OF CONDUCT

When relationships are framed as contracts, morality consists solely of everyone having his or her rights respected. Harm consists in violating someone's rights. A rights orientation suggests that moral behavior is no more than a matter of following the rules. While the rights/contract formulation describes the bare essentials of what ought not to be violated, it hardly embraces a full moral approach to the conduct of human relations. Ladd (1982) gives the example of viewing the immorality of the Holocaust in terms of the Third Reich having taken away the rights of Jewish people not to be gassed. Or take his example of the starving person. If I have food and she doesn't, then, under rights-based thinking, I should give her food because she has a right not to be starving. This construction fails to define moral conduct in terms of how I ought to behave: I ought to share food because it is the good and right thing to do; it is my human obligation.

Rights-based thinking is inappropriately minimalist in its ethical approach to the conduct of intimate human relations (Hardwig, 1984). Likewise, the application of a rights-based view of human relations to clinical work offers no moral basis for the conduct of clinical relations (Ladd, 1982; Veatch, 1984). That the patient and I should each have our rights secured is a minimal but not defining condition of the relationship. Standing alone, the rights orientation offers a sorry view of the doctor-patient relationship, implying that, when they are most vulnerable, people need to be protected from the people dedicated to caring for them.

CONTRACT AS RHETORIC

RIGHTS AND RESPONSIBILITIES

Discussion of the contractual notion of the doctor-patient relationship is replete with the language of responsibility.[6] Unfortunately, the word is used in two confusing ways: responsibility as obligation, and responsibility as culpability. Under paternalism, the doctor had all the power, all the privilege, all the obligation (except financial), and all the responsibility (culpability) for the outcome. The move to the contractual view of the relationship allows the culpability to be shared. One ethicist calls this the "central moral and practical dilemma" facing doctors and patients: "to balance the rights of patients and the responsibilities of physicians—and the rights of physicians and the responsibilities of patients" at a time of changing values (Siegler, 1981).

Doctors writing about contract are eager to define all patient responsibilities as obligations—for example, to share decision-making and to ask questions. This shift in emphasis occurs not because shared decision-making is empowering or because information is essential, but because if responsibilities (obligations) are shared, culpability is shared as well. If the outcome is not ideal, a portion of the fault lies with the patient (defined as responsible for his or her self-care), who is increasingly held accountable for preventing his or her sickness, getting well, and staying healthy (see, for instance, Meyer, 1992). Although one advocate for the contractual model explicitly denies that a contract is an attempt to "abrogate physician's responsibility by placing the patient in a self-care situation" (Brody, 1980, p. 720), the very language of duties and responsibilities refutes his statement. Another ethicist worries that patient autonomy may serve as an excuse: "[The physician's] conscience may not be quite so acutely tuned to implicit Hippocratic responsibilities if he or she has already discharged explicit obligations by maximizing the subject/patient's autonomy. The current fashion to avoid an unpopular paternalism may become a socially approved if unconscious excuse to avoid traditional responsibilities" (Morison, 1984, p. 45). Implicit in the understanding of contract is the doctor's ability to withdraw from the contract when a patient is not "responsible."

The rights and responsibility framework does not acknowledge the fact of oppression. Oppression damages the ability of some persons to make good assessments of what they need and what choices they have. "It misinforms and mystifies them about the choices they do have and their consequences, it damages their general ability to choose, and it ensures that unrealistic and needlessly limiting associations are created in them, both by manipulation and by the unintentional influence of others" (Wendell, 1990, p. 36). Oppression limits some people's self-confidence by shaping their sense of themselves and their potential. In practical terms, it prevents patients who are in some way restricted from full personhood in society (for instance, a woman being beaten by her partner) from exercising those rights that the contract model would claim (Wendell, 1990). Wendell argues that oppression, by putting such limits on certain people, reduces their responsibility for their actions. In contrast, others, whose "fears and desires are based on realistic associations formed in an atmosphere of diverse opportunities for experience and social tolerance," bear greater responsibility (p. 36). The disempowering effect of oppression on many persons who become patients requires that any discussion of rights and responsibilities address power relations.

OBSCURING POWER RELATIONS

Advocates of the contractual notion of the doctor-patient relationship see it as a universal concept, a moral ideal of the relation between equals. In reality, however, doctors invoke the idea of contract when they feel their power-over challenged or threatened—when they are having trouble with the relationship or when they need to make explicit the demands and concerns of each party (Quill, 1983). Advocates of contract hold that it can allay the "mutual mistrust and even suspicion that currently poison so many patient-doctor relationships" (Gillick, 1992, p. 83). Contract can serve as the route to improved communication and clear guidelines "by forcing doctors and patients to confront areas of potential conflict in advance" (p. 85). Preventing and resolving conflict becomes important because conflict represents a challenge to the doctor's power-over. In other words, although it is upheld as an ideal form of relation, doctors appeal to contract when relationships are conflictual.

To address such conflicts, as well as contemporary disenchantment with and distrust of doctors, some advocates propose explicit contracts as a way to resolve differences between doctor and patient. Brody, for instance, calls for physicians to adopt an "empathetic attitude in which they assume the patients' internal frame of reference, attempt to perceive the world as the patient sees it, and consider the patients' value system" before they respond to a patient's suggestions—a worthy objective. However, after they reach a decision, "a contract can be signed by both parties to reinforce the results of the negotiation" (1980, p. 720; see also Gillick, 1992). The need for this written contract is unclear. Brody states that the contract serves as "an effort to ensure the preservation of the patient's values as the basis for treatment decisions" (p. 720). However, the requirement that a contract be mutually signed lends a legal cast to the process and implies that signing may serve less to underline the patient's values than it does to enforce compliance; the pressure for signing suggests that those who refuse to sign are untrustworthy. The transition from contract as ideal to contract as conflict resolution, to contract as signed document, makes it clear that the contract itself is an instrument of power, to be invoked when there is no relationship or when the relationship is antagonistic. Initially a supposed arrangement between equals, it emerges as a tool of engagement in the hands of the more powerful to enforce compliance.

Doctors invoke the idea of contract exactly when power-over is threatened by patients' expectations or behavior. Certain problems seem to set the stage for doctors to propose an explicit contract with a patient: irrationality (psychiatric patients); failure or refusal to comply with the medical regimen (patients with chronic illness); or anticipated conflict with patients they perceive as demanding or controlling (and therefore threatening), such as drug-seeking patients, or patients who insist on specific medical workups. For instance, Quill offers the example of using a contract to define the terms of his relationship with a man who demanded narcotic analgesics and repeated medical workups for chronic pain. Previous physicians had found this man to be "a troublesome patient" (1983, p. 228). Contract served as a way to circumscribe their connection: the doctor agreed to provide the narcotics, refused to pursue further workup, and insisted on regular office visits. Thus, although medicine appeals to the idea of contract as a way to prevent abuses and guarantee equal footing, it actually uses contracts when patients challenge medical authority and, by extension, existing power relations.

FOSTERING FURTHER LEGALISM

The language of contract situates the doctor-patient relationship in legal language and implicitly in a legal context. Terms like "contract" and "informed consent" bear legalistic connotations (distinct from their legal interpretations) for both doctors and patients. Patients perceive that the use of such language derives from doctors' defensiveness about litigation; doctors preoccupied with the possibility of being sued view the use of these terms as protective. In a reversal of the goal of protecting patients against paternalism, doctors may also view contracts as guaranteeing their rights in relation to patients. Despite insurance company evidence that failed communication is a far more likely cause of litigation than medical negligence (Green, 1988), medical strategies to avoid suits focus far more on documentation and accountability than on strategies to maintain successful relationships.

The theory and practice of informed consent offers a case in point. Upon entry into a hospital or before surgery, a patient signs a form giving permission for the hospital or doctor to do the necessary procedures. This signing is consent, and it relieves the hospital or doctor of the charge of battery. But it does not constitute *informed* consent, a term that implies that the patient, understanding the risks, benefits, and alternatives, has made an educated decision. Used by attorneys and insurance companies, however, the term is used to promote doctors' defensibility, not to ensure joint decision-making (Green, 1988).

A variety of standard practices support the idea that informed consent is not a process between doctor and patient but rather a legal maneuver. First, the written materials patients are expected to read and sign are unintelligible and legalistic—that is, they are designed by lawyers with the intention that they will be read by other lawyers if legal action ensues. Consent forms are not intended to give readers (patients) a clear idea of risks, benefits, side effects, and alternatives to tests or treatment. (Tests of readability of standard consent forms place them at the thirteenth-grade reading level, with at least 22 percent at the postgraduate level [LoVerde, Prochazka, & Byyny, 1989].) Second, the signing of a form after the decision has been made—that is, just before surgery—and sometimes even after a procedure (for example, after the insertion of epidural anesthesia during labor) conveys to both patients and health care professionals that the purpose is legal and not educational (Green, 1988). Patients understand that their signing serves to complete documentation or to protect against later legal complaint, not to confirm their understanding. Framing the doctor-patient relationship as a contract contributes to patients' understanding that legal defensibility is the doctor's primary concern.

Contracts will continue to legalize medical relationships because contracts are the stuff of legal work. Despite protestations to the contrary, lawyers are sure to insist on making their contribution to shaping the defensible doctor-patient contract: "While lawyers may well wish to work with physicians on designing a prototype contract, there would be no need for legal counsel in the routine completion of contractual negotiations, any more than there is a need for a lawyer to draw up a living will, health care proxy, or business contract" (Gillick, 1992, p. 85). The reality, of course, is that people do seek lawyers to make their living wills, health care proxies, and business contracts. Doctors anxious about litigation are likely to check with their lawyers or the lawyers of their employer before signing any documents. Lawyers are likely to apply the language of legal contract to such documents, a process destructive to the intent of informed consent. Patients will perceive such documents in a similar light to other legalistic medical documents. Thus, the explicit application of contracts to clinical relationships will guarantee that those relationships are increasingly perceived as legal entities. Further litigation, not improved communication, will be the result.

CONTRACT AS COERCION

NEGOTIATION AS CONTROL

Contract advocates consistently call for negotiation to mediate the interaction between doctor and patient. In their way of thinking, negotiation is both a skill and a process. The very popularity of the concept of negotiation between doctor and patient deserves attention: it is a testimony to the penetration of contract language into the doctor-patient relationship, as well as an admission of the adversarial and embattled position in which doctors see themselves. Negotiation, with its overtones of fairness and legality, has been widely acclaimed as the paragon of interaction and as a result has received relatively little criticism.

Negotiation does, however, deserve careful examination, both as an ideal and as a practical construct. At best, negotiation permits patients some measure of control by requiring that they be allowed to express their needs for understanding, for diagnosis, and for treatment. Conceptually, negotiation assumes that the parties are autonomous and that their interests are potentially, if not actually, conflictual; negotiation is the strategy to resolve their explicit differences. (Note the congruence of these assumptions with those of the contractual model.) Although not necessarily equal in power, the parties to a negotiation, who frequently have no prior knowledge of each other, are assumed to have equal ability to negotiate.

The use of the term and the application of the process of negotiation shows how rhetoric itself can be turned into a force for coercion. At the rhetorical level, we hear: "Negotiation is a process between two persons with relatively equal power willing to be influenced by one another" (Quill, 1983, p. 229). This language clouds clinical reality. Doctors and patients, as we have seen, are hardly equal, and doctors' willingness to have their decisions influenced by patients is variable. Even patients who are skilled in acting on their own behalf may be unable to negotiate fully at a verbal level in the clinical setting and may thus demonstrate their concerns and interests through actions, such as not taking medicines, refusing tests, or seeking alternate opinions. Doctors are advised to elicit the patient's view and explanation of his or her illness in order to engage in a productive negotiation that will result in patient cooperation. The goal is not to get inside the patient's perspective (Schwartz & Kahne, 1983). Finding out what the patient wants, thinks, or believes is not an end in itself but rather the most efficient way to serve the doctor's ends. Negotiation emerges as a *tactic* the doctor can employ to attain his or her objectives. Thus, negotiation, overtly proffered as a form of cooperation, covertly serves as a tool for the physician. Prized as the ideal form of interaction because of its presumption of fairness and autonomy, negotiation, with its underlying assumption of a contractual relationship, cloaks the latest version of a physician-dominant relationship.[7]

CONTRACT AS BEHAVIOR CONTROL

In clinical settings, the idea of contract has devolved into a method for controlling behavior that staff wish to change (Boehm, 1989). Particularly with psychiatric patients but occasionally with medical patients, "contracting" is a fashionable method for managing what is perceived as difficult behavior. The clear purpose is control. For example, contracts are considered useful to manage psychiatric inpatients diagnosed with borderline personality disorders (Bloom & Rosenbluth, 1989). But contracts negotiated by staff members still angry at a patient are likely to be punitive and to contain unnecessary and excessively rigid limits on the patient (Miller, 1990). Since behavior that makes others angry is typical of patients carrying this diagnosis, the possibility that such contracts will indeed be negotiated by angry staff is quite likely. Taussig (1980) gives the example of a woman hospitalized on an inpatient medical unit for polymyositis (an inflammatory muscle disease) who refused to go to physical therapy. She felt she had no time to herself to rest during the day. The staff "contracted" with her for time to herself if she would cooperate. She had to bargain for free time to rest, as if her time were not hers to begin with. Calling it a contract hides the coercive nature of the agreement by implying that she is a freely participating party when, of course, she is at the mercy of the hospital staff in almost every respect. This sense of contracting offers patients the illusion of autonomy and freedom while actually taking it away from them.

The use of contracts to control behavior is based on principles of behaviorism. In contrast to animals, however, human beings demand to know what is being done to them.[8] Contracting is the method that medical staff use to inform patients about the rules that will be applied to their behavior. Staff apply the principles of operant conditioning and positive reinforcement to manage patients. Human beings, unlike animals, may be allowed to choose their "reward." For instance, human contact is regarded as a commodity to be bargained for; a patient's reward for desired behavior might be fifteen minutes with a staff member, thus turning human relations into commodities or bargaining chips (Taussig, 1980). In these applications of the idea of contract to behavior control, the contract is not based on any prior relationship between clinician and patient but rather is predicated on their lack of relatedness. Nor does contracting encourage the formation of relationships; rather, it renders patients into objects to be manipulated.

A FEMINIST CRITIQUE

The above critiques of the autonomy-contract-negotiation model of the doctor-patient relationship have not identified the gender bias in these concepts. It is clear that the old authoritarian vision of the doctor-patient relationship was highly gendered; that is, it described a relation marked by stereotypical masculine attributes: dominance, control, rationality, and objectivity. Less clearly spelled out is that the prescribed antidotes—patient rights, patient autonomy, and a contractual view of the relationship—likewise emerge from a gendered perspective. The admittedly masculinist practice of paternalism in medicine was supplanted by an equally male-dominated image of personhood and relationship: autonomy and contract.

The standard critique of paternalism in medicine rests largely on two related ideas: first, that the treatment by the doctor/authority/parent of the patient/passive subject/child violates the patient's *autonomy*; and second, that in relationships in which one party has more power than the other, the one with less power will be used, abused, or taken advantage of. These ideas draw on a masculinist tradition—they take manhood as the ideal form of what people are like and how they should relate to each other. The (male) individual appears as a "theoretically isolatable entity":

> This entity can assert interests, have rights, and enter into contractual relations with other entities. But this individual is not seen as related to other individuals in inextricable or intrinsic ways. This individual is assumed to be motivated primarily by a desire to pursue his own interests, though he can recognize the need to agree to contractual restraints on the ways everyone may pursue their interests. (Held, 1987a, p. 124)

If contract is a masculinist answer to medicine's problem with power-over, what is the feminist solution?

Two feminist philosophers—Annette Baier and Virginia Held—have detailed the problems with the contractual view of human relationships, particularly with respect to women (Baier, 1986; Held, 1987a, 1987b). Baier points out that contract presumes an equality between the parties and explicit expectations. Contract exemplifies a "limit case of trust . . . designed for cooperation between mutually suspicious risk-averse strangers" (1986, p. 251). Contract offers no room for trust, which she defines in terms of vulnerability to the goodwill of the other: "Trust . . . is reliance on others' competence and willingness to look after, rather than harm, things one cares about which are entrusted to their care" (p. 259). Trust may have no specific moment of beginning, and its growth may be slow and imperceptible. It does not require verbal acknowledgment. In contrast to the notion of contract, which requires adult parties who are equal in power, Baier offers infant trust as an example of noncontract-based trust. Relations between children and parents are not and cannot be contractual. "Parental and filial responsibility does not rest on deals, actual or virtual, between parent and child" (p. 244).

What Baier calls "the male fixation on contract" (p. 247) originated with men who did not view relations with women, children, slaves, the sick, the dying, or the mentally incompetent as warranting serious consideration. The men who wrote the moral treatises on trust relied on women to look after their households, raise their children, and even care for their needs, but they did not expect women to have a viewpoint on trust. Such men "were in the morally awkward position of being, collectively, oppressors of women, exploiters of women's capacity for trustworthiness in unequal, nonvoluntary and non-contract-based relationships" (p. 249). Needless to say, they did not make those kinds of relationships the center of their understanding about trust, even though trust is more essential to such relations than to those between equals.

At the time when the idea of the social contract was developed, women and family relations were outside the contractual domain, which included only "equal men." "The total or relative exclusion of women from the domain of voluntary contracting has then been thought to be either inevitable or appropriate" (Held, 1987a, p. 118). Contract calls for a model of relationship foreign to many women, one based on a legal, political, or even commercial definition rather than one from women's experience. The themes of autonomy and contract appear irrelevant to women's typical relations with others. "[Contractarians] managed to relegate to the mental background the web of trust tying most moral agents to one another, and to focus their philosophical attention so single-mindedly on cool, distanced relations between more or less free and equal adult strangers, say, the members of an all male club" (p. 248). The web of trust she refers to is the network of dependent human relations essential to survival from infancy to adulthood, in sickness or health, and among family members, who are inevitably vulnerable to each other in myriad ways. Women's relations with men and with children are not definable in terms of the contract, and thus women are excluded from consideration in contract theory. If philosophers are going to deal with women and children and the sick, aged, or infirm, they cannot claim that the rights and duties of free adults are the core of all moral relationships (see also Grimshaw, 1986). In medicine, contract theory treats the enormous inequality between doctor and patient as nonexistent and irrelevant. And medical ethics operates as if the oppression of women did not exist, in both medicine and society (Sherwin, 1992). The presumption of equality cannot work for relations between those of such disparate power; it is "at worst an offensive pretense of equality as a substitute for its actuality" (Baier, 1986, p. 249).

Similarly, Virginia Held agrees that contract is an inappropriate model for human relations:

> To see contractual relations between self-interested or mutually disinterested individuals as constituting a paradigm of human relations is to take a certain historically specific conception of "economic man" as representative of humanity. . . . If what it is to be human is thought to be a disposition to be a rational contractor, human persons creating other human persons through the processes of human mothering are overlooked. (1987a, pp. 113, 120)

The idealization of the rational contractor discounts the viewpoint and position of women. Held points out that for most of history, bearing and raising children has been a noncontractual and nonvoluntary affair.

Even when a woman can make a choice to have a child, the responsibilities are not voluntary. Furthermore, she cannot choose the child she gets, and children have no choice over their parents. "The ties that bind mothering person and child are affectional and solicitous on the one hand, and emotional and dependent on the other" (p. 125). Held argues for replacing the paradigm of "economic man" with the paradigm of mother and child, for replacing the contractual view of human relations with one that draws on an understanding of the relations between mothers and children to understand all human relations (p. 114). Both Baier and Held see unequal and noncontractual relations as typical of the relationships in women's lives. The inequalities cannot be legislated away by contract. Definitions of moral conduct need to be based in such relations exactly because they are between unequals. "A complete moral philosophy would tell us how and why we should act and feel toward others in relationships of shifting and varying power asymmetry and shifting and varying intimacy" (Baier, 1986, p. 252).

By appealing to a vision of morality based in maternal-child relations, I am not advocating a return to paternalism; neither am I recommending that adults treat each other like children or that doctors infantilize patients. I am certainly not saying that all relations between mothers and children are ideal. Rather, I am saying that the kind of relationship that ideally develops between the mothering person and child, with its inexplicitness of expectation, its inequality of the parties, its basis of trust, and its uncontractibility, is a more appropriate model for clinical relationships than contracts between cool, distant, equal, and disinterested parties. Empowerment would be the goal in these unequal but mutual relations (see chapter 10). In fact, Held is careful to clarify that she is not referring to the mother-child relations in a patriarchal household where women are subservient and women and children are vulnerable to the abuses of a male figure. She also makes it clear that men can engage in mothering as well. Likewise, a vision of doctoring based on the morality of mothering would not valorize domination, which Held upbraids as a degenerate form of mothering.

The disappearance of beneficence from the contractual view of relations does not correspond with the realities of women's practices in the world, such as caring for children, students, and sick people. These activities require a motivation beyond contract; Baier calls this motivation trust: "Whereas contracts make explicit the services (or service equivalent) exchanged, trust, when made express, amounts to a sort of exchange of responses to the motives and state of mind of the other, responses, in the form of a confident reliance" (p. 258). Feminist visions of the moral conduct of clinical work, like that of mothering, put an obligation on the caring person to accept the other for himself or herself (Malterud, 1990; Noddings, 1984). This kind of receptivity is alien to the language of contract.

Contracting derives from a rules-based approach to conduct. It upholds "keeping to the minimal moral traffic rules, designed to restrict close encounters between autonomous persons to self-chosen ones" (Baier, 1986, p. 249). Explicit contracts allow for explicit penalties when contracts are breached. Gilligan's (1982) work suggests that boys and men may be more comfortable with a morality grounded in such rules while girls and women look to the care of relationships in their approach to morality. Hare-Mustin (1987) argues that the appeal to rules may have less to do with gender than with power; those in power invoke rules and those without power appeal to caring. For instance, women appeal to caring in relation to men but invoke the rules in their dealings with children. Indeed, a woman physician offended (or threatened) by confrontation can become an ardent advocate of explicit contracts (Gillick, 1992); a male physician committed to a relational model may eschew them (Stoeckle, 1992). Usually, however, following the typical gender and power lines, doctors (mostly men) invoke contract and rules in relation to patients. Nurses (mostly women) and disempowered patients (disproportionately women) are more likely to raise the issue of caring in clinical medicine. (In a parallel fashion, family medicine, less prestigious than other medical specialties, also places caring at the center of its values and criticizes more powerful fields for their lack of caring.)

As a contrast to the rights and rules orientation of male moral development, the work of Gilligan, Ward, Taylor, and Bardige (1988) suggests an alternative ethical organizing principle, one that is more often demonstrated in the conduct and decision-making of women: care of the relationship and for the feelings of others. Gilligan formulates these two themes as gender-connected—men with the ethic of justice, and women with the ethic of care. Her formulation—which has become extremely popular in lay circles, perhaps because it supports gender stereotypes of men as rational and women as caring—leaves her open to the charge of essentialism: that women *are* this way and men *are* that way. Such generalizations can be used to discourage women from entering the scientific and academic realms and to restrict them to activities considered emotional or relational, such as teaching, nursing, or family work. Nevertheless, Gilligan's work legitimized in public circles the morality of caring for relationships.

Some feminists object to discussions that set up justice and care as an either-or choice: caring without justice supports paternalism; justice without caring is heartless and inhumane. Held, for instance, opts for a "both-and" solution, pointing out the feminist demands that the values of justice and equality be extended into the family and that the (post-patriarchal) values of care and concern be extended into the wider society. Some feminists warn against institutionalizing caring as an ethic because caring as women have done it and continue to do it occurs under oppressed conditions. Calling on women to continue caring as an ethical imperative is a way to lend moral justification to the immoral arrangements in some women's lives—for instance, when they are battered, unsupported in child care, or under- or unpaid for caring work. Although medical ethicists have actively argued about justice versus care, the issue has not penetrated into medicine itself (Carse, 1991; Sherwin, 1992). The contemporary preference for the contract model of relationships guarantees that the ethic of rights and justice will overshadow the ethic of caring until feminism challenges medicine at this level of ideology.

The militarist overtones of the idea of negotiation are also problematic. When negotiation stands for "conflict resolution through mutual concessions" (Ruddick, 1987, p. 251, citing W. B. Gallie for the term), it derives from an understanding of peace that assumes mutual conflict and self-interest: "Partners moved by fear and frustration, concede and compromise in order to be left alone in safety" (p. 252). This vision of peace is inherently unstable, for it can always be rocked when one party thinks it can gain by resuming the conflict. Medicine's choice of contract and negotiation as the models for peace in a relationship as personal as the clinical relationship reflects an underlying acceptance of competition to dominate as the central motivation of the parties. In contrast, when the model of maternal practice is the basis of peacemaking, other, by now familiar assumptions apply: that differences in strength are given; that power shifts over time and in different situations. "Peace is not a precarious equilibrium in which everyone is somewhat warily left alone. . . . Peace is a way of living in which participants counting on connection demand a great deal of each other" (Ruddick, 1987, p. 253). Peace in the doctor-patient relationship will require just this kind of connection.

The current critique of the paternalistic doctor-patient relationship is based on a set of assumptions that can be understood as gendered—specifically, as masculinist assumptions about human beings and therefore about the doctor-patient relationship. The assertion that persons are separate and autonomous is congruent with the belief that separateness and autonomy are the goals of human development. A doctor-patient relationship between autonomous parties is an example of a relation in which unequal power results in domination and therefore requires limits to prevent abuse. Such limits include structuring the relationship as a contract in which each party has rights and duties. Contract theory appeals to rules to establish the moral basis of conduct. Negotiation emerges as the highest form of relation possible within the contract model. Negotiation assumes equal parties and conflicting interests. Rather than being engaged and affected by their relationship with each other, the parties compete to get their way and arrive at a compromise. Thus, contract is a modality proposed by those in power to mediate interactions between themselves and others. It is an example of one way of being in the world that may not fit those out of power, who are often women. The contractual view of the doctor-patient relationship does not allow women's perspectives on themselves and their experience to shape the clinical relationship.

Medicine does not recognize itself as a gendered activity; nor does it acknowledge that its ideology reflects a vision of activities and relationships conducted primarily by men. Like vampires who cannot see themselves in mirrors, medicine cannot "see" the gendered bases of both its dilemmas and its proposed solutions.[9] Thus, medicine's response to the criticism of domination, or power-over, has been to advocate contract, which at bottom is itself an equally gendered vision of relationship. Jordan et al. (1991) describe this view of human relations as "competing subjectivities" rather than intersubjectivity. If persons are not separate and autonomous at their most developed, however, if power-over is not an acceptable dynamic for the doctor-patient relationship, if contracts offer an impoverished approach to medical relations, what alternative is there?

Physicians could join with feminists in regarding persons as primarily connected to others, with differing degrees of interdependence and relatedness (Jordan et al., 1991; Miller, 1976). Following self-in-relation theory, medicine might accept relatedness, instead of autonomy, as the goal of development, and it might come to regard unequal relations as typical of clinical relationships. Doctors might see that the moral conduct of such relations could be modeled on the ideal practice of mother-child relations (or teacher-student relations), in which trust rather than contract is the binding tie. The next chapter examines different kinds of knowing and suggests that "connected knowing" is more appropriate to clinical relationships than the "separate knowing" privileged by the contractual view. Using connected knowing as a way to learn about other persons during health and illness, clinicians could replace contract with mutual realization as the goal of clinical relations (Whitbeck, 1983).

CHAPTER 7

Ways of Knowing in Medicine

> Our scientific methods, as women, as feminists, require see-
> ing things as they are: whole, entire, complex. Our work
> requires that we see things in context, that we understand
> and explain our eventful, complex reality within and as a
> part of its matrix. It is only within its matrix that experience,
> reality, can be known. And this matrix includes the knower.
>
> Barbara Du Bois, "Passionate Scholarship" (1983), p. 111

HOWEVER MUCH doctors may wish to stand apart from the families they work with, the position of neutral observer is not
open to them. As a "knower," the physician carries out actions
and makes interpretations that reflect a standpoint. In medicine, the
prevailing standpoint is that knowers are and should be separate from
what they know about. Based on the assumption that human beings are
fundamentally separate, the knowledge that such knowers can glean
presumes that separateness. Separateness does not acknowledge itself
to be a standpoint, but, of course, it is. A view of human beings as fundamentally in-relation allows us to consider the different kinds of
knowing that result from the presumption of human connectedness.

Let me begin with an example. Some years ago, a family practice resident was having a difficult time establishing a relationship with a former state hospital patient, or at least having some difficulty liking the
patient. To promote the possibility of a connection between the resident
and the patient, I suggested that she try to get to know the patient better by reviewing with her the events leading up to her first hospitalization. The act of gathering this history, I thought, might help the resident
see the patient as a person, and the act of telling it might strengthen the
patient's connection with the doctor. I was aware that the approach
might not work, since not all patients can respond to it, especially if
trust is a major problem or if their survival depends on suppression of
their feelings. However, starting from where the resident had posi-
tioned herself, I thought there was not a lot to lose.

The resident informed me later that day that the patient refused to talk. Several weeks later, she received the following letter in the mail (I have changed the dates and places for privacy reasons):

Dear Dr. Y.,

I know you want to know me better, and I agree with you all the way. The reason I'm writing to you is because I have a very hard time to express myself in person, sure hope you don't mind, I find it's easier to write about myself on paper, than trying to talk about it.

I was born in Vermont, Barre, lived with my grandparents for many years. Was raped by my grandfather at the age of 9. My grandfather and grandmother had 15 children.

I was having problems (which can't remember) while living with my grandparents. I went to live with my mother in Pittsfield at the age of 9. In my family there was 5 of us, my Mom, my Dad, my sister, my brother and myself. Lived with my family about 4 or 5 years. I was having problems in school, that's when they called my Mom in, then they went to another room where I couldn't hear them, I don't remember how long my Mom was gone. But when she (my Mom) came back, she didn't look too happy. She (my Mom) then took me home.

That's where it all began, I was only home a few days, when my Mom received a call I don't know who it was from, I was never told.

The following day my Mom took me to a place and turned me over to the State. She (my Mom) told me that she couldn't do anything with me, and that I needed some kind of help. She then turned and walked away, I wanted so much to run after her, my mom, but didn't, I really don't know why.

I went to the Children's Unit in the State Hospital, was there until I turned 16 years old. On the day I turned 16, I went to Springfield State, where I spent many years. In the many years, I was in the hospital, became very involved with a guy, I liked very much, and figure he liked me also. One thing lead to another, I'm sure you know what I mean. Within a few months I [decided] to go to the doctor's. Sure enough I was pregnant 3 months. I was so happy, that I couldn't wait to tell my boyfriend, I figure he was going to be as happy as I was, but little did I know, he wasn't happy at all, because the following day, when I wake up I find that he was gone. By the way the guy and I was going together about 8 months before I got pregnant.

Shortly after that I ended up back in the Hospital.

Where I was told, I would be given a two month trial period, (because of the past times I had tried to commit Suicide), to prove to the hospital people that I could [handle] myself in a [grown-up] way. I was so happy about their Decision I ended up crying, and thanking the Lord for what I had to do to prove to them that I could do anything.

The next months while carrying my baby, went just fine. No thanks to the people at the hospital, because I was being watched at all times.

The day finally came it was May 12, 1968. I was in a room, off the Dayroom with others, I felt something, don't know how to expect it. Ran to the toilet right across from the Nurse's office, call a nurse because something was happening but didn't know what. The nurse came running in, and ask me what was wrong. I told her I didn't know, but I was afraid. She [took] one look at me, and then told me that my water had broken. That was May 11, 1968 in the A.M., that afternoon I was brought to a Medical Ward, where they could keep a better eye on me, I don't mind saying I was afraid.

I was there only a short while, when a doctor came to check me out. He told me, that [I] was dilated, three fingers at that time.

It must have been getting close to the time for my baby to be born because the doctor transferred me to the Hospital where I was to have my baby, I was in contractions all the night. The following Day I was brought to the Delivery Room to have my baby.

By the way, I wasn't suppost to have my baby for at least a couple more weeks. It was supost to be a June baby. Anyway it was time for my birth.

[It] was time already, [it] finally happen my baby was born. It was a boy—blond hair and blue eyes, weight 6 pds. 5 onc. He was in Good Health, the only thing He had is what they call a lazy jaw, I was the one who told them about it. Because when they brought him in, for me to feed, I notice that he was drinking the milk that was in the bottle, and it was all around his little mouth, and his sleep wear. That was the only and last time I saw [my] son.

A few days after my birth, I went back to Springfield State. I wasn't back that long when the Head Nurse of the Ward I was on, told me I had an appointment with the Head of the Hosp. I meet with the Head of the Hosp. where he had told me, I would have a meeting the following day.

Anyway I went to the meeting the following day with a nurse by my side. I figure she was going to stay with me, spoke for me, and etc. Anyway, she didn't. We went to a big room where the Door was closed. On the door it said Conference Room. She knock, and opened the door, there was so many people there, I didn't know half of them. Anyway after the different ones ask me questions, the Head Doctor said to me, that the Court and himself decided to put my son up for [adoption]. He told me it was the court or myself who would put my son up for [adoption]. Many things were turning around in my head,

I decided to put my own son up for [adoption]. I figure no way is the court going to do this. So I signed my name on a piece of paper. Shortly after that the meeting was over. When I walk out of that room I was never so heartsick in all my life as I was at that moment. All I could do is cry.

Shortly after this I tried to kill myself, by covering the bandage I had on my left arm from cutting myself with a razor blade. I covered the bandage with lighter fluid, then put it on fire. I got very scared, and call for help, the nurse on duty came running in and saw me. She put out the fire (I don't remember how) and help me up off the floor and brought me into the Nurse's Office.

She call the opertion [supervisor] for help and told her what had happen.

Within Seconds that was, God only know how many (I don't recall) people came to the Ward, where the Nurse and I was.

All I remember was it was very painful. One of the people who came in, took one look at my arm, then call the doctor on call. He came and told the Nurse, what he wanted done, also told her it was a very bad burn. Second and third degree burn right down to the bone.

Anyway's at times there is a burning, or whatever its call, in my left shoulder.

Sure hope this information is helpful.

Linda Smith

P.S. There will always be a part of me, that left, when I had to put my own son, up for [adoption].

Subsequently, the resident reflected in an interview on her relationship with the patient after she received the letter:

Dr. Y.: I was getting bored seeing her every month. I felt like I needed to see her every month because she had tried to overdose on her anticonvulsants. I feel like I need to keep in good contact with her, and I was getting bored just seeing her every time and seeing basically how she was doing because nothing was happening in her life. So I said that I wanted to know a little more about her, and I asked her about her family first, and who was in her family, and then I asked her when she had first gone to the state hospital. And the more questions I asked her the more withdrawn she got. And she would answer me in monosyllables ("Why do you want to know that?"), defensively. She was sort of angry at me when I first went in to her that day because she had been waiting a while and she just got more and more angry and more and more withdrawn. But I sort of kept on until I got a little bit.

And I told her at the end that I thought it was helpful and that I realized that it was hard for her to talk about it. When she left I wondered if I had stirred everything up, because she was real depressed. She was manic-depressive—and mostly depressed—and has had multiple suicidal gestures.

L.C.:   How did you feel about having tried that?

Dr. Y.: I felt worried that I had stirred too much up. She was obviously having a reaction to my questioning her. I was afraid that the next call I was going to get about her was that she had made another OD attempt. But I didn't worry *too* much about it. But that was in the back of my mind definitely.

So then I got this letter about a week later. I had had a series of letters from somebody else that had just driven me crazy because I didn't know what to do with them; they had all come marked "personal." "Personal." So I had a sinking feeling about it really. Here's this person, she's going to say this stuff to me, and then I'm going to have to *do* something. So then I read this letter, and it was the most incredible letter I had ever had from anybody. One of the most incredible things I had ever read—it was so alive. She was so alive in it, much more alive than she ever is in person. I felt as if I was living it practically, it was so strong, the description. I cried . . . when I got to the point at the very end when she said that a part of her had died or had been lost when her son was taken from her. There was just so much strength there it was pretty amazing.

For this doctor and this patient, the letter—that is, the requested telling of the patient's story to the doctor—irrevocably changed their relationship and deepened their commitment to each other. Both the process and the content transformed the clinician's way of knowing. It was no longer possible to remain separate or disconnected. Its effect rippling outward, this powerful communication went on to change my own relationship with the resident and, more broadly, my understanding of how physicians grow in their work with patients.

SEPARATE VERSUS CONNECTED KNOWING

We owe the distinction between separate and connected knowing[1] to the work of Belenky, Clinchy, Goldberger, and Tarule, authors of *Women's Ways of Knowing* (1986), who set out to find out how women come to learn about the world. They interviewed hundreds of women, some several times over a period of years, asking how they describe themselves, how they see themselves in relationships, how they see themselves in the world, how they come to learn and to know, and how they see, identify, and solve moral problems. The authors describe a sequence of ways of knowing, ranging from the strategies of women who are socially and politically disempowered—battered and homeless women—to those of fortunate and articulate women—privileged college students and graduates.

Much of what transpires in medical education fits into a learning stage that Belenky et al. call "procedural knowing." In this kind of knowing, typical of academic settings, students learn the methods of argument and analysis of each discipline. Form is more important than content; how you set about it is more important than the position you take. In contrast to "subjective knowing," which is often used by women with less power, procedural knowing is suspicious of excessive personal involvement in interpretation. Much of medical education goes on at this stage: trainees learn the essentials of clinical methods but are discouraged from claiming the importance of their own or the patient's unique personal contributions to solving common clinical problems.

Differential diagnosis (the process of deducing the patient's most likely diagnosis, using all the available facts and literature) goes on at the subsequent stage of "separate knowing." Based on "critical thinking," "objectivity," and "reason," separate knowing actively excludes the self. Separate knowers willingly confront authorities using rhetorical skills and highly polished arguments. (The women in the Belenky study who applied this kind of knowing felt a particular emptiness and pointlessness in their success.) In contrast, "connected knowing" is built on the belief that "trustworthy knowledge comes from personal experience rather than the pronouncements of authorities. . . . Separate knowers learn through explicit formal instruction how to adopt a different lens—how, for example, to think like a sociologist. Connected knowers learn through empathy. Both learn to get out from behind their own eyes and use a different lens, in one case the lens of a discipline, in the other the lens of another person" (Belenky et al., 1986, pp. 112–13, 115).

Belenky and her colleagues found that through connected knowing a woman learns about another person or about a written work or an art form by taking it into herself, finding the ways in which she can see the world from the point of view of the other. The other is no longer "out there" but also within. Connected knowers seek to find out about the other person's experience; in medicine we do this by trying to find out what the other person is experiencing and how he or she is perceiving the world. In these terms, the empathic activities of clinical work go on at the level of connected knowing, while other kinds of clinical activity—problem-solving or contracting, for instance—stay confined to separate knowing. (Most medical research falls into the realm of separate knowing as well.)

Although my discussion is drawn from a study that focused on women (Belenky et al., 1986), I am not claiming that only women think as connected knowers. However, separate knowing is more compatible with men's socialization, and connected knowing is more consistent with women's socialization to view relationships as the central activity in their lives. Despite these forces, I suspect that many men in primary care fields like family medicine and pediatrics think as connected knowers but feel uncomfortable or even guilty about it. After all, men are even more strongly socialized to think that rational, emotion-free objectivity is the only proper lens through which to look at the world.

The distinction between separate and connected knowing has parallels in other disciplines. For instance, Jerome Bruner described what he called paradigmatic versus narrative modes of thought: "The one seeks explications that are context free and universal, the other seeks explications that are context sensitive and particular" (1985, p. 97). Bruner's paradigmatic mode (what some call the logico-scientific mode) is based on categorization and the methods by which categories are linked to form systems; based on consistency and noncontradiction, this mode tests hypotheses to arrive at empirical truth. In contrast, the narrative mode works in two "landscapes" simultaneously: the landscape of action (the play, the agent, the goal) and the landscape of consciousness (what the actors know, think, or feel). While believability is the touchstone of narrative, falsifiability is the standard of the scientific method. I shall return to this distinction.

What the clinician does when he or she sees a patient in the office, particularly in primary care settings, is often closer to constructing a believable account in Bruner's narrative mode than it is to proving an empirical hypothesis in the paradigmatic mode. This is not to say that clinicians do not spend a lot of time trying to match those stories with pathologically defined conditions: for example, fever, cough, green sputum, and rales in lungs equals pneumonia. But many accounts do not match any previously outlined medical diagnosis. The conflict between these modes accounts, perhaps more than anything else, for the mismatch of expectations created when the doctor is searching for a specific hypothesis in the scientific mode and the patient is seeking to be heard and believed in the narrative mode.[2]

However, the narrative mode can also serve to constrain the patient's story. The narrative mode is limited by the listener's framework of expectation: when the listener thinks he or she knows what the patient is going to say and therefore does not allow the speaker's story to stand on its own ("These people, they always complain about. . . ."). The listener's stereotyping and a priori interpretations restrict his or her understanding of the speaker and may allow the patient's age, race, class, or sex to constrain what the listener can hear. For instance, British male general practitioners explained the symptoms of midlife women in terms of menopause and the "empty nest"; their ability to understand and treat their patients was constricted by the inherent sexism in their assumptions about women (Barrett & Roberts, 1978; Roberts, 1981). Such listening bias in a doctor constitutes an abuse of power.[3] In contrast to this bias, the hypothetico-deductive approach seems unbiased and just, even though its capacity for distortion and lack of care for the speaker or storyteller is also enormous.

In family medicine, Anton Kuzel (1986) draws a parallel distinction between rationalistic inquiry (the traditional scientific method) and naturalistic inquiry (investigation within the natural setting of whatever or whomever is to be studied).[4] The two forms of inquiry recognize different forms of trustworthiness: for instance, the rationalistic mode uses the criteria of internal and external validity; the naturalistic mode depends on credibility, or what Reinharz (1983) calls plausibility. The investigative stance differs in the two approaches: objectivity, with all its implications of distance and separateness, is central to the rationalistic mode; what Kuzel calls "reflexivity" is the stance of the naturalistic observer, who consistently examines the contribution of his or her own perspective and interpretation to the investigation at hand.

Also within family medicine, G. Gayle Stephens (1985a), in the tradition of Foucault, draws the distinction between seeing and hearing, two avenues that lead to different understandings of patients. Twentieth-century medicine respects the primacy of what can be seen; the capacity to generate visual images of the body has expanded exponentially in the past twenty years. At the same time, clinicians' abilities to hear patients have probably not grown and may even have atrophied. Vision, compared with touch, for instance, promotes a sense of separateness between knower and known and encourages a sense that the knower is autonomous and free to choose (D. R. Gordon, 1988). Listening and hearing, in contrast, allow the clinician's imagination to become open to the imaginings, hopes, and fears of the patient. In hearing and listening, the doctor takes the other into herself or himself. This is the sensory correlate of Kuzel's reflexivity.

These contrasts between different ways of finding out about the world—separate versus connected, paradigmatic versus narrative, rationalistic versus naturalistic, seeing versus hearing—are tensions, not polar opposites or rigid dichotomies. What they have in common is the recognition that certain ways of finding out about and knowing the world have held the dominant position in academia, not only in the natural sciences and social sciences but in the arts and humanities. In medicine, the prevailing viewpoint remains the positivist conception of science, and separate knowing dominates clinical activities as well as research. Academic success requires achievement in the dominant mode of separate, rationalistic knowing. Those individuals (often women) and primary care fields (like family medicine) most comfortable in the connected, narrative, naturalistic, and listening modes are also those with the least prestige. In pursuit of academic credibility, we may forfeit our customary way of knowing and turn instead to what appears to be the more "scientific" way of knowing in writing and research.

In discussing how family medicine might reclaim legitimacy as a discipline of connected knowing, I will focus on four distinct ways of thinking to show how the typical work of family medicine represents this kind of knowing: context, time span, believability, and empathy. Finally, I will describe connected knowing at work in ordinary practice: in life history work and in what I call "the family approach at each moment."

CONTEXT

Separate knowing is necessary but not sufficient to many of the activities of clinical work. For instance, I cannot treat a urinary tract infection properly if I do not know what organisms are likely to be causing it and what antibiotics are likely to be effective against those organisms. But already this example pulls me away from the context. Perhaps a woman tells me that she has burning on urination, but further inquiry reveals that she is worried about having a sexually transmitted infection because her boyfriend is staying out all night. Or perhaps urinary frequency is her main complaint, and her underlying concern is pregnancy. Without finding out about her main concern, I may not perform the necessary examination or even the correct laboratory test. Although I may have all the ingredients of separate knowing about urinary tract infections, if I cannot connect with the patient's basic concerns, I will find myself looking in the wrong direction.

In naturalistic or connected knowing, the context is central to understanding the situation or the person. (Despite the trendiness of the word *context*, I prefer it to more obscure terms like *ground* or *surround*. *Context* conveys the concrete, detailed particularity of any clinical moment.) We cannot get a good fix on something until we have a feel for its surroundings. Appreciation of context allows a clinician to comprehend a person's unique situation, illness, or recovery. Individual, family, or N of 1 studies followed over long periods of time exemplify the research that has been done in this framework. (N refers to the number of subjects in an experiment. An N of 1 study is an investigation that evaluates one person's response to the experimental condition.) In contrast, rationalistic or separate knowing relies on removing a phenomenon from its context, isolating the elements, with the goal of establishing a useful generalization, law, or rule. In looking for common elements or associations, this approach strips away differences. Controlled trials are the paramount example of this way of thinking.

The doctor-patient context and the patient's family context are familiar settings to clinicians. But context, as I use it, also includes the social and political dimensions of clinical work. Doctor and patient may take these contexts for granted, or both may be ignorant of the historical features that shape their apparently inevitable context. Take, for example, abortion and fertility control. A contextual approach situates women's reproduction in terms of their less powerful status in relation to men and to the society that makes laws determining their ability to control their own fertility. Decisions by individual women take place within a local and specific context, but these are shaped by social and political factors (see Sherwin, 1989, for a discussion of why case discussions in medical ethics need to be informed by a feminist understanding of the surrounding social and political context). For instance, if, because of political pressure, abortions are not funded for women on Medicaid or women who work for the federal government, then the political context is pressuring such a woman to carry a pregnancy even if she would otherwise choose not to. Similarly, if female sterilization has been the only socially sanctioned and culturally acceptable form of contraception for fifty years, as has been true in Puerto Rico, a woman's decision to be sterilized emerges from a context in which all the women in her family may have "chosen" *la operación* as the final way to manage their fertility.[5]

Every clinical moment has a political and social context, but I will offer two examples that touch on broad issues. The first example comes from psychotherapy: Comas-Diaz (1987) describes a second-generation Puerto Rican woman who was successful in her work and wished to advance in it, but her husband was dissatisfied that they had two girls and no sons. He did not support her work ambitions and made clear his desire for another child right after her promotion. She did not want more children. She felt she could not get support from her mother because her mother suffered from *ataques* (literally, "attacks") and even discussing it might cause her to have an *ataque*. (See Guarnaccia, Good, & Kleinman [1990] for a discussion of the culturally specific meaning and function of *ataques* in Puerto Rican families.) Her husband did not want to engage in therapy, although he "allowed" his wife to do it. She terminated therapy when she became pregnant. This example points out that the cultural pressures for performance as a wife, mother, and daughter may push a woman in directions she herself does not wish to go. The influence of marital as well as family power dynamics is part of the context here, as well as the patriarchal preference for male offspring.

The other example comes from a study of mothers of chronically mentally ill adults (Cook, 1988). Even after their children have become adults, these women continue to function as mothers and to do family maintenance as part of the gendered division of family labor. They take more responsibility for their offspring and feel more anxiety, depression, fear, and emotional drain than their husbands do. Their continued involvement with and concern for their adult children results, predictably, in their being scapegoated for causing or exacerbating their children's problems.

The context of families with a mentally ill adult child includes the social blame the mother receives for "failing" to raise a healthy and acceptable child, her own self-blame, and her ongoing feeling of responsibility as a mother for the care of her chronically ill offspring. These women's view of themselves is shaped by social constructions of gender and mothering.

TIME SPAN

Narrative or naturalistic knowing relies on observations made over a prolonged period of time. When doctors have not been present in the pasts of their patients, they can use tools like the genogram or life story to explore their pasts. In family medicine, our present work is predicated on maintaining our connections over a long enough time span to participate in the unfolding of the individual and family narrative. Stephens has highlighted the importance of this historical perspective for individual patients in his work on "clinical biographies" (1985b) and "careers of illness" (1986). The prime example of research focused on families within a community is F. J. A. Huygen's monumental work (1982) tracing the family medical histories of hundreds of Dutch families for up to four generations. In contrast, the attention span of most North American research is very short; for example, a recent retrospective study on the "natural history" of palpitations looked at patients with a mean age of forty-three for a mean period of forty-one months, a very short period in the life-span approach (Knudsen, 1987). While all clinical work must pay some attention to the role of time, as in the "history of the present illness," the dominant view in clinical research is far more cross-sectional than longitudinal.[6]

BELIEVABILITY

Narrative is about "the working out of human intentions in a real or possible world" (Bruner, 1985, p. 106). One way to assess a narrative is for believability. In clinical work, practitioners must initially listen to and accept the story the patient tells us about himself or herself, not approach the patient's statement as a scientific hypothesis to be disproved. We ascribe believability, or plausibility, to the account of a child who tells us that he or she has been sexually abused. We must act based on our belief that the narrative is true. Our job is not to disprove the statement but rather to begin our work based on the likelihood that it is true. (Briere points out the destructive effect of disbelieving a patient's report of sexual abuse in contrast to the minimal harm that comes from accepting what may be "a distorted or technically false disclosure" [1989, p. 54].)

In contrast, rational knowing adopts disprovability as a basic measure of truth. The means of evaluation include "the operations of causes, structural requiredness, reasoned correlation" (Bruner, 1985, p. 106). To test hypotheses in this framework, the rational knower attempts to disprove them. Both the judicial system and scientific, hypothetico-deductive systems attempt to disprove hypotheses. Belenky et al. state: "Presented with a proposition, separate knowers immediately look for something wrong—a loophole, a factual error, a logical contradiction, the omission of contrary evidence" (1986, p. 104).

Certain clinical situations seem to require a posture of disprovability rather than believability toward the patient. Perhaps there is some opposition between the patient and an outside authority, as in disability assessments and compensation claims. Or a clinician is assessing whether a parent's account of a child's injury is an attempt to hide abuse. Doctors also adopt a stance of disprovability when confronted by patients seeking pain medications. Wary of creating or colluding with addiction and anxious not to be duped, doctors approach with suspicion patients who want narcotics or other drugs that might be salable. The result is an opposition that rarely results in a productive relationship (see Quill, 1983, for the application of contractual thinking to this kind of opposition). In contrast to ordinary clinical encounters, in each of these situations the doctor is ultimately answerable to an administrative or legal authority. The doctor becomes the agent of those authorities, not the patient's advocate. Legalistic standards of verification replace an appreciation of the patient's credibility within a relationship. Not surprisingly, clinicians who define their work within a relational context are uncomfortable with the doubting posture evoked by these situations.

Belenky et al. (1986) found that the women in their study were uncomfortable with doubting; they saw it either as a game or as something threatening to their relationships with others in the sense that someone might get hurt. Doubting requires a particular suspiciousness of a person's involvement in his or her own story and of one's own personal responses to it. Doubting relies on the removal of self, or objectivity. Believing, in contrast, felt real to the women Belenky and her colleagues interviewed, "perhaps because it is founded upon genuine care and because it promises to reveal the kind of truth they value—truth that is personal, particular, and grounded in firsthand experience" (p. 113). Believing means that you accept as valid another person's experience in shaping his or her way of looking at the world, even if you do not share their experience or viewpoint. The person's subjective interpretation is important in your understanding of him or her.

I am not taking the position that the doctor should believe every factual claim a patient makes. If a woman says her husband beat her and her husband denies it, the doctor cannot believe that both are telling the truth. I am saying that doctors should approach patients as if they were believable without challenging, minimizing, or trying to catch them out. It is helpful here to draw a distinction between the believability of a narrative and the believability of a person. Narratives often make sense within the context of existing power relations; the believability of a person emerges in the context of a relationship. When a patient is vulnerable to powerful others, not telling the truth or "faking" may be more "believable." For instance, a pregnant fourteen-year-old, when asked about a past history of sexual abuse or rape, may deny any such experience. A negative answer does not, however, mean that it did not happen, only that at this time, in this context, she cannot recognize or acknowledge that it did occur. My respect for her answer lets her know that I think she is a believable person. She is not telling a lie; she is answering with what she can accept as the truth. Likewise, the teenager who, in front of her insistent mother, denies that she is having sex is a believable person—even though her narrative may not be truthful. When I see her alone, my job is not to determine if she is lying, thereby perpetuating the powerlessness she feels; rather, my goal should be to create with her a safe and confidential relationship that respects her needs for information about contraception and infection and enables her to make wise choices.

What I know about parents of teenagers, what I know about teenagers on the brink of sexual activity, and what I know from past visits about the mother and daughter in the last example lead me to maintain a stance toward each of them as believable while containing the tension of their contradictory narratives. The thought is intolerable to the mother that her daughter could be having sex. Knowing this, the daughter can only deny it. The very intensity of their relationship makes each position more credible. For the clinician, discerning true and false is not the issue but rather understanding the stories within the context of patients' lives—and in this case, perhaps someday fostering the ability of both mother and daughter to hear clearly the other's story. Knowing patients well within the context of their family relationships, the clinician comes to understand that people are truthful in complicated ways.

Various elements create the history that leads patients to bring a problem to the doctor: fear about the meaning of a specific symptom, intolerance for the severity of a symptom, and shame over a symptom are only a few of the feelings that precipitate office visits. Fear and shame may also lead people to avoid doctors or to deny the unacceptable origins of their symptoms in physical or sexual abuse. Clinical practice based on believability assumes that the narrative a patient tells about himself or herself makes sense, and that the clinician's job is to understand the story the patient tells, to put together his or her picture of what is happening. A child's revelation of sexual abuse offers one such example. A woman brings in her ten-year-old daughter, who states that her stepfather has been sexually abusing her for some time. The mother, who is a caseworker for the welfare department, is extremely upset and angry. She has already been to the police and to the court to file a restraining order. She herself was sexually abused, and she chose her work to be able to do what she could to prevent it from happening to other children. The intern who examines the child finds no physical evidence of sexual abuse but is certain based on the child's terror that the story is accurate. I know from indirect sources that the intern herself is a survivor of an emotionally abusive relationship and that she has an infant daughter. She asks for help from me in writing her record so that the lack of physical findings will not work against the girl's story. The intern is already thinking about the scrutiny of her record in court and wants to make sure that it is helpful to the girl.

This example has many levels. The mother believed her daughter and acted on that belief immediately. Likewise, the intern had no doubt about the child's history. I believed the intern's assessment of the girl's believability. The intern was worried that a court would try to disprove her assessment because of the lack of physical evidence; she implicitly recognized the distinction between her stance of believability and the usual legal application of disprovability. Although I assured her that courts are now well aware that sexual abuse may leave no physical findings, I knew that her worry was appropriate. In a courtroom setting, despite the girl's believability, the lack of physical findings might be used against her in an effort to disprove her story. Contributing to the intern's anxiety that the child would not be believed was her own vulnerability as a survivor of abuse and her personal history of having been disbelieved about that abuse.

This example highlights the difference between a stance that rests on believability and a stance that places a "burden of proof" on the storyteller. The application of connected knowing by the listeners (the mother, the intern, and me) led us to believe the child's account. Within the complex set of relationships created among us, we all found the child believable. The stepfather, his lawyer, and perhaps the judge may try to disprove her. The standards for verification are very different for the two sets of knowers. As this example shows, believability is often tied to advocacy. Patients subject to abuses of power bring their stories of vulnerability to clinicians every day. Those stories become part of the relationship. Advocacy means arguing for the believability of those stories.

EMPATHY

The last set of distinctions I would like to make between the separated and connected ways of looking at the world centers on their different interpretations of the word *empathy*. When we practice connected knowing, we find ourselves caring about the person we are learning about; we take the other's experience into ourselves. As in the narrative, naturalistic, and hearing modes, we attempt to let the other in, to allow the other to speak to us, to listen actively to the one speaking. This contrasts with the stance of the rationalistic separate knower, for whom feeling is suspect and who would argue that if you care too much you cannot exercise rational judgment. Dissection and other visual modes of finding out about the world are examples of separate knowing, from which caring is best removed. For rational knowers, science and caring are two separate activities; they are often separated by gender as well (White, 1986).

Definitions of empathy—a form of human connectedness essential to clinical work—vary depending on whether separateness or connectedness is the primary underlying value. For instance, Kohut, who placed empathy at the center of the psychoanalytic process, could still say:

> [Empathy] is a value-neutral tool of observation which (a) can lead to correct or incorrect results, (b) can be used in the service of either compassionate, inimical, or dispassionate-neutral purposes, and (c) can be employed either rapidly and outside awareness or slowly and deliberately, with focused-conscious attention. We define it as "vicarious introspection" or, more simply, as one person's (attempt to) experience the inner life of another while simultaneously retaining the stance of objective observer. (1984, p. 175)

Kohut appears to be taking pains to assure the reader of the separateness involved in empathy, in the service of arguments about the scientific basis of psychoanalysis.

Another psychoanalyst, Roy Schafer, defines empathy as "the inner experience of sharing in and comprehending the momentary psychological state of another person. . . . The shared experience is based to a great extent on remembered, corresponding affective states of one's own" (1959, pp. 345, 347). To "share" the feelings of the other, the therapist looks inside himself or herself. The "shared experience" occurs in each person separately. Empathy is an *inner* experience of the clinician, not the joint creation of mutual participation. These definitions of empathy reveal two assumptions: first, that human beings are separate from each other, their thoughts and feelings disconnected from human relations. Second, objectivity should be privileged and feelings avoided and distrusted because they are incompatible with the conduct of medicine as a "rational" activity.[7] Thus, even in a discussion of the meaning of empathy, which most people take as paradigmatic of connectedness, the legacy of separateness exerts strong pulls. The assumption of human separateness underlies our grammar and vocabulary and shapes our ability to think about what it means to join with another.

In medical settings (remote from feminist interpretation), the meaning of empathy continues to be based on the assumption of human separateness. Even in the patient-centered method, the meaning of reciprocity is to put one's self in the other's place. The doctor attempts to elicit the patient's perspective, "to enter the patient's world, to see the illness through the patient's eyes" (Levenstein, McCracken, McWhinney, Stewart, & Brown, 1986, p. 26). However useful this maneuver may appear, separateness again underlies the corresponding view of empathy. Gilligan, wrestling with the same problem, noticed that, "despite the transit to the place of the other, the self oddly seems to stay constant" (1986, p. 240). The self does not change. When autonomy and detachment are the values that define a person, new knowledge refers back to the self, not to the relationship.

Despite the presumption of separateness in medical and psychiatric descriptions of empathy, the concept remains troublesome for separate knowers in medicine. Although empathy is considered essential to the caring clinical relationship, it is problematic because it implies feelings, and feelings are untrustworthy in the world of separate knowing. To avoid this contradiction, the separate knowers' construction of empathy relies heavily on technique. Medical definitions and descriptions of empathy focus on the cognitive aspects to the exclusion of feelings. Efforts to teach empathy reconstitute it as a "communicative behavior" that trainees can practice through the use of empathic statements. For example, Novack defines empathy as "sharing in another's emotions or feelings as if they are one's own" (1987, p. 351). This sounds as if empathy includes responsiveness to the patient's feelings, yet when he elaborates, it becomes clear that empathy in his mind is a cognitive task that is useful in strengthening the relationship and facilitating the patient's disclosures:

> Empathy involves accurately identifying a patient's feelings then communicating this to the patient: "I understand how difficult it is for you to be going through this illness"; "It sounds like your Mom's illness has been a real burden to you." Empathy also involves eliciting and responding to the meaning of the illness for the patient. (E.g., "I can understand your worries about this angina, especially since your brother died of a heart attack.") In addition to strengthening the bond between doctor and patient, expression of empathy can aid the diagnostic process. After experiencing physicians' empathy, patients are

often encouraged to reveal their most difficult problems. Communication of empathy is a skill that can be effectively learned. (p. 351)

Here empathy means identifying the feeling and reflecting it back to the patient, not joining the patient or transcending his or her separateness in any significant way. Empathetic statements become an observer's summation of what appears to be the other's condition, derived from a position of separateness. This kind of empathy requires no change or transformation in the clinician, who can "understand" in the sense of accurately identifying feelings yet is not required to make an affective response. Clinicians comfortable with separate knowing can learn to make qualified statements—such as "I can understand how that might make you feel"—that keep the patient's (and their own) feelings at a distance.

The strategy of identifying the patient's feeling and framing it into a statement may be a skill that can be "effectively learned." It conveys that the listener has been paying attention, and this in itself is important. However, the absence of any internal experience of the other's reality or of any sense of joining together calls into question the trustworthiness of the practitioner. Empathetic statements may induce the patient to confide intimate details, yet how can the patient know that the practitioner "really means it," that he or she is "not just saying that"? To "really mean it" requires that the practitioner join the patient's feelings.[8] The possible lack of genuineness attributable to a clinician who is "just saying that" raises the possibility that the version of empathy described by separate knowers could be used in the service of harm (Gardiner, 1987; Lang, 1994). Although most doctors are unlikely to use empathetic statements to harm patients, the use of empathy as a tool does not require that the doctor genuinely care for the patient. Some doctors may use such statements just to get through the visit; others may use them to take advantage of patients' vulnerability. These potential uses show that such statements are not empathy but a stand-in for empathy.

Declarations of empathy by the clinician toward the patient—"I know just how you feel"—are also potentially intrusive and coercive (Code, 1994). Because of the power difference between the parties, claiming to know how another feels "can readily expand into a claim that I will tell you how you feel, and *I* will be right, even though you might describe it differently, for your perceptions are ill-informed, and my greater expertise must override them. . . . In women's confrontations with authoritarian expertise, exchanges of this sort are common" (p. 84). Code's analysis reminds us that empathy itself must be put into context. A professional's failure to consider differences in power, class, race, and gender makes "putting oneself in another's position more an act of arrogance than of altruism" (p. 89).

The distortion of empathy as a purely cognitive tool is matched by the equally pernicious and distorted idea that it is purely a matter of feelings. Moreover, contrasts between thought and feeling shape up along gender lines. Empathy-as-feelings is devalued as part of women's allegedly "natural" caregiving. Empathy and the other skills women develop

> are judged valueless when they merely emanate from what women do; yet are promoted to the status of scientificity and professional attainment when men "discover" them. . . . As a female practice its knowledgeable, rational dimension disappears into the chaos of inchoate affectivity; as a male-defined professional accomplishment it is a peculiarly effective, nuanced mode of knowing. (Code, 1994, pp. 83–84)

This highly gendered approach to empathy as either cognitive (when some men do it) or emotional (when women do it) is destructive. It keeps the male knower cut off from his feelings, and it keeps women's knowing in the apparently less valid category of "feelings." To arrive at another view of empathy, one less dependent on stereotypes about thought and emotion, we need to consider empathy within connected knowing.

In self-in-relation theory, mutuality is central to the meaning of empathy, even when the relationship is asymmetrical, as in psychotherapy. Jordan moves away from Kohut's ideal of objectivity and pushes against the assumption of human separateness.

> When empathy and concern flow both ways, there is an intense affirmation of the self, and paradoxically, a transcendence of the self, a sense of the self as part of a larger relational unit. The interaction allows for a relaxation of the sense of separateness; the other's well-being becomes as important as one's own. This does not imply merging, which suggests a blurring or a loss of distinctness of self. (1991b, p. 82)

Jordan takes care to distinguish her definition of empathy from fusion, weak ego boundaries, and other characteristics often derogatorily applied to women's capacity for empathy.

For connected knowers, empathy requires a taking-inside of the feelings and world of the other. In contrast to masculinist descriptions of empathy as "projection into the other," within connected knowing empathy is a form of reception: "I receive the other into myself, and I see and feel with the other" (Noddings, 1984, p. 30). Noddings describes this process as a motivational shift: by putting oneself at the service of the other, one becomes *engrossed* in the other. This engrossment consists of both feeling and thinking. Receiving the other "without evaluation or assessment" comes first. Problem-solving comes later. "As we convert what we have received from the other into a problem, something to be solved, we move away from the other. We clean up his reality, strip it of complex and bothersome qualities, in order to think it. The other's reality becomes data, stuff to be analyzed, studied, interpreted" (p. 36).

Noddings enlists her rational powers "in the service of [her] engrossment in the other" (p. 36). She describes the connection between the abstract and the personal: "We keep our objective thinking tied to a relational stake at the heart of caring" (p. 36). Such a blend of thinking and feeling, of objectivity and subjectivity, is no mean feat. The self-in-relation theorists hold that the practice of empathy requires not only a balance of thought and feeling but a well-differentiated sense of self, flexible ego boundaries, and appreciation of how one is both the same as and different from the other person (Jordan, 1991b). Empathy involves a movement back and forth, a sense of being separate as well being in-relation. Because empathy involves momentary changes in self-boundaries, it allows the possibility for change, and thus empathy "always contains the opportunity for mutual growth and impact" (Jordan, 1991b, p. 82).

What is provocative about the connected knower's definition of empathy is how its practice creates a transformation in the knower. Noddings talks about "allowing ourselves to be transformed" (1984, p. 34). For example, my personal discomfort with the physical enormity of a 25-year-old man who weighed 355 pounds prevented me from hearing how much he hated himself and his life. When I was able to let myself imagine what it must have been like for him to grow up as the oldest son of two depressed parents who each felt sicker than the other, when I could let myself feel how profoundly uncared for he had felt, when I could sense how trapped he felt between his parents, his in-laws, his marriage, and his church, I could finally get beyond my prejudices to allow his pain in. Indeed, being vulnerable to such a transformation may be a prerequisite to empathy (Brody, 1992a). Not only does the person cared for feel heard and received, the one caring is changed. We might say, then, that a the separate knower's view of empathy tells us how to take another's point of view temporarily by sitting in his or her seat; a relational view of empathy tells us how to move our own seat next to the other's, or how to negotiate the arrangement of our chairs.[9] A relational understanding of empathy requires that persons change in response to each other; they cannot remain unaffected by their encounter. The transformation of the knower through empathy is unique to connected knowing and utterly foreign to empathy viewed from the standpoint of rational or separate knowing.[10]

These four ways of thinking about patients—context, life history perspective, believability, and empathy—are strong strands in the fabric of connected knowing. Deliberately adopting these approaches will result in connected knowing in the care of patients. To foster the adoption of these ways of thinking, I will flesh out two of them in detail: using life history work with patients, and taking a clinical approach grounded in one particular element of context—the family.

LIFE HISTORY WORK

Nowadays most clinicians—be they doctors, nurse-practitioners, or social workers—do not have the advantage of extended practice over long periods in one setting. They rarely get to know patients for more than a few years. The geographic mobility of both patients and clinicians, as well as changes in insurance coverage, guarantee disconnected care over time.[11] Most life histories are therefore collected by clinicians who have not been a part of patients' lives for very long.

From a literary point of view, patients' stories and clinicians' translations of those stories can be viewed as a form of narrative (Hunter, 1991). The idea that the patient's story constitutes a narrative is gradually gaining credence in medical circles, and physicians are coming to recognize that the telling and hearing of those stories lends a depth and humanity to medicine unavailable in routine clinical work (Brody, 1988; Kleinman, 1988; Shapiro, 1993). Analysis of the stories of elderly patients with hip fractures reveals that their recovery is directly related to their perceived role as actors in their own narratives (Borkan, Quirk, & Sullivan, 1991). For a variety of reasons, however, including time constraints, clinicians do not routinely consider the usefulness of patients' narratives or life histories in clinical work. Yet narratives are a unique and potent force in the service of connected knowing in patient care.

What I mean by a life history is a narrative of events from the patient's experience, not a commentary on intrapsychic events. The questions to be asked are factual and nonthreatening. I begin with "Where were you born?" followed by questions about how the patient's mother and father met, migration from other places, birth order of siblings, and so on. I construct a genogram as a connected project. For many people, movement from place to place is an important way of organizing events and should be chronicled. If necessary, the life history can be "collected" over several visits. Especially with patients who have long-term problems and see doctors frequently, the usefulness of the life history overrides objections that it is too time-consuming.

Eliciting a life history from a patient serves several purposes. It offers a wealth of information that credits the patient with a breadth of experience not usually included in the medical history. It can uncover a variety of complex and difficult life experiences the patient may no longer consider important, and thus it can serve as a bridge for the clinician to the powerful events that have shaped the patient's life. It is more than technique: learning about a person's past sets the stage for a personal, as opposed to a professional, relationship. The clinician's interest in the life history is a clear expression of his or her interest in the patient as a person, not as a "case." The very process of telling the story to a concerned listener creates an engagement that can energize the relationship. The patient may perceive the telling of the life history as a particularly meaningful moment in his or her medical career and may form a more immediate and lasting attachment with the inquiring clinician.

For clinicians, the life history is useful with chronically ill patients, patients who have many symptoms that never improve, patients with no diagnosable disease, and patients with chronic mental illness—in short, those patients with whom clinicians have difficulty forming or enjoying relationships. When trainees (like Dr. Y. described earlier) complain about not being able to get attached to or like a given patient, I recommend that they spend several office visits collecting a life history from the patient, a process that usually solves the problem. In the example of Dr. Y., the tactic of eliciting the life history during office visits did not succeed. Perhaps the reason Dr. Y. had found the relationship so tedious lay in the patient's self-assessed difficulty in expressing herself "in person." What doctor, however experienced, could have known that this patient would be so much better able to express herself in writing than in speech? Reading the patient's story in a letter (rather than hearing it) completed Dr. Y.'s act of asking for the life history. The effect was the same: the relationship was transformed by connected knowing.

The life history is the historical equivalent of the home visit. All clinicians recognize that seeing patients in their homes adds immeasurably to our understanding of who they are. Like the home visit, the life history is a dramatic way to change the doctor's view of the patient. In the life history, the patient provides us with a brief tour of his or her past, just as we might be shown around the house. We make internal observations as we proceed from place to place, noting interesting items out of the corner of our eye, saving it all up for later consideration. We might conclude with the parakeet, or the photos on the mantle, or the stairs to climb. Just as the home visit ineluctably changes the relationship, the construction of the life history also has irreversible effects on the relationship. Like Dr. Y., the doctor who receives, hears, and collects life history information can never be discarded as just another doctor, and the patient who is known to have lived certain experiences can never again be viewed only as the person with, say, a somatoform disorder.

FAMILY AS CONTEXT

One application of contextual thinking in medical practice is "the family approach at each moment." By "family" I mean the personal context important to the patient.[12] By "at each moment" I mean to direct attention to the constantly changing configurations of intimacy and power. I do not intend to sanctify the nuclear family or heterosexual unions; the patient's understanding of family, not mine, is what is important in this approach. Although family is one—and only one—context in which human beings live their lives, I choose to focus on the family context because of its crucial role as a setting in which health and illness are played out. I could also choose the overlapping contexts of gender, race, and work, and indeed, these inform the family context. Since patients share clinicians' recognition that family is a primary context, and are not likely to be surprised or offended by questions about family, I have chosen to focus on the family as one important area for contextual thinking in medicine.

I will put forward an approach to the whole family "at each moment" in three areas—the office practice of well-child care, episodic care, and care for pregnant adolescents. I have chosen these areas because they are common clinical experiences; nurses, social workers, pediatricians, and a variety of other clinicians engage with patients in these areas in similar exchanges. These descriptions draw on my personal experience and depend to some extent on my preferred style of talking with people. However, this approach is more than just a matter of style: it is a consistent attempt to situate any given interaction within the larger context of family.

THE WELL-CHILD VISIT

Despite clinicians' best efforts to involve fathers in prenatal care, labor and delivery, and well-child care, mothers continue to shoulder the vast responsibility for child care, including the task of bringing children to the doctor for routine visits. (One benefit of widespread unemployment is that fathers are often available to make daytime office visits.) Grandmothers occasionally accompany their daughters to an office visit in late pregnancy or in the postpartum period, but later on they play a more invisible role. Yet all of the family members are active in the intergenerational challenge of raising a new baby.

Many times I have asked a young mother what she was feeding her two-month-old only to learn that she was overfeeding the baby with cereals, fruits, vegetables, and meats, as well as juice or formula. However noncritically I attempt to educate her about the proper nutritional balance for an infant of this age, my lecture goes unheeded. I will always be indebted to my colleague who pointed this out to me when we were residents. Cryptically he quipped, "You can't fight Grandma."

He knew from his family that what young mothers feed their babies has more to do with what family members advise than with any recommendations doctors offer.

Moreover, if we tell the young mother to hold off on feeding the child meat, and this is the advice her mother-in-law has been giving her, we have suddenly lined up against the mother herself in the family battleground. If we know what various parties have been advocating before throwing in our advice, at least we know what we are doing. My more general inquiry into infant feeding now includes questions like: "What does your mother say about feeding the baby? Your mother-in-law? What did your sister do? What do you think is right? What do you think I am going to say? How are you going to decide?"[13] In the example above, a successful strategy might be:

> Well, different people in your family have a piece of the truth. You are right to want to offer your baby a balanced diet. Your mother-in-law is right that we usually wait until six months to start meats. Different generations of mothers learn different ways to feed their babies. Even different generations of doctors have said different things. Given what all the people in your family think, how could we work out a plan for the next two months that will keep everyone happy?

This approach lets the mother know that I am aware that she may feel caught between family members in her effort to learn to feed her child. At the same time, I am acknowledging that all infant care, especially food, is a family affair. In this way, the well-baby visit becomes an exploration of the family system, not just an infant checkup. I am using a contextual way of thinking to situate her and her baby in the world.

When both parents come for well-baby visits, the doctor gets the chance to observe the father's involvement with the child. This chance to communicate directly with the father offsets the doctor's tendency to make an alliance with the mother against him and other family members simply because the doctor sees the mother most frequently. When the father does not or cannot attend, the doctor can still ask, "What are the baby's father's concerns right now?" or, "Is there anything about the baby your partner/boyfriend/husband is worrying about at this point?" Should these questions turn up important concerns, the doctor can ask the mother to have him call or stop in after the visit, rather than using her as a messenger. (These same questions can be asked if the mother is parenting as part of a lesbian couple or together with her mother or grandmother.)

When the father or other parental figure does come in for well-child visits, it is important to ask him directly if he has any concerns of his own about the baby. When young parents come in together, I sometimes also ask, "Do you ever argue about how to raise the baby?" After the giggling and sheepishness are over, some important, previously unvoiced questions usually come out. This approach of taking each family member seriously, whether present or absent, conveys respect for each of them and a recognition that despite their family bond, each still experiences conflictual demands and obligations. It also shows that differences are to be expected and can be recognized and negotiated, not ignored or ablated. This understanding about individuals in families may appear basic but nevertheless is rarely conveyed as part of well-child care.

Sexual abuse prevention is another aspect of well-child care that requires a family perspective. The family is the most common location where children (especially girls) experience sexual abuse; it is also the most likely place where the abuse will be disclosed. Family members often know whether anyone in the family has a reputation for molesting children. Often these awarenesses are not openly discussed. I do not expect children to divulge to me, a relatively distant adult authority, in a routine exam, a past experience of sexual abuse, even though I often ask. Far more helpful is the preparation of the child and the family for its possibility.

When children are between three and five, I begin a discussion of this topic by asking the parent, usually the mother, "What have you told your child about sexual abuse prevention?" Responses range from "I told her never to let anyone touch her down there" to "They had a program on that at school." I ask the child what he or she would do if anyone ever tried to do that, and I try to help them work their way to a "Say no and try to get away" answer. I ask them who they could tell. Most children answer, "My mother." I then ask the mother whether she would believe them. It is important to support the mother for believing the child and for not responding with either anger or punishment. I remind her that if the child expects to be punished, he or she will not be able to confide in her.

At this point, I often interject a quick question for the parent: "Did anything like that ever happen to you?" In a yes-no form, this question lets me know whether the parent may have complicated reactions to the discussion and to the possibility of a disclosure by the child. The question is also limited enough that its import is not usually apparent to the child. If the mother says yes, I ask if she would like to talk about it later. Some mothers start talking right then and there. If this happens, I try to focus on the issue of disclosure—whether she did, and if so, what happened. I then tie her experience with disclosure to her child's ability to disclose any similar experiences. I turn back to the child to ask, "If your mother wasn't around, or didn't believe you, who could you tell?" Usually he or she mentions one or two other adults. I remind both mother and child that the people who touch children are usually not strangers and stress the importance of disclosure even if the person is someone in the family.

If there is a boyfriend or stepfather in the family, I ask the mother whether she feels comfortable leaving the child with him and whether she thinks there is any risk. If possible, I try to verify at another time her comfort with her partner. I remind mothers that as their children (particularly girls) get older, they are particularly at risk from nonbiological father figures in the home. (This is not to minimize the significance of father-daughter incest, only to recognize the higher likelihood of molestation by other males in the home.) If the mother has a history of childhood sexual abuse, I try to determine whether the perpetrator is still in the family and whether the child ever spends any time in a household where he or she might be exposed to this person. Frequently I have found that the grandfather, uncle, or older brother who abused a woman or her sisters is someone she still must see at family events. Supporting her ability to protect her children from a known perpetrator is part of my role in strengthening her mothering.

This may seem like a digression from the subject of well-child care, but sexual abuse occurs with far greater frequency than most medical conditions for which doctors routinely screen in the well-child exam. Thinking about the family as context acknowledges that it is often the context of child sexual abuse. In the setting of prevention, asking mothers about their own experience helps them make a connection between their recollection of childhood vulnerability and their child's current vulnerability. More often than not, I have found this discussion helpful in understanding the mother's childhood experiences in her family of origin in a way not usually open to me during her own health care visits. Any way that I can help equip a mother (or any nonabusive parent) to protect her children from abuse (and to respond supportively to them if it happens) has a stronger chance than any other intervention of reducing the vulnerability of her children to further victimization.

Episodic Care

The episodic visit is even less likely than well-child care to be situated within the world of the family. In acute illness, the medical model reigns unchallenged; stripped away are issues of context and life history. Empathy and believability do not appear relevant to the critical matter at hand. It is only after multiple visits for the same unremitting but undiagnosable symptom that the possibility of "something going on in the family" is raised. When an illness provokes episodic visits, neither the family nor the doctor puts the family context squarely in the center of the transaction. Yet this is precisely the time when the clinical method should be informed by a sensitivity to the family context. Critics might retort, "But what about the simple sore throat?" Of course, as Freud is reputed to have said, "Sometimes a cigar is just a cigar." But more important, in work with families, when is a cigar not a cigar? Or when is a "simple sore throat" the inconspicuous entryway into the labyrinth of the family system?

In our practice with mixed-income multigenerational families, when a mother brings in a child with a sore throat, she may have multiple agendas. I hear the history, examine the child, do a throat culture, agree on treatment, and do patient education. I often ask the mother what she thought the sore throat was and what she expected of me. I may learn that she was worried about strep or recent exposure to scarlet fever. I may be able to place the meaning of symptoms in the context of the whole person. But I may also find out that the mother brought the child in because if she had not and the child got sicker, she would have faced criticism from her mother or sister or mother-in-law for not acting sooner—for not being a "good mother." Or if her husband were to come home from work and find the child still sick, he might have become impatient and angry and insisted on taking the child to the emergency room, with the resultant delays and frustrations. So the mother may bring in the child with the sore throat to fend off the pressures of her family. This agenda is rarely, if ever, articulated by patients without prodding by a trusted clinician.

Yet the clinician can elicit this agenda simply and nonthreateningly by asking, "What do other people in your family say about this or want done about this?" Once we acknowledge the multiple influences on decisions about going to the doctor, we can begin to untangle the reasons behind any given episodic visit. Parents—or mothers and grandmothers, as another example—have talked to each other before heading for the emergency room. In our culture as well as others, patients "consult" a variety of resources before entering the medical care system (Kleinman, 1980; Zola, 1972). The process of informal consultation and the decision itself to go to the doctor reflect certain family dynamics that the physician could recognize but more often does not.

Take the example of a child with a fever. What to do? The young mother calls her mother, who tells her to give the child baby aspirin. The child remains fussy and febrile. The father tells the mother to call the doctor, who meets them in the emergency room. There the doctor diagnoses an ear infection, gives an antibiotic, and switches the child to acetaminophen. The father concludes that the grandmother was wrong and feels vindicated in having insisted that the mother call the doctor. The mother feels uncomfortable with the wedge that has been further driven between her spouse and her mother, as well as stuck in the middle. Later, mother and father fight over issues tangentially related to the grandmother.

Alternatively, the doctor asks the couple in the emergency room, "What have you tried so far?" The mother replies, "My mother told me to give baby aspirin." The doctor could say, "You were right to try to control the fever. You did as best as you could with what you had at home. You have managed this as well as you could up to now. I would prefer acetaminophen over aspirin in this kind of an infection. Will you be able to get some on your way home?" The result is that existing tensions in the family are not exacerbated and may be lessened by contact with the doctor.

Because episodic care is often an example of stranger medicine—doctor and patient are strangers to each other—a deliberate effort to develop connected knowing in this setting may be even more important than a visit when doctor and patient know each other well. With no previous shared experience to help situate the patient or child within a family context, the doctor providing acute care has few cues to situate his or her assessment of the problem or its treatment. Sensitivity to the family context, as I have described it here, requires no more time but rather a different focus to the doctor's questioning and a different way of thinking about patient responses—in other words, trying to "think family" (Sluzki, 1974). It calls for an openness to the stories that precede our moments with a patient, an awareness of the complexity of context, a historical sense of the patient in the course of family time, and a readiness to be empathetic toward the person in front of us. It is a different kind of knowing from the usual approach to episodic care.

ADOLESCENT PREGNANCY

Clinical work with teenagers presents a special challenge and offers unique rewards to the clinicians who work with them. Despite admonitions about how important it is to be nonjudgmental with teenagers, the responses of individual physicians to individual adolescents are still likely to be determined by the personalities involved. During a visit with a given adolescent, a practitioner often finds it difficult to set aside personal feelings about smoking, drinking, drug use, unprotected intercourse, and running away from home. Doctors may preach acceptance and limit-setting to parents but can be just as likely as parents to be critical, judgmental, and rejecting. Pregnant adolescents represent a particularly difficult but rewarding challenge because of the unique setting of teen pregnancy at the intergenerational crossroads.

What I mean by "intergenerational crossroads" is that the adolescent pregnancy is the time when the new generation is formed: the child becomes the parent, and the parent the grandparent. However bitter and recriminating, or loving and accepting, or infantilizing and fantasy-ridden this process may be, the intergenerational meaning is inevitable. Interactions with any individual in the family have immediate reverberations throughout the family. Praise or criticism, recommendations or admonishments, any statement open to interpretation, all will be subject to intense scrutiny by family members as a measure of judgment about them. The family system is in so much flux that each moment is highly charged with family meanings. Clinicians choosing to work with pregnant adolescents and their families must carefully pick their way across an obstacle course strewn with boulders of stubbornness and potholes of family legacy. Each pathway is unique; caring for a pregnant thirteen-year-old requires the creation of a set of alliances different from those accompanying the care of a pregnant seventeen-year-old.

With a thirteen-year-old, the physician must first work through for himself or herself the girl's and the family's choice about keeping the pregnancy or terminating it. If the clinician is seen as championing an option that the family cannot tolerate, the family will be forced to go elsewhere. This is equally true of the choice to abort as it is of the choice to keep the pregnancy. (Later the same is true about the choice to release a baby for adoption or keep the child.) When a thirteen-year-old chooses, within the context of her family, to keep a pregnancy, the doctor's relationship to the girl and to the family is crucial. Given the needs of a girl this age for schooling, peer relationships, and physical and social maturation, the project of caring for her during pregnancy involves building an alliance with the adults in her family, who, in reality, will be caring for the infant a significant amount of the time. (A realistic assessment of the girl's experience of physical and sexual abuse within the family is also essential. Not all the adults in her family may be trustworthy.) The reliable adults must be engaged in the task of permitting the girl to grow up even as she carries out a task they (and the doctor) associate with adulthood. The doctor's relationship with these adults, be they parents, aunts, or grandparents, is therefore central, as is the steady consistency of his or her relationship with the girl herself. Nevertheless, the girl's relationships with teachers, social workers, and peers are usually more important than her relationship with the doctor; doctors need to know how to depend on these support networks to get education and assistance to the young teen. In other words, doctors need to develop an appropriately limited view of their own role.

Different ages offer different challenges. The care of the pregnant seventeen-year-old, for instance, requires on appreciation of her growing self-reliance. She may demand to be seen as an individual on her own terms, with the right to make relationships and choose her own course in life separate from the wishes of her family. Her pregnancy itself may reflect her wish to plot her own course. When there is overt conflict between the young woman and her family, the clinician must convey his or her respect for the adolescent and allegiance to her growing abilities to make her own decisions. At the same time, clinicians may have to translate this process for parents who are deeply angry and rejecting toward their daughter. Some adolescents may need to see a different doctor from their family doctor, as a gesture of independence from their family of origin. The new doctor must still situate the young woman's actions within the context of her family. Other pregnant teens may continue seeing the same doctor, actively choosing the consistency of a known parental figure at a time when relationships with their parents are tumultuous.

Not only is caring for the child who is becoming a parent one of the most challenging tasks in clinical work, it also exemplifies what is crucial about the approach to the whole family at each moment. The practitioner who lines up on one side in a struggle between one generation and the next, or on behalf of one individual against another, is taking a risk. Such an alliance may result in the breaking off of some relationships; some family members, as well as the clinician, may be expelled. The rapidly shifting sands of adolescent pregnancy may leave the teenager and parent reconciled by the time of delivery and the clinician stranded on a sandbar. Clinicians need to assess whether such a risk is warranted.

One moment when the clinician must take a clear stand is when it is discovered that the teenager has been the target of physical or sexual abuse in the family. This finding compels the clinician to strengthen his or her alliance with the adolescent in an effort to protect her and possibly her siblings' safety. Depending on the identity of the perpetrator and on how separated the teenager is from her family of origin, a move to protect the teenager almost inevitably results in the immediate exclusion of the doctor from any further dealings with the parents. Even though the teenager may later reconcile with her parents, this avenue will not be open to the doctor who takes a stand about abuse. Nevertheless, when a teenager has been abused, it is more important to act swiftly and unambiguously on her behalf than to attempt to "keep open the lines of communication" with her parents. The abused teenager needs to see and hear clearly from responsible adults that abuse is totally unacceptable. In abuse cases, actions speak louder than words. More often than not, pregnant teenagers do *not* initially disclose a prior history of sexual abuse, even when it has happened. However, the practitioner's stance (that such abuse is not acceptable and not her fault) enables the teenager to disclose at a later time when she feels safer.

Success in clinical work with pregnant teenagers can be measured by the satisfactory evolution of the young woman into motherhood, her ability to develop an adult-to-adult relationship with the baby's father or other partner, her parents' growth into their identity as grandparents, and the entire family's ability to accept the infant as a new person in the family, with a status of his or her own. While the early part of this process may be marked by rejection and conflict, the later stages are frequently characterized by reconciliation of the young woman with her mother or both parents, reacceptance in the parental home, and support in the labor, delivery, and postpartum experience. The following example shows how each generation's satisfactory passage through the transitions resulted in a new, less symptomatic family equilibrium.

Elba, the oldest daughter in a Puerto Rican family headed by a single mother, became pregnant at seventeen. Her mother, Maria, was widely regarded in the extended family as incompetent because of a seizure disorder. The oldest of many cousins, Elba had been a mother figure in the whole family. She was now gaining her full adult status by starting a family of her own. Maria's episodes of *ataques* became more severe (Guarnaccia et al., 1990). The doctor somewhat helplessly watched as the grandmother-to-be worsened at the same time that the mother-to-be was demonstrating her competence by coming to all her prenatal appointments, learning about pregnancy, delivery, and baby care in the teen pregnancy program, and in general becoming a model teen mother. At the time of delivery, Elba chose to be accompanied by Maria in the delivery room rather than by the baby's father. After the baby was delivered, the doctor handed Maria the scissors to cut the cord as part of the customary natural childbirth routine. She accomplished the task and gladly greeted the arrival of her first grandson. Later on, Maria boasted of her new competence as a person who knew about babies because of her important role at the birth. She became active in the care of her grandson while Elba finished school. In the first few years of her marriage, Elba was able to return home for support when the young father became abusive. As the marriage stabilized and both grandmothers supported Elba's ultimatum about no physical abuse, Elba was able to aid her mother financially. Office visits for Maria lessened remarkably, as did her complaints about seizures and nerves.

In the years following a teen pregnancy, the new mother usually achieves the status of adulthood in the eyes of the family. Families themselves usually stretch and shift to incorporate the daughter, and perhaps her partner, as adults and to accept her baby as the next generation. In Elba's case, taking the family approach meant thinking in terms of the extended family as well as following Elba's lead in choosing her birth support. Including Maria in the birth process facilitated her transition to her new role as a grandmother and perhaps contributed to the improvement in her health and self-esteem.

PUTTING THE KNOWER IN THE CONTEXT

I have told the story of Elba and her family from the point of view of a neutral observer. This stance does not include my position as a knower. Over the years I have taken care of Elba, her children, her mother, her two younger sisters and brother, her brother's wife, and seven of her nieces and nephews. From literally hundreds of encounters I have gained a sense of how their extended family works, and they have a comparable sense of how I work as a doctor and what they can expect from me. I am a familiar part of their health care—a known person in their lives, their childbearing, and their episodes of sickness. The relation of the knower to the known is a crucial element of context: there are many nuances to the multifaceted relationship I have with this family, and my position as their doctor for almost two decades bears on what I can know about them, and what they can know about me.

As a connected knower, I know that any action I take as a clinician plays an implicit role inside the family. For this reason, it is crucial that I be explicit about the values underlying my actions. The power relations surrounding my work dictate that my actions may be influential in ways unknown to me. Doctors are variously aware of this fact; therapists are more so: "Any kind of therapy is a way of intervening into a family. Whether one works with an individual or with multiple members of a family, from the family therapy point of view the reality of mutual interdependence still remains. The remaining question is whether one works directly with the family in an implicit or explicit manner" (Ransom & Grace, 1979).

Traditionally, physicians, even family physicians, have worked primarily with individuals. The recognition has been slow in coming that each step or action they take conveys an implicit stance toward the family. The possibility that doctors' involvement with individuals may contribute to family distress and perpetuate family problems has been rarely considered. But doctors are not neutral or uninvolved at the family level; they take an active, albeit unknowing role in families through their primary work with symptom bearers. Because the organization of medical work is predominantly with symptom bearers, and with mothers as the primary caretakers of children, the actions of doctors tend to perpetuate existing family dynamics around illness and promote "careers of illness" (Stephens, 1986). Said in another way more typical of family therapy, a clinician may get "locked into binding coalitions" (Penn, 1983) by virtue of the individual approach toward the symptomatic family member who makes extensive use of the medical care system.

The fact that women go to the doctor more frequently for themselves and their children has the practical result that the doctor has far more contact with mothers in young families and with women more than with men. The tendency for women to view themselves as defective (Greenspan, 1983) and to take the blame for their children's ills may also predispose them to become the identified patients. In the care of children, the doctor typically tells the mother what is going on and what needs to be done and expects her to act on this information and perhaps relay it to the father. As a result, the father is excluded from the communication and may perceive the mother and the doctor in alliance with each other, sometimes against him. Through ordinary work, the clinician's actions may unintentionally contribute to a depiction of the mother as weak, defective, and overly involved with a sick child, and the father as distant and excluded. This characteristic portrayal appears in rigidified form repeatedly in the case histories of psychosomatic families that abound in the family therapy literature. Unless medical clinicians look at how their work with individuals plays into ongoing dynamics in the family, they may perpetuate symptoms they are attempting to alleviate. In other words, everyday work with patients assumes and promotes certain family constellations that may create symptoms in the first place.

Physicians must be particularly aware of alliances created by their gender. When a mother complains to the doctor about fatigue, anxiety, depression, and physical symptoms, the sympathetic doctor, recognizing the reality of her stressful situation in the family, enters into an alliance with her. The effect of this alliance may be problematic for both men and women doctors, but in different ways. Here the gender of the knower (the clinician) is part of the context of clinical work. The woman doctor, sensitive to what she sees as a woman's issues, may underline the portrayal of the man in the family as unfeeling, uncommunicative, and distant. The women thus line up against the man, who is further distanced from the important communications within the family by the doctor visit. Understandably, he may later find it difficult to trust the woman doctor, whom he sees as his wife's ally against him. This alliance is especially tricky for clinicians who recognize the oppression of their women patients but may not recognize the divisive effect their stance might have on their patients' families. If a woman patient asks for support in remaining in an unbalanced, oppressive relationship, the doctor's own values make her ambivalent about providing such support. If the woman clinician takes a position against the man or against the relationship and the woman then chooses to stay with him, the clinician may in effect force the woman to choose between her relationship and her doctor.[14]

The position of the caring male physician is no less complicated. It is not uncommon for a woman patient to tell her troubles to and get support from a male physician, who, perhaps in contrast to her husband or boyfriend, is warm, sympathetic, and understanding. The doctor may unintentionally begin to personify the ideal husband or father in the eyes of the woman patient. Despite the absence of any sexual intimations, this cross-gender relationship has the effect of excluding the woman's partner from the doctor-patient relationship, which the partner may view, at best, as the province of the woman and their children and, at worst, as a sexually threatening liaison. Jealous and violent men may accuse the woman of sexual involvement with the doctor and may even threaten the doctor himself. Even in less highly charged situations, the male partner may find it difficult to engage with the idealized male physician.

When abuse is not an issue, clinicians must examine the customary stance of working primarily with women and try to engage the usually excluded man in a way that is respectful of his concerns. One way to do this is to ask him to call the doctor after a given visit to elicit his concerns and to give him directly whatever medical information was conveyed. In a phone call to a family, both parents can be asked to get on the line, or each can be spoken with in turn. An active effort to include the father can work against the tendency to view mothers as primarily responsible for the family's health and sickness. Such an effort serves the woman's well-being by recognizing that children are a shared responsibility rather than hers alone.

Nevertheless, women's position of vulnerability in families requires constant vigilance from clinicians. Every clinical act is played out in the theater of the family, where power inequities may be a particularly dangerous backdrop for women. A clinician's act may support a woman's confidence and enhance her strength, or it may narrow her options and contribute to her vulnerability. Although the position of sole responsibility for children is often a crucial feature of women's oppression in the family unit, a doctor's attempts to distribute some responsibility to the man without assessing the potential for abuse may create trouble. Bringing the father into communications about the children's health may imply to the mother (and father) that the mother is failing at her "job." In an abusive relationship, an apparently simple request can become a focus for further criticism and abuse from the man. Both male and female physicians must therefore examine the potential for abuse in every clinical situation.

I am not advocating clinical neutrality; rather, I am advocating for an alliance with the woman's empowerment. Mindful of the potential for abuse, the doctor needs to clarify for himself or herself, and for the patient, certain issues: in what way is she being strong, taking charge, making decisions, acting on behalf of her children, garnering support, and being supportive to other people? Using the answers to such questions, the practitioner can support the woman's relational skills, including her mothering, her connections with her family and friends, and her contribution to the doctor-patient relationship. By listing her competencies, the clinician can buttress the woman's strength.

Another way family physicians become implicitly involved in coalitions in families is on behalf of the overtly more powerful forces. Doctors frequently react to the squeakiest wheel. For example, an alcoholic single mother, sober for the previous eighteen months, sent her fourteen-year-old daughter by herself to see the doctor for a problem of two months' duration. The doctor arranged some tests and talked with the girl. With her permission, the doctor called the mother, while the daughter listened, and reviewed the plan. Three days later the tests were not yet back. The grandmother called the doctor to say that the girl was at her house and that she was vomiting and in pain. The doctor decided that hospitalization was required at this point and told the grandmother and the girl on the phone. Then the doctor called the mother and informed her of the new decision. She acquiesced. Behind the scenes, the grandmother called the mother and admonished, "You see, I told you, you haven't been taking care of her properly. If I hadn't called the doctor, she'd still be sick and in pain." The result: the doctor's intervention served to undermine the mother's struggle against her alcoholism and seemingly endorsed the grandmother's view of the mother's incompetence.

In family systems language, the mother was "triangulated" by the coalition between her mother and her daughter, now joined by the powerful force of the doctor. In medical terms, this teenager was strongly suspected to be suffering from inflammatory bowel disease that had rapidly deteriorated before diagnosis and management could be accomplished on an outpatient basis. Only by paying attention to the entire family at the moment of deciding to hospitalize the daughter could the doctor have avoided the unfortunate appearance of making an alliance with the grandmother. Combating the tendency to respond first and primarily to the person who appears to be in charge requires an actively watchful stance on the part of the doctor.

In families with seriously ill or chronically ill children, every effort must be made to say everything to both parents and to elicit opinions from each family member rather than dealing with one, usually the mother, as the main link to the family. Otherwise, doctors tend to increase the likelihood that the mother will become mired in the care and responsibility for the sick child; by doing so, they unknowingly remove the father further from the child, despite the probability that he is just as worried as the mother about the child. Doctors, through their work with mothers, symptom bearers, and identified patients, can actively sustain an unhealthy dynamic. Keeping the entire family in mind at the moment of any clinical action is an example of contextual knowing. Work that proceeds from connected knowing can avert some of the suffering human beings experience as members of families.

For many practitioners—usually women, but men as well—connected knowing is a basic way of looking at the world. Family medicine makes some particularly strong claims on connected knowing as uniquely characteristic of the field (Carmichael, 1976; Stephens, 1982). Yet separate knowing appears to be an inevitable requirement of the world of science in which we live and work. Connected knowers feel obligated to prove themselves scientific. For instance, one family practitioner titled his complaint "Desperately Seeking Science" (Goldstein, 1990). This conflict raises the question: how can clinicians steadfastly maintain the practice of connected knowing while working in the scientifically dominated world of medicine?[15]

The effects of applying separate knowing to medicine are clear: instrumentation, specialization, and depersonalization. Connected knowing is usually practiced because a particular clinician is personally inclined to, not because medical practice or institutions foster such a viewpoint. Connected knowing requires that we question the assumptions and frames of knowledge of our practice and our institutions. In clinical work, we can use approaches informed by connected knowing to situate the events in patients' lives in both a historical and family context.

In the Belenky et al. (1986) study, women moved beyond the dichotomy between separate and connected knowing by integrating what the authors called "constructed knowledge." These learners were able to integrate what they came to understand intuitively and through their own experience with what they were able to learn from others. Using self-knowledge, a constructed knower uses himself or herself as "an instrument of understanding" (p. 122). What does it mean to be an instrument of understanding in clinical work? For me, constructed knowledge means I can unify various aspects of myself—doctor, mother, daughter, lover, thinker, activist—in my work. Constructed knowledge of clinical work allows us to recognize, attend to, and respect our contribution as persons to our work with patients, to accept and value ourselves as active instruments of knowing and healing. The next chapter examines the clinician's decision to contribute personal information to the relationship with the patient. In this exploration, we discover how clinicians committed to constructing mutual knowledge bring their own experience to long-term relations with patients.

CHAPTER 8

Doctors-in-Relation

CONNECTED KNOWING in clinical work requires that the clinician engage fully, as a person, with patients. What do I mean by "engage fully, as a person"? One form of this engagement is the recognition of mutuality between clinician and patient, of the personal contribution each makes to the relationship.[1] Connected knowing allows us to consider how doctors might act as "beings-in-relation." It offers us a way to think about practitioners' efforts to heighten mutuality and sheds new light on why doctors might tell something about themselves to patients. Telling the patient about oneself is a special case of being-in-relation. Perhaps for this reason psychotherapists and feminists have paid particular attention to the implications of self-disclosure.

"Self-disclosure" is the term commonly used to describe the act of talking about oneself with another.[2] Early understandings of the role of disclosure in relationships came from the field of experimental psychology (Chelune, 1977, 1979). Sidney Jourard (1968, 1971), the existential psychologist who initiated the study of disclosure, saw self-disclosure as both a sign of a healthy personality and a way of becoming a fully functioning individual. Subsequent investigators (Cozby, 1973; Davidson & Duberman, 1982; Lavine & Lombardo, 1984; Sollie & Fischer, 1985; Taylor & Hinds, 1985) focused on all facets of the question, Who divulges what kind of information to whom under what conditions? Under experimental conditions, researchers investigated such variables as the effect of positive and negative disclosures of high and low intimacy by persons of high and low status (Brooks, 1974; Chaikin & Derlega, 1974; Hoffman-Graff, 1977) and the possible relevance of the level of disclosure to one's suitability as a counselor (Lombardo, Franco, Wolf, & Fantasia, 1976). Jourard's discovery of the "dyadic effect" or "disclosure reciprocity" has remained a solid finding: a person is likely to disclose in a setting of disclosure by another person and at the same level of intimacy.

Experimental work suggests that women are more likely than men to self-disclose (Cozby, 1973) and more likely to feel better afterward (Mark & Alper, 1985). Social and cultural expectations may enable women to be more self-revealing, especially with other women. Assumptions about gender on the part of both patient and clinician may affect what each tells the other about herself or himself. Just as women patients may find it easier to be open with women clinicians, women practitioners also find themselves self-disclosing to women patients in areas of shared life experience, such as childbearing (Candib et al., 1987; Fenster, Phillips, & Rapoport, 1986).[3]

SELF-DISCLOSURE IN PSYCHOTHERAPY

Modern psychotherapies originated in the Freudian tradition of psychoanalysis, which was predicated on the assumption of the therapist's neutrality. Freud saw psychoanalysis as the scientific study of the patient's psyche played out in the form of the transference. The analyst was required to be as much of a blank slate as possible in order not to contaminate the process with the analyst's own material. This material, the countertransference, was thought to represent unresolved issues from the therapist's own analysis. Later revisions of the idea of countertransference came to see it as a useful and healthy aspect of therapeutic work (Epstein & Feiner, 1979). Self-disclosure, particularly of one's response to the patient's work, initially appears to be a form of countertransference.

Against the backdrop of the strong ideological prohibition against any kind of disclosure, except for specific applications of countertransference, contemporary psychotherapists from a variety of disciplines have begun to examine the issue of therapist self-disclosure (Anderson & Anderson, 1989; Auvil & Silver, 1984; Baldwin & Satir, 1987; Fenster et al., 1986; Mathews, 1988; Palombo, 1987; Silverstein, 1991; Stricker & Fisher, 1990). Newer examinations of self-disclosure suggest that it cannot be subsumed under the category of countertransference. Rather, specific categories of self-disclosure can be defined: historical, emotional, relational, philosophical, and fantasy (Kooden, 1991). Underlying these discussions is a shared appreciation that the point of such disclosures can be to help the patient and further the goals of his or her therapy, rather than to meet the therapist's needs.

Family therapists often use self-disclosure of historical personal experience as a technique—for instance, a therapist reveals how she herself resolved an escalating conflict with an adolescent (Duhl, 1987) or took on a symptom present in the family (Garfield, 1989). Self-disclosure may be used as a method to show empathy, build trust, or "undercut the idea of the omnipotent therapist" (Kramer, 1985, p. 294). In such examples, the therapist talks about himself or herself as part of an explicit therapeutic strategy. The therapist is making implicit use of "disclosure reciprocity."

Self-disclosure in psychotherapy is not just a matter of strategy, however; it is embedded in the therapeutic process. Because the person of
the therapist is present in the therapy, a certain kind of disclosure is
always present. For instance, Carl Rogers reports that a patient said at
the end of therapy: "I don't know a thing about you, and yet, I have
never known any one so well" (Baldwin, 1987, p. 45). Beyond this way
of being oneself as a therapist, at the deliberate and verbal level a therapist chooses when and whether to disclose certain experiences to certain patients at particular moments in the therapy. Specifically, while
the patient is struggling to resolve a particular issue, it may be counter-
productive for the therapist to reveal his or her way of resolving it.
Perlman (1991), a formerly married gay therapist, gives the example of
his decision to withhold his background from a bisexual married man
in the midst of making choices about his sexuality. Prematurely revealing his own resolution of that issue might have foreclosed the patient's
options and activated his homophobia. For different reasons, Brown
(1991b), a lesbian therapist, reports her choice to postpone discussion of
her own preferred childlessness with a lesbian patient struggling with
infertility. Clearly how and when and what to disclose are essential
aspects of therapeutic work.

Gay and lesbian therapists and women therapists may also use self-
disclosure in the service of becoming a role model to the patient
(Kooden, 1991). Perceiving the therapist as a role model does not dictate that the patient make the same choices as the therapist.
Nevertheless, working with a clinician who shares social experiences of
oppression, discrimination, or harassment and seeing how that person
has faced those challenges affords a patient a chance to see what kinds
of healthy choices can be made. Women family therapists are particularly likely to choose styles of self-disclosure in which they share verbal
and nonverbal reactions to the therapy, past and present personal
issues, and expressions of emotional connectedness. Moreover, women
with more experience are more likely to choose such a style, suggesting
that women therapists' own adult development facilitates their ability
to use themselves therapeutically (Shadley, 1987).

FEMINIST APPROACHES TO SELF-DISCLOSURE

Asymmetry in the revelation of personal material is typical of relationships between nonequals. Personal information flows toward the
greater power or status (Goffman, 1967): the researcher investigates the
participant, the teacher learns about the student, the doctor knows
about the patient's personal life in great detail. In such structured relations, the party with less power knows little about the other as a person.[4] Feminist approaches to such situations when both parties are

women uphold the centrality to the underlying process of the personal experience of each of the women involved. Tapping personal experience is a way to show how all women experience, in various ways, oppressive conditions—that is, to show the relevance of generalized oppression to the life of each person.

Feminists have examined self-disclosure in situations that involve the transfer of information from one person to another (research and teaching) and in service relationships (psychotherapy and social work). In each setting, developing a relationship turns out to be crucial for the process at hand, and self-disclosure often is an ingredient of building that relationship. Even those who set out to gather information, such as sociologists, find themselves forming relationships and have to assess what they reveal about themselves to the people they study because of the implications for the relationship. These explorations are important for the understanding of self-disclosure in medical relationships, since learning about people, getting and sharing information, and helping others are all part of clinical work.

FEMINIST SOCIAL SCIENCE RESEARCH

Mutuality is a foreign concept in traditional research, which assumes neutrality and noninvolvement between researcher and participant. Feminist social scientists point out that objectivity in research is in fact a myth; the claim of objectivity—that is, lack of personal involvement—has been used to hide power arrangements in academia and politics as well as in research projects. Feminist researchers argue for acknowledging a position of partiality or involvement and stating one's self-interest and commitments up front. This approach to research makes some kinds of self-disclosure a primary ethical obligation. Feminists also call for a methodology informed by women's experience—as researchers and as those who are studied. Part of this methodology requires paying attention to the relationship between the researcher and the participant, real persons with rich and complex lives that they bring to bear on the research experience. Personal self-disclosure emerges as part of the relationship born of the research encounter.

Ann Oakley, an English sociologist, using an intuitive appreciation of reciprocal disclosure, found that the women she was studying revealed more accurate and intimate information when she became known to them. She carried out a longitudinal study of women during their first pregnancy, childbirth, and the postpartum months (Oakley, 1980, 1981). "In most cases, the goal of finding out about people through interviewing is best achieved when the relationship of interviewer and interviewee is non-hierarchical and when the interviewer is prepared to invest his or her own personal identity in the relationship" (1981, p. 41).

In her analysis, Oakley argued for an open exchange of experience about motherhood between the researcher and the researched. Rather than responding evasively to questions posed to her about her life, as sociologists are taught to do, she answered truthfully, in a spirit of mutual exchange with women who had disclosed the details of their lives to her. Oakley's work suggests that when the research relationship goes on over time, an appropriate, nonexploitative way for a researcher to learn about people's lives is to respond openly to questions about his or her own experience. Oakley discards the notion of the supposedly objective interview (commonplace in medicine as well as sociology) with "the recognition that personal involvement is more than danger-ous bias—it is the condition under which people come to know each other and to admit others into their lives" (1981, p. 58). Researchers (and doctors) who want to learn about people's lives must regard their work as a reciprocal project. Although the clinician and the researcher have different goals, the implication of Oakley's work for clinicians is that sharing experiences can promote a more genuine and less hierar-chical relationship.

Among feminist researchers, mutuality with the women who partic-ipate in their studies and empowerment of those women are explicit goals. Examples of such mutuality and empowerment include allowing research subjects to review and modify written drafts of manuscripts (Billson, 1991), producing a version of the findings accessible to lay readers (such as Ann Oakley's *Becoming a Mother* [1980]), and giving participants control over the uses to which the research may be put (Mies, 1983). I do not mean to imply that the achievement of such goals is common or easy. A review of psychological research published in two journals oriented toward women's concerns, *Psychology of Women Quarterly* and *Sex Roles*, found that even in these journals positively dis-posed toward feminist concerns authors found it very difficult to achieve the goals of mutual participation, egalitarianism, social action, and personal relatedness between researcher and participants (Walsh, 1989).

The assumption of shared gender (both parties are women) underlies the feminist goal of mutuality in research. "Knowledge of the other and knowledge of the self are mutually informing, because self and other share a common condition of being women" (Westcott, 1979, cited by Billson, 1991).[5] However, shared gender alone cannot overcome the dis-trust created by racism and class differences. Riessman (1987) points out the ease with which a white interviewer sensitively drew out the story of a recently divorced white woman—and her utter failure to make sense out of the experience of a Puerto Rican woman who had also recently divorced. Black women may be suspicious about the pur-pose of research and distrustful of a white interviewer, even a woman. The only power the black woman may have is the ability to refuse par-ticipation or to provide unrevealing material. The onus falls on the (usually) white interviewer to bring up the issue of racial difference and thereby acknowledge the enormous differences in life experience between herself and her subjects (Edwards, 1990). The obstacle presented by class and race differences to achieving mutuality is potentially offset by the researcher's willingness not only to acknowledge openly the importance of those differences but to make close personal connections through longitudinal research. Self-disclosure is an almost inevitable feature of such long-term conversations.

The intimacy born of the long-term relationship between the feminist researcher and the research participants does not overturn the existing power relationship and in fact may exacerbate it. Stacey (1988) points out how the research may perpetuate or take advantage of that power differential. First, the fieldwork itself is an intervention in the lives of the participants, "a system of relationships that the researcher is far freer than the researched to leave. The inequality and potential treacherousness of this relationship seems inescapable" (p. 23). Since the ethnographic method depends on attachment and engagement with the researcher, it puts the participants at risk of manipulation and betrayal. Second, the exploitative nature of research seems almost unavoidable; the researcher, after all, is using the relationship to gain information: "The lives, loves, and tragedies that informants share with a researcher are ultimately data, grist for the ethnographic mill, a mill that has a truly grinding power" (p. 23). Even the death of an informant during a study, while a loss, can be conceived of as a "research opportunity" (p. 23).

Despite these dangers, feminist research often offers real support to participants, "a form of loving attention, of comparatively non-judgmental acceptance, that they come to value deeply" (Stacey, 1988, p. 26). A researcher who chooses to explore the lives of the socially disenfranchised may provide welcome social contact and support (Cotterill, 1992; Hoff, 1988). Accompanying this real benefit, however, is the attendant risk of desertion and loss of the researcher after she has become an important figure in the lives of her subjects. Clearly the close engagement of feminist researchers with those whom they study creates ethical problems that require careful attention to the power dynamic. Research, after all, is a "privileged activity" (Ribbens, 1989).

FEMINIST EDUCATORS

The classroom is another setting where persons with different degrees of power engage in ongoing conversations with each other. Women's studies teachers use self-disclosure to show that what happens in one's life is worthy of study and can contribute to important understandings about women's position in society. As with psychotherapy, feminist educators agree that the purpose of personal disclosures is to enhance students' understanding. For example, one professor described to her students her experience of having a botched illegal abortion in 1972, prior to *Roe v. Wade* (1973), a time when most of her students had not yet been born. The students responded that the personal disclosure made real what had been to them a distant and abstract issue. Another faculty member disclosed her experience of having left a battering relationship, another her near rape and strangling, another her recent diagnosis of breast cancer. (This discussion took place on an electronic discussion forum among women's studies faculty.)[6] Because women's studies courses often require reading women's personal histories, keeping a journal during the course, or integrating personal experience into political discussion, the practice of faculty self-disclosure is consistent with a high level of mutuality and reciprocity between teacher and students.

These educators do not deny the power relations between themselves and their students. They acknowledge the drawbacks of such disclosures—the difficulty of ascertaining any given student's ability to deal with the disclosed material and the possibility that it might be too painful for some students to tolerate. Some students might not take such disclosures seriously and might see them as diversions, as not what a "real" teacher would do. Because students may see self-disclosure as something associated with women's practice (like other behaviors related to intimacy, sharing, and emotions), they may derogate the content and the person disclosing. This interpretation could undermine women faculty in exactly those areas where they are seeking credibility.[7] Additionally, the practice of self-disclosure makes some teachers, who know that personal disclosures may be used against them by hostile students or administrators, feel professionally at risk. Nevertheless, the very extent of self-disclosure among women's studies educators suggests that most of these teachers attempt to reveal themselves as real and genuine in the course of their work within a complex hierarchy of personal and political relations. Self-revelation in this setting can transform the power dynamics of the teacher-student relationship.

FEMINIST PSYCHOTHERAPY

Like their counterparts in research and teaching, feminist psychotherapists also work toward the goals of mutuality and egalitarianism. Self-disclosure is one means of reducing the power discrepancies and openly acknowledging shared oppression. However, some kinds of disclosure arise not from the therapist's choice to reveal herself but from her visibility in a small community. The marginality of feminist and lesbian therapists often compels them to live and practice in a small social world in which they, their lovers, and their patients may all take part in common activities. As with other token professionals (for instance, clinicians of color), many aspects of their behavior—participation in political events, level of fees charged, social life—are subject to public scrutiny (Brown, 1991a). The constant visibility results in overlaps between personal and professional roles. For explicit feminists, principles of feminist therapy "in some ways encourage or enable such overlap even when it is not already in place" (Brown, 1991a, p. 325).

The overlap between personal and professional life may support the principle of egalitarianism by equalizing the power between therapist and patient; however, it may also erode necessary boundaries between patient and clinician. Sharing membership with a patient in an oppressed group, combined with the clinician's professional isolation and personal neediness, may make it very difficult for the lesbian clinician to maintain boundaries to benefit the patient or the therapeutic relationship (Brown, 1991a). Assessment of self-disclosure becomes a subtle matter in this setting; it depends on the therapist's motives, the kind of material, the timing, and what Brown calls "the frame that has usually contained the therapy" (1991a, p. 327). The feminist therapist must ask herself, "When is a behavior an expression of feminist therapy principles of egalitarianism, empowerment, and consciousness-raising, and when does it represent a visible break in the frame?" (Brown, 1991a, p. 327).

The risks of mutuality in feminist clinical practice parallel the risks in feminist research. Although patients and psychotherapy clients differ from research participants in that they come to the clinician in search of attention, acceptance, and treatment, the relationship between practitioner and patient has parallels with that between researcher and participant. Intimacy and mutuality can both reduce the power inequality and aggravate it. The proposal for mutuality and intimacy between researcher and participant raises concerns about the potential for exploitation (Stacey, 1988): the research may exploit the subject for information that advances the researcher's career or changes her position in the community; the clinician's intimacy may take advantage of the patient's trust to meet the practitioner's emotional or social needs. Though both clinician and researcher need their counterpart to complete their task, both remain in unequal relationships with them. Thus, the goal of mutuality and reciprocity accepts fundamental ethical vulnerabilities in relationships that cannot be equal.

FEMINIST SOCIAL WORK

When inequality is marked and the professional and the client have little in common, mutuality is more difficult to imagine, yet the ethical obligation of the more powerful to promote egalitarianism is even more obvious. In the field of social welfare, Ann Withorn argues for enhanced mutuality between the worker and the users of the system, with the goal of reducing the power imbalance. She advocates divesting power by giving away as much information as possible: "Workers should support the development of as much power as possible with clients and abandon those aspects of their power which can be given away. One can divest power by sharing all information about procedures and options, by sharing personal and political expectations, and by attempting to treat people as potential comrades, as equals who can be allies" (1984, p. 109).

Withorn's idea of the user of social welfare services as a potential comrade to the social worker implies a sense of mutuality and reciprocity: both have something to gain; they are potential allies in a larger struggle to change the system. Withorn requires personal transformation on the part of the worker: "An essential element of political practice may well be one's ability to identify with service users and to link one's own experiences with theirs" (1984, p. 85). Since workers control the resources the users want, the first move to change the relationship belongs to the worker. Workers may need to make whole series of moves before distrust can be broken down. "Workers must acknowledge their power, but also attempt to break its grip on the interaction by specific acts and attitudes, as well as by sharing and self-disclosure" (p. 103). Withorn is careful to warn against sharing personal experiences before trust develops. "False assumptions of connectedness serve no purpose":

> Telling personal experiences can also emphasize class, race, or cultural differences before enough trust exists for such differences to be useful. . . . The task is to build honest relationships based on shared experiences (around the human service interchange) and shared values. Asserting the presence of a relationship by an overly generous disclosure of one's life may embarrass, bore, or anger clients. (p. 109)

Nevertheless, the ideals of feminist social work are difficult to put into practice. Published studies of social service programs for families reveal little clinical application of feminist principles (Walker et al., 1988).[8] It emerges that it is personally difficult for practitioners to work consistently in feminist ways: to take the perspective of those in need, to relinquish power and prestige, and to maintain the "double vision" of being part of an elite yet oppressed within that elite. These same difficulties arise when trying to apply feminist principles in medical practice.

This review suggests that self-disclosure by the more powerful person in settings of unequal power can enhance mutuality. However, if a trusting relationship has not already been established, disclosures may backfire, especially in the presence of differences in race and class. At the other end of the spectrum, when the two parties in an unequal relationship share membership in a small or marginal community, self-disclosures by the more powerful may confound preexisting ambiguities in the boundaries of the relationship. As always, in relationships characterized by intense trust, perhaps engendered by mutuality, the less powerful are vulnerable to exploitation.

SELF-DISCLOSURE BY DOCTORS

Despite their obvious personal contributions to the relationship, medical practitioners rarely discuss the extent to which they share personal life details with patients. With the exception of one study of nurse-practitioners (Coolidge-Young, 1989), studies of communication in clinical work with patients have not looked at offerings of personal information by physicians (see, for example, Byrne & Long, 1976; Fisher & Todd, 1983; West, 1984). Since doctors regularly engage in relationships that can endure for decades, during which they themselves go through enormous changes, it is not surprising that they would convey significant information about themselves to patients in the course of their mutual exchanges. What does this practice mean for the relationships they establish with patients? How does it relate to issues of gender and power in the relationship?

The tradition of the doctor's reticence with patients about her or his own life originates historically in at least two views of the relationship. First, in the positivist conception of medicine as science, the doctor plays the role of a neutral scientist studying the patient and the patient's illness. The purportedly objective position of the doctor does not permit the disclosure of personal information. Despite contemporary uncertainty about the overarching idea of scientific neutrality in the doctor-patient relationship, the stance that accompanied neutrality remains a habit in practice. Thus, silence is taught as part of professionalization; combined with expertise, it sets the doctor above the patient. The doctor's ability to withhold information maintains the power discrepancy (Henley, 1977).

The second source of medical practitioners' habit of maintaining silence is the legacy of psychoanalysis, a very narrow version of the doctor-patient relationship. Like psychotherapists, physicians have historically been mandated to silence about themselves in their work with patients. Modern theorists on the doctor-patient relationship have followed in Freud's footsteps. Michael Balint (1969; 1972), for instance, trained originally as a psychoanalyst, construed the doctor's response to the patient as a form of countertransference. Balint's seminars with British general practitioners in the 1950s pointed out how the doctor's personal material usually hindered progress in the clinical relationship. In modern medical practice, the countertransference is now viewed as a creative way to understand doctor-patient interactions (Stein, 1985). In this tradition, self-disclosure by the physician is considered an act of countertransference. The doctor deliberately chooses to reveal personal material as part of the treatment. Nevertheless, such self-disclosure is not a part of standard teaching.

However orthodox their training and tradition, some doctors do make themselves more accessible to patients. Eschewing white coats, titles, and big desks, these clinicians encourage patients to refer to them by their first names. One British general practitioner talked about frequenting the local pub to reduce the social distance between himself and his patients (Jefferys & Sachs, 1983). Rural doctors writing about lifetimes of practice in small communities emphasize the experiences they have shared with their patients: living their lives in common with their patients, personal joy and tragedy are community emotions (LaCombe, 1990). Rural life itself may have a leveling effect. Although the doctors have a valuable public role, they have no more privacy than any other member of the community. Writing after a heart attack, one physician lamented: "After my catheterization and bypass (performed in an adjacent community), half the people in the hospital and a significant number of my patients and friends knew the anatomy of my coronary circulation better than I" (Seaver, 1987, p. 32). Of course, the public nature of the physician's life in a small town is not the result of deliberate disclosure on the doctor's part but rather a reflection of small-town life. Nevertheless, choosing to live in a small community where his or her personal life is inevitably quite public reflects a doctor's willingness to be "known" to patients.

In psychotherapy, therapist disclosure promotes client disclosure (Chelune, 1979). The parallel implication in medical relationships is that patients will be more likely to disclose to clinicians who are open with them. Indeed, in an experimental study, college student patients disclosed more psychosocial information to a self-disclosing nurse-practitioner than they did to a nurse-practitioner who was not self-revealing (Coolidge-Young, 1989). The converse may also be true: practitioners may be more likely to share personal life details with patients who have shown trust by revealing themselves.

I began thinking about the issue of what doctors say about themselves to patients during a study in which a group of (white, heterosexual) women colleagues and I considered the effect of our pregnancies and childbearing on our doctor-patient relationships. We noticed that this life-change event had led to increased sharing of personal experience with patients (Candib et al., 1987). I was struck by the fact that disclosure was spontaneously described by all the group members. Similarly, psychotherapists found their pregnancies to be a time when, contrary to their usual practice, they were likely to reveal personal information about themselves (Fenster et al., 1986). I set out to discover the extent to which my colleagues—family physicians, both men and women—talk about themselves with patients. I found that disclosing personal information was a fact of life, regularly practiced, often in specific circumstances, with very clear goals and some commonly agreed-upon warnings. None of the doctors with whom I discussed self-disclosure considered it unusual or unethical, although most agreed that it was not something taught in school or learned from books.

As a feminist, I share with feminists in other disciplines an interest and familiarity with self-disclosure; as a doctor, I share with other physicians a training in the strong proscription against it. I want to state at the outset that the most common reason doctors are not self-revealing to patients is that they sincerely believe their function is to help the patient, not talk about themselves. Even physicians who have not been exposed to psychoanalytic thinking manifest an understanding of the potentially negative role of the countertransference in their fear that their disclosure of personal experience might be a disguised appeal for help, sympathy, intimacy, or nurturing. In this view, whatever yearning the doctor may have for the patient to take care of him or her must be distrusted and silenced. As a result, while the respondents in my informal study were comfortable disclosing experiences that they had already resolved, they generally agreed that it was inappropriate to divulge current problems. For instance, one doctor whose daughter had a worrisome facial mass requiring surgery asked, "What should I tell them when they ask about her? Certainly not that she needs surgery and that we're terrified." She concluded that it is not fair to share one's own fear or one's need for comforting and reassurance.

This belief is founded on acknowledgment of the inherent imbalance in the doctor-patient relationship: the patient comes to the doctor for help; the doctor's privileged and powerful position is not to be abused. The physicians with whom I spoke would agree with this description of the power discrepancy and the resulting obligation not to take advantage of patients. Yet each of them had revealed significant and sometimes intimate life details to patients. These disclosures were not out-of-character abuses of power but rather examples of active caring.

METHOD

Since doctors are generally expected to maintain friendly but professional attitudes in their clinical relationship (Jefferys & Sachs, 1983), they may understandably be reluctant to admit to having transgressed this standard by sharing personal life details with patients. When being studied, they could be expected to offer "public accounts" (Cornwell, 1984) of their work in an effort to "manage their appearance"—to put their best foot forward. Interviews by strangers would tend to elicit the public accounts. On the other hand, in the privacy of close relationships with other physicians, it is sometimes easier to make admissions of disclosures to patients, or "private accounts." With this in mind, I chose to raise the topic with physicians I knew well.

I collected information in hallways, over lunch, between patients, after Balint group, on the telephone, at parties, or wherever else the subject could be broached. Our Balint group is a weekly meeting of faculty family physicians focused on the doctor-patient relationship. Basing our group on the work of Michael Balint (1969, 1972), we have been meeting for over twenty years. Since the participants had to be willing to share with me not only the fact of their disclosure but also the material disclosed, the sample is an intimacy sample in addition to being a convenience sample—in other words, people I knew well who were convenient to interview. The group of respondents consisted mostly of family physicians from various age groups and practice settings who knew me quite well. I purposely sought out individuals with substantial practice experience beyond training, since I felt that they were more likely to have made significant disclosures.

It is important to note at the outset that the telling disclosures are those made by individuals who have been trained not to disclose. In other words, the disclosure of the medical student who blurts out to the patient, "Oh, yes, I had the same diarrhea last week," is the expression of a young person as yet untrained and unsocialized in a professional role. The disclosures in this study, on the other hand, represent personal life details shared with patients by experienced physicians presumably socialized to keep their personal and professional lives separate. These physicians also had more established relationships with patients.

THEMES

The Physician as Model

In these examples, the doctor shared personal experiences using himself or herself as a model. Sometimes the doctor revealed positive aspects of self for the purpose of instruction or guidance; sometimes the doctor disclosed potentially negative information in order to encourage patients in a course of action. The similarity of the doctor's role to that of a teacher or parent is apparent. One fifty-year-old physician stated that he regularly shared descriptions of how he had managed particular times in family life. He gave two examples. When mother, father, and baby come in for the ten-day postpartum office visit, he uses himself as an example of what fathers can do at this time, explaining how he helped his wife at this stage of parenthood. This physician added that this works only when the father is present; expecting the mother to relay such a message to the father ("Dr. Diamond says you have to . . . ") would function divisively (see the discussion of the family approach in chapter 7).

In the second example, this physician regularly explains to adoptive parents that their children may become preoccupied in their teens with the identity of their birth parents and the desire to find them. From his own experience he can forewarn the parents about how frightening the search is for the teenager and about how important parental support is during the process. Explicit in this very specific form of anticipatory guidance is this doctor's open acknowledgment of his own anxieties in raising adopted children. His function as a role model for adoptive families has a broad foundation. For many years, both he and his wife, a social worker, have been actively involved in the adoption process. They have facilitated the release and adoption of many children over a twenty-five-year period. In their openness about their large family of adopted and birth children, this couple serves as a role model for patients and neighbors in their community. Another physician stated that as part of well-child care, she asks parents what they are doing for their own relationship. She regularly recommends that parents go away overnight, and she offers her own experience of needing to make space in her life with small children to attend to her relationship with their father.

The practitioners I studied did not discuss the possibility that their use of themselves as role models might be alienating to patients whose lives differed sharply from their own. They did not bring up class bias as a problem with their recommendations. They appeared to have chosen heterosexual families with two parents (similar to themselves) for their advice. Although these examples might be used to support the idea that doctors fail to deal with so-called nontraditional families, the doctor with the large family of adopted and birth children has in fact supported his single daughter's struggle to raise a child on her own. A lesbian mother in my sample, while usually guarded about her personal life with patients, found that her passage through pregnancy, childbirth, and motherhood offered her a common ground with patients who were unaware of her sexual orientation.

This willingness to be forthcoming about one's family life is a way of showing reciprocity. Although asymmetry of power is maintained in doctors' presentation of themselves as experienced in family matters, they are also revealing themselves as similar to their patients. The prominence of life-cycle themes in their responses suggests that events associated with these themes are the most common and acceptable material for disclosure (Shadley, 1987). Almost every informant who was a parent mentioned talking about the experience of raising children. Perhaps being a parent is one of the most traditional and credible roles for physicians, whose style of relating to patients may be parental as well. I do not mean "parental" in a paternalistic, authoritarian, or controlling sense, but rather in the best senses of nurturing, guiding, and comforting. By referring to their own experience, doctors are attempting to emphasize the universal aspects of the parenting experience: the concerns of parents about their children and their need to attend to their adult relationships.

Some respondents stated that they shared personal information with patients in order to make their own position credible and thus to lend further weight to whatever advice they might be giving: for example, "I know because my two-year-old had the same thing." One internist with hypertension offered that he regularly tells his hypertensive patients about his own experiences with antihypertensive drugs. He thinks this offering of personal material makes his recommendations more credible and leads to better adherence to the medical regimen. One physician reported using the story of his own family doctor's role during his wife's serious illness to convince people about the important function of a family doctor: "My family doctor helped us figure out how to use the medical care system, which specialist to call, and stayed with us through all the ups and downs." He uses this description to encourage patients to let him help them make their way through the medical maze. This doctor's momentary revelation of himself as a person who has needed help shows him joining in the experience of patienthood, with all its attendant uncertainties.

The Physician and Relationships

The unifying theme in these disclosures is the explanation that the sharing served to advance the relationship. Sharing life experiences with patients consistently contributes to intimacy and mutuality between doctor and patient. By intimacy I mean the creation of an atmosphere of closeness in which deeply personal thoughts and feelings can be exchanged. (The highly charged and one-sided disrobing and touching of the encounter can obviously engender fantasies of further physical intimacy for both doctor and patient, but this is not the sense in which I am using the term.)

Many physicians disclose experiences from their personal lives to show empathy for the feelings of patients undergoing similar or relevant experiences. Worrying about family members is a typical example. "I know how scary that can be, my daughter needed surgery too." (This statement differs in tone from statements made to identify feelings or to appear empathetic, for example, "I can see that you are feeling scared about your child's surgery" [see chapter 7].) Experiences of common illness, such as low back pain, were also frequently disclosed to patients. All physicians who mentioned low back pain stated that they openly empathized with the experience of slow and halting recovery and the attendant anxiety and depression. Although common troubles in parenting were the events in family life most frequently mentioned, one physician whose father had been seriously ill one thousand miles away also commented that he could share that experience with patients who worried about the illness of parents living far away. The empathy in these examples shows the doctor's recognition, in open statements of similarity, of the patient's pain, both physical or emotional. Defining the task of the doctor as recognition—of the patient, of the person, and of the illness—is described in poetic (but masculine) terms by John Berger in *A Fortunate Man* (1976):

> This can be achieved by the doctor presenting himself to the patient as a comparable man. It demands from the doctor a true imaginative and precise self-knowledge. The patient must be given the chance to recognize, despite his aggravated self-consciousness, aspects of himself in the doctor, but in such a way that the doctor seems to be Everyman. This chance is probably seldom the result of a single exchange, and it may come about more as the result of the general atmosphere than of any special words said. (Berger & Mohr, 1976, p. 76)

Presenting oneself as a "comparable woman" appears to come easily to physicians who become mothers. Participating in the common project of raising children allows for mutual recognition. Patients frequently ask about one's children, whom they may never have seen, as a way of giving attention back to the doctor and at the same time recognizing that the doctor has another role as a parent. Such recognition is central for the development of mutuality (Kuykendall, 1983). Two physicians offered their own experiences of depression to patients as a form of recognition. One stated that the very nature of the disease leads the depressed person to discount any effort by the physician to reach out. The doctor brings up his or her experience to reach through the cloud of hopelessness with an expression of commitment to the patient's care. "I want them to know when I tell them to call me, I really mean it." The other stated that the advice or encouragement given from the position of personal experience carries a more convincing vocabulary; the patient can accept it as authentic.

These extraordinary self-exposures show the doctor's sincerity, as evidenced in the act of shedding the mantle of authority in order to reach out to desperate people. A further example was offered by a colleague who shared her own deep personal loss with a patient who had similarly suffered. One son of the patient had died in a car accident, and another son had become quadriplegic from a separate accident. The usually reticent doctor revealed to the patient that her mother and brother had been killed in a car crash. On reflecting on her motivation for this rare disclosure, my colleague stated that such losses are so catastrophic that the survivor feels that no one can understand. She also described the patient as someone who had been bearing her burden silently and alone. Her disclosure, she felt, served the purpose of reaching out to an isolated and grieving human being. In mutuality, the doctor revealed herself as a person who knew the depth of such losses.

A physician in his midthirties told me the story of his visit with an inarticulate patient who spent an entire session complaining about the pains rambling through her body. He had a hunch that she was worried about infertility, although she did not bring it up spontaneously. When he asked her directly, she started to cry. It turned out that she had had some kinds of testing but did not understand the results or implications. He was able to offer her his own frustrating experience of infertility. His gesture of trust—that he could tell her something deeply private—showed his confidence in her. It served as the bridge over the differences in class and education that had impeded their work together.

The physician may show trust in a patient by revealing intimate and potentially stigmatizing evidence of human frailty. For example, several respondents stated that they had disclosed their own experience of the usefulness of therapy in encouraging patients to enter psychotherapy or marital therapy. One physician stated that she had shared her experience of attending Al-Anon with her patients who were also children of alcoholics. Having done so, the doctor could openly address the symptoms of excess feelings of guilt and responsibility experienced by adult children of alcoholics and addicts.

In these examples, the doctors disclosed personal experiences with the explicit goal of convincing the patient to do something difficult or challenging. To encourage patients to take a desired course of action is a conventional activity in the doctor-patient relationship. To reveal a history of psychiatric treatment or family alcoholism is not. In trusting the patient with the knowledge of his or her own personal difficulty, the physician attempts to reduce the isolation, shame, stigma, or embarrassment the patient may feel about the problem. The doctor is also demonstrating the treatability of conditions thought to be shameful.

In these disclosures, each physician was careful to mention the importance of context: the disclosures took place in the course of long-term (five to ten years) relationships with patients. When the material disclosed is highly stigmatized, the revelation may also create a secret bond of trust: one recovered physician in my sample revealed to an alcoholic patient a personal history of drug addiction, cutting through the distance between doctor and patient by sharing his secret. Such a revelation is the equivalent of giving a "sign" (Goffman, 1963): it shows that the doctor has been initiated, that both parties are members of the secret society, and that the preliminaries can be discarded. The capacity for making a very personal admission is certainly suggestive of the high degree of mutuality in such relationships. It was also characteristic of the recovery of this particular physician, whose experience underlines that such disclosure is predicated upon the safe context of the long-term doctor-patient relationship.

When Sharing Goes Awry

As clinicians, doctors accept the risks associated with the use of drugs and surgery—why not with disclosure? I received a number of examples from nonphysician friends of inappropriate disclosure by physicians. An English professor reported that every time she sees her doctor for her hypertension, he tells her about his father dying because he neglected his high blood pressure. She suspects that the doctor has never resolved his own feelings about his father's death: "It was clear to me that he needed to 'work on' his grief!" Another woman reported that every time she takes her child to the pediatrician, he spends more time talking about his own child than inquiring about hers.

In these examples, the repetitiousness of the physicians' disclosures suggests their obliviousness to the context of the patient at hand, as well as lack of insight into their own need for attention. Withorn offers a similar example reported by a welfare recipient: "I guess he was being nice to me, but the more he talked about his wife and her problems and how they were like my worries the madder I got. Who was he to assume anything about my life? And how could he think that his prissy little wife with a husband and a job of her own could be anything like me?" (1984, p. 109). Such examples buttress the orthodox position that disclosure is inappropriate. Are there common characteristics of disclosures gone awry?

Disclosure can be destructive to the budding doctor-patient relationship. One physician recalled having revealed her homosexuality to a young woman patient with whom she had a tentative social connection. At the same time, the doctor was starting to work with another patient on issues related to her abusive marriage. The first patient revealed the doctor's sexual orientation to the second patient, who then left the practice. When the doctor does not know the patient very well, she or he is more likely to make unfounded assumptions. One doctor who practiced in a devout Christian community, assuming that he and a crying patient shared the same religious beliefs, initiated a prayer session during an office visit. The patient later became angry with the doctor for taking advantage of his emotional state. Such an example does not represent disclosure of specific life events but rather shows a physician using a strategy from his own spiritual life to address a patient's problems. In these instances, unfounded assumptions about the patients' values and beliefs hold great potential for backfiring.

One example from my own experience occurred while I was covering for another doctor. I was asked to refill a prescription for barbiturates for a patient who carried the diagnosis of somatoform disorder. The patient, a former pharmacist, practiced polypharmacy, taking innumerable drugs in varying combinations. I explained to her that I did not refill barbiturates because they are addictive, and that I was familiar with such problems among medical professionals because my father had been an addict. The patient subsequently threatened to sue the practice because she felt that I had accused her of being an addict. In retrospect, I see that my self-disclosure to the pharmacist may have reflected my unresolved anger at my father for abusing the privileges of being a doctor. In an interaction where control issues were already highly conflictual, the pharmacist probably identified the anger underlying my unwillingness to prescribe addicting substances for her and reacted with a threat. Here again, the disclosure of highly stigmatizing material occurred outside the context of an established doctor-patient relationship.

When the doctor has a palpably negative reaction to a patient, self-disclosure is likely to be unproductive. An example of such a disclosure is offered by Miriam C. Chellingsworth, a doctor with multiple sclerosis. She describes her negative feelings toward a patient with the same illness who she felt was inordinately focused on her symptoms.

> Whenever the paediatrician talked to her, she experienced tingling in her hands in addition to her usual dysesthesias. She described the latter as "terrible." "I know," I said, "they're awful." "You don't know, you can't know!" "I do know. I have them too; I have MS." I immediately regretted my impulsive remark. Her whole attitude changed to one of pity for me rather than for herself. I find pity difficult to cope with at the best of times; it makes a doctor-patient relationship impossible. (1987, p. 93)

In another example, a lesbian physician reported the experience of suturing a laceration near a patient's eye in an emergency room. The patient began making homophobic comments during the repair, and the physician stated point-blank that she was a lesbian and that he had better watch out! She later regarded this disclosure as an error. While the first story suggests that the physician may not have resolved all her own issues around her multiple sclerosis, the second underscores the harassment from patients experienced by physicians from vulnerable groups (Phillips & Schneider, 1993). Self-disclosure in the setting of such vulnerability may be particularly unwise.

With particular kinds of patients, some doctors expressed fear of disclosure. Several respondents described patients they viewed as extremely dependent, who seemed to try to make the doctor a part of their lives and to spend all of their office visits talking about the doctor's family. The doctors' feeling of invasion made them extremely wary of any personal revelations. Nevertheless, they reported, such patients had an uncanny knack for finding out a great deal of personal material. These doctors saw such patients as threatening them with fusion; rather than becoming more available, the doctors withdrew. This scenario suggests that doctors may use disclosure to control distance—being more open when they value intimacy as a goal, but closing off any avenues for patients to learn more about them when they perceive intimacy as threatening. This finding supports Goffman's (1967) observation that only the more powerful in a relationship is allowed to initiate intimacy and thus, in this case, to control it.

Several physicians mentioned the occasional feeling of being coerced to disclose. When patients ask, "What would you do?" or, "What did you do?" they may not be asking for the doctor's personal experience but rather attempting to force the doctor to make a decision for them or to take a public stand. (Cotterill reports the same sense of being put on the spot in her research about in-law relationships when a subject asked her after the interview, "Will you tell me something now quite truthfully and as honestly as you can? What do you think of Henry and I as in-laws?" [1992, p. 603].) From these examples it emerges that disclosure may jeopardize the relationship when doctor and patient have not yet reached a tacit agreement about control. Put another way, when patient and doctor do not share assumptions about the relationship, one party or the other may construe the intimacy and reciprocity implied by disclosure as threatening.

It is possible, of course, for some doctors to use self-disclosure as yet another way to exercise control in the relationship. The fact that the doctor survived, resolved, or triumphed over a difficulty places the patient in the presence of someone strong who conquers his or her problems. The result may be unwanted: "If he tells only the good things that he has already resolved, [patients] may see him as smug, unreal, or condescending" (Kramer, 1985, p. 294). This way of using self-disclosure shows that it does not necessarily make the doctor appear more human and more accessible as a person. Alternatively, the fact that the physician has survived and resolved the problem, or come to live with it, offers patients the awareness that they too will be able to draw on their own strengths to survive the acute discomfort of their current situation. The problem that doctor and patient have in common can be viewed as survivable or perhaps bearable. The closeness of the relationships in which the physicians I surveyed practiced self-disclosure suggests that, at least for them, this description is more fitting.

Self-disclosure as Healing for the Doctor
Despite the fear of "unloading" on patients, the theme of healing tentatively filtered into the responses of the physicians I questioned. Some were more comfortable expressing this feeling in terms of "learning from patients." One clinician talked about how much she learned from patients with children older than her own. Another commented, "Patients can be therapeutic indirectly for us. Empathy for them deepens us." Three psychotherapists who had had a parent die in the past few years told me about informing patients about these deaths at the

time. All were convinced that patients would know something about them was different and that patients should be allowed to know the source of the therapist's distress. Their disclosures permitted patients to offer words of comfort—a circumscribed way of giving back to the therapist.

The scant literature on physician illness, an area where doctors might engage in self-disclosure, offers little description of how their journeys into illness have affected doctors' relationships with their patients. In a book of essays about doctors' illnesses, Mandell and Spiro's *When Doctors Get Sick* (1987), many physicians reported that their experience of suffering deepened their understanding of patients. Some were quite open with patients, and others were reticent. Some with obvious physical sequelae (such as an amputation) mentioned their patients' acceptance of and accommodation to whatever changes they needed to make in the style and technique of their practice. A few reported that their specific experience was helpful in advising patients undergoing similar illnesses. The opportunity to talk more meaningfully to very sick children and young adults about death was especially important.

> During the months following the diagnosis of Hodgkin's, I wore the diagnosis on my sleeve. I felt that it was good for me and good for the children in oncology clinic for me to speak to newly diagnosed patients with Hodgkin's so I could tell them what to expect. . . . Once, at Christmas time, I sat down with a courageous little 9-year-old with end-stage cardiomyopathy who waited in vain for the availability of a suitable heart for transplant. We spoke frankly of our fear of death and the need for hope. I think she supported me as much as I did her.
>
> More recently I discussed my illness frankly with a 20-year-old with life-threatening arrhythmias. The side effect of the investigational antiarrhythmic agent became so severe that he decided he could no longer endure it. We discussed the issue of longevity versus quality of life, and I felt myself able to communicate at a different level than I could have a few years ago. (Kleinman, 1987, p. 315)

The physician in my group with a history of addiction regarded his disclosure to an addicted patient as personally therapeutic: it was another step in his journey away from the abyss. The idea of healing oneself through healing others is central to the concept of the "wounded healer":[9] "Making one's own wounds a source of healing, therefore, does not call for sharing of superficial pains but for a constant willingness to see one's own pain and suffering as rising from the depth of the human condition which all men [*sic*] share" (Nouwen, 1979, p. 88).

The ability to recognize from one's own experience of pain the universality of suffering is a central theme in John Berger's description of John Sassall, a British general practitioner who became depressed in the course of years of practice. He became unable to concentrate or to meet the demands of his work. Sassall's illness led him to abandon the accepted code:

> But he can only partially overcome his conviction of inadequacy by admitting it. And so, to those of his patients who are in a state to be able to accept his confession, he admits his crisis. He throws himself on the mercy of their tolerance. He depends on the fact that their demands are minimal. The circle is complete. And, as often, the completed circle is the seal of conscientious suffering. (Berger & Mohr, 1976, pp. 146–47)

The roles reverse; the doctor reveals himself as a suffering human being. Such sharing cannot be recommended in routine medical practice, yet we must try to comprehend it. Berger's portrayal of Sassall tells us why such sharing might occur: a lifetime of general practice in a small community sometimes creates relationships that transcend the classic boundaries between doctor and patient. But the healing of the doctor does not take place only because of an abstract joining with humanity. Rather, the doctor's vulnerability, in the context of a relationship, enables the patient's own healing powers to emerge (Miller & Baldwin, 1987). With some trepidation, I will offer an example from my own practice.

Fourteen years ago, I began taking care of Margaret O'Donnell, then a fifty-year-old receptionist married to a retired man nineteen years older. They had married a few years earlier, after the death of his first wife. From time to time she mentioned her husband's gradual aging and increased dependence on her. When I first met her, I was single and living alone. Subsequently, I came to live with and have two children with a man nineteen years older than I am. Mrs. O'Donnell's experience took on a new relevance for me. My first pregnancy prompted many questions from longtime patients about my spouse; to Mrs. O'Donnell I confided the coincidence about the nineteen-year difference in ages between us and our partners. More important, I let her know that I saw her as a resource for me in understanding how my life might be in the future.

Seven years ago, her husband had a sudden stroke and died. Initially, she made more visits to see me, but they tapered off as she gradually became accustomed to her life alone. For myself, I learned that the loss I dread can be survived. And I have acknowledged to her from time to time that working with her has been healing for me. Although it is not entirely clear to me how my disclosures have affected our relationship, I sense that she feels appreciated for having offered me something valuable. (Upon reading this paragraph in manuscript, she wrote, "If I have helped you in any way, that makes me happier to think that I was able to help 'my doctor and dear friend.'")

SELF-DISCLOSURE IN RELATION

Initially, the questions surrounding self-disclosure appear complex and risky. Yet the clinicians with whom I spoke did not seem to find the process mysterious. The picture of the doctor-patient relationship that emerges from their stories is of a highly personal interaction between two individuals "with a history and a future" (Ransom & Vandervoort, 1973). The predisposition toward mutuality in the work of these doctors reveals an underlying relational view of the doctor-patient relationship. Thus, what one tells the patient about oneself in long-term work is a specific example of being-in-relation. Being-in-relation, for a doctor, as in any other relationship, means knowing when to introduce one's own point of view and experience and when to attend to the needs and concerns of the other.

The doctors with whom I spoke believed that their disclosures fostered a sense of intimacy and reciprocity with patients. Carmichael proposes what he calls the relational model to describe the quality of this connection; for him, the word *family* in "family medicine" pertains not to the unit of care but rather to the kind of relationship established between doctor and patient. He characterizes the elements of the family relationship as affinity, intimacy, reciprocity, and continuity. "Essential to [intimacy] is a degree of openness and willingness to acknowledge one's vulnerability to others. Exposing one's unprotected parts in a family relationship is not submission but evidence of trust." Reciprocity is "a sharing between members that gives rise to an interdependence. The reliance on each other is not from weakness but is accomplished to attain greater strength" (1976, p. 562).

Valuing closeness and reciprocity, we can see why, in a relationship already characterized by affinity and continuity, doctors would choose to talk about themselves with patients. Offering personal news or responding to appropriate questions are spontaneous gestures that show the practitioner to be an ordinary person. Within this context, patients' questions about a doctor's personal life or habits may serve as a way to determine whether the doctor understands and can be trusted. Such disclosures, even with all their potential to confuse boundaries and aggravate the power difference, also have the potential to enhance intimacy and reciprocity by showing that the clinician engages personally in the relationship. The disclosures offered above strongly support Carmichael's relational model of the doctor-patient relationship, which presaged the more complex appreciation of the clinical relationship in self-in-relation theory. This theory offers an understanding of why mutuality is essential to clinicians: it reveals them as relational beings, not isolated individuals or entities. The practice of empathy benefits both parties and transforms the clinician as well: "The movement toward the other's differentness is actually central to growth in relationships and also can provide a powerful sense of validation for both self and other. Growth occurs because as I stretch to match or understand your experience, something new is acknowledged or grows in me. . . . I am touched by your experience" (Jordan, 1991b, p. 89).

Self-disclosure reflects physicians' commitment to grow and stretch and to be touched in their relationships with patients over the years. Disclosing personal experiences to patients entrusts them with privileged information that itself conveys respect and may make it easier for them to share both their positive and negative experiences in return. The clinician who sees herself or himself within a relational context need not assume an absolute bar on self-disclosure but rather can discover with his or her patients the appropriate level of self-disclosure with each one, with each patient's family, and within the community. Such disclosures take place within a "flexible frame" of therapeutic action, consistent with the doctor's understanding of himself or herself within a wider personal and community context (Brown, 1991a). Nevertheless, the ethical commitment underlying such disclosures must be to the empowerment of the patient.

Shared experience can be a source of empowerment for both patients and physicians with illnesses and disabilities. The spread of self-help consciousness to physicians may result in a new form of sharing from doctor to patient: doctors with disabilities are emerging from silence to form organizations such as the Society of Handicapped Physicians. The potential for reciprocity through mutual sharing between such physicians and patients with similar disabilities is theoretically very strong. In this chapter, however, I have focused not on physician illness or disability but on the kind of sharing by physicians that emerges in the context of two people coming to know each other in ordinary care—that is, care by unremarkable physicians in the course of their daily work with patients over the years.

Self-disclosure by doctors engaged in long-term relationships with patients shows how the use of oneself as a person can foster intimacy and reciprocity—two themes in a relational understanding of doctoring. Revealing oneself to another is then one step in a process of mutuality. When the clinician is committed to the empowerment of the patient, disclosures can bring about mutual realizations, for both doctor and patient. Such doctoring can be seen as typical of feminist practice—a coherent, cooperative activity rather than a self-other opposition (Whitbeck, 1983).

The doctor who shares the experiences of growing and suffering with patients becomes more of a human being in their eyes. Major events in the doctor's life, such as pregnancy and childbirth, the death of a parent, and common illness, make her or him credible as a real person who faces the same life events as patients, despite differences in class or education. Patients' responses of joy, sympathy, or well-wishing demonstrate a giving-back, a reciprocal caring for the doctor. Sharing the stigma of sickness, disability, emotional illness, or addiction in the context of an ongoing relationship reveals the doctor as an authentic person, unafraid to reveal his or her reality to another human being. As a manifestation of intimacy and reciprocity, the doctor's disclosure is a powerful force for growth in the relationship. As we see in the next two chapters, new visions of caring and power in clinical work are essential for the relationship to serve patients' empowerment.

CHAPTER 9

Caring-in-Relation

I HAVE BEEN PRACTICING in one place for twenty years. It is clear to me that the meaning of caring for patients I have known during those years is different from the caring that goes on when I meet a person for the first time, or the meaning of caring as an abstract idea. I would like to talk about the meaning of caring in the context of long-term clinical relationships as I have known them, then look at the relevance of that discussion to clinical caring in other situations.

The researchers who study doctor-patient communication often mix data on first encounters and later encounters between doctors and patients and rarely look at the length of relationship as a variable in clinical conversations (see Roter, Hall, & Katz, 1988, for a review of this area). However, when Bertakis and Callahan (1992) compared conversations with established patients and those with new patients, differences emerged. (New patients were those who had not been seen at the clinic for over two years and who were seeing the physician for the first time; established patients were seeing their primary care physician.) On return visits, doctors spend more time chatting, counseling, and discussing health promotion activities. They are also more likely to review prior findings in the patient's history, exam, and laboratory work and to spend more time talking over previously recommended treatments and their effects than they do with new patients. They are less likely to structure the interactions, and they spend less time discussing family history or the use of alcohol and tobacco (Bertakis & Callahan, 1992).[1] The doctors in this study were second and third year family practice residents who could have known their patients for three years at the most. How much greater might the differences be in much longer term relationships? I must surely be different with a patient I have known for almost half my life, and patients themselves say that they feel different with a doctor they have known for many years, sometimes their whole lives.

Mrs. Power, a woman I had known for fifteen years, recently died at home from lung cancer that had spread to her brain. When I first knew her, she had already had three back operations for chronic pain. During our first years, we worked on how to manage her back pain without codeine or tranquilizers. After the diagnosis of her cancer, she had made it clear that her main issue was to be able to live free of pain. Over a six-week period, Mrs. Power remained alert but gradually became more and more bedridden and more dependent on morphine. The hospice nurse made daily visits, arranged for all of the medications and supplies she needed, and spoke with me almost every day. I made house calls twice a week, usually once on the weekend. Twice I brought my nine-year-old daughter, Addie. On one visit Mrs. Power gave her a bookmark she had embroidered. Addie, in turn sewed Mrs. Power a tiny cloth bag and placed a polished stone in it. She brought Mrs. Power this gift three days before she died.

At one point during the six weeks, I spent two days at a national meeting where I met with Naomi Remen, an internist who works with cancer patients in California. Mrs. Power was on my mind, and I made time to talk to Naomi about the new things I had learned about her since attending her at home. I had found out that for years Mrs. Power felt rejected, manipulated, and used by her ninety-two-year-old mother. Now, at the point of dying, Mrs. Power and her husband had finally been accepted into housing for the elderly, in the same building as her mother. And now she was dying. Her miserly mother was thriving at ninety-two, and she was dying. It was all so unfair. Mrs. Power, and to some extent her husband, were preoccupied with their anger. I was feeling somewhat guilty for not having known all this about my patient, despite having known her for so many years. Her years of back pain made sense in view of her enormous anger. I must have conveyed my sense of inadequacy to Naomi. For whatever reason, she offered this suggestion: "I give people my phone number and tell them they can call me in the middle of the night when they get scared. I also tell them, when I leave, 'I'll be thinking about you.'" I took home these two pieces of advice.

On my next visit, I asked Mrs. Power, who had proudly shown me her oil paintings decorating her bedroom, if she would paint me an impression of her mother. I remembered to tell her husband that he could call me at home. The next time I visited, they proudly showed me the small canvas that she had completed with the help of her daughter-in-law. Swirling, dark khaki-colored curves surrounded a blackness in the center. That, she told me, was her mother's pocketbook! I asked her then if she thought that being so angry at her mother had anything to do with how hard it was to recover from her back problem. She said, "Of course, feeling so mad all the time." We were all proud of that painting—me for thinking of it, Mrs. Power for completing it, her husband because it enabled her to vent, finally, her anger and get on with saying goodbye.

The time grew nearer. Naomi had told me that in China the same specialist is both obstetrician and oncologist. It makes sense. As with attending births, attending this death had a rhythm. I was a part of that rhythm, and it was a part of me. One evening Mr. Power called, urgency in his voice: "Please, can you come over now?" At their apartment, I found that she was moving in and out of consciousness. She surfaced briefly to acknowledge me, then withdrew again. She had probably had a seizure and rolled her eyes, frightening him. I stayed a while and promised to return when he called. I knew it would be soon. I called in the morning, and she was stable. She was still holding in the evening. At 6:00 o'clock the next morning the phone rang. She was gone. I went over and pronounced her. I sat with Mr. Power and his son and daughter-in-law for a while in the early light. I called the other son, who lived at a distance. We sat in the living room, and she lay in the bedroom. It was like before, only different. They were relieved and sad, yet glad about how they had done it. They planned the wake for that evening. Later that morning, a woman from the funeral parlor brought me the death certificate to sign. Cause of death: lung cancer and terminal anger?

I brought both my children to the wake. Addie was very sad. She looked thoughtfully at the photograph of a happy Mrs. Power on the casket and then sat quietly feeling the loss. My almost five-year-old son Eli brought his Legos and asked lots of questions about what would happen to the body. He looked at the photograph and placed his Legos on top of the casket. It looked as if he wanted to give her a present too. Mr. Power looked over at me and laughed. We did a lot of hugging, and I took the children home.

Yes, it was a lot like a delivery. And, as with births, I am changed by it, perhaps more so because I was more a part of this passage than I am with some births. The visits, the cloth bag, the painting, the phone calls, the Legos—connecting points among persons-in-relation.

My daily encounters with patients are embedded in my relationships with them. A man comes in with new visual symptoms. As he talks, I remember attending the delivery of his only child fourteen years before. For reasons unclear to me, his wife and daughter now go elsewhere for their health care. Somehow the "fit" with our clinic is better for him. I remember making a house call on his blind eighty-year-old mother. I can clearly remember innumerable conversations with him. This time we puzzle together over the possibility that his new symptom holds some serious portent. I order tests that turn out to be normal. The symptoms gradually disappear. Several months later, he reminds me that it is time to make another house call on his mother. This time I meet his sister, who lets me in. I learn more about the family. In this uneven and almost haphazard way, my relationship with this patient grows and strengthens. Time is an essential ingredient. Over the years, of course, many patients have moved, many have gone through changes in insurance coverage, which controls where they may obtain medical care, and others have been discouraged by the cumbersome telephone and appointment system at our health center. Some may have found my personality or my personal style (of dress or speech or practice) a poor match for their expectations. Some may have found a specialty model of health care more to their liking. For others, my part-time status—essential to me to be able to write—may have been the final difficulty that pushed them to go elsewhere. But with that group of patients whom I have known for twenty years I have sustained relationships characterized by caring—mutual caring, in fact, although here I will concern myself only with my caring.

It is caring within the context of these long-term relationships that I wish to explore. Mayeroff uses the term "devotion" to refer to the aspect of caring that extends across time to "a novel and unforeseeable future" (1965, p. 466). Devotion, he says, is not optional; it is a necessary ingredient in caring, as it is in friendship. He is not alluding to "slavish" devotion; rather, he means commitment in the face of uncertainty. A clinician's devotion is clearly not a one-way connection. Years of knowing each other create the possibility that a relational kind of medicine, perhaps not acknowledged at the outset, may develop. Unfortunately, there are few narratives of a physician's long tenure in a specific community. (Huygen, 1982, and Berger & Mohr, 1976, are exceptions.) As a result, the theme of caring-in-relation is largely undeveloped in medicine. When caring is addressed, human separateness, not relatedness, is a basic assumption.

CARING IN MEDICINE

In 1926 Francis Weld Peabody, an upper-class, Harvard-trained Boston physician, gave the public lecture that is the source of his much-quoted statement, "The secret of the care of the patient is in caring for the patient" (1927, p. 882). Peabody felt that medical care in the hospital was disease-focused and impersonal, but that at the patient's home it cannot be.

> The treatment of a disease may be entirely impersonal; the care of a patient must be completely personal. The significance of the intimate personal relationship between physician and patient cannot be too strongly emphasized, for in an extraordinarily large number of cases both the diagnosis and treatment are directly dependent on it, and the failure of the young physician to establish this relationship accounts for much of his ineffectiveness in the care of patients. (1927, p. 877)

Peabody's plea can be viewed as a hearkening back to a more "feminine" nineteenth-century vision of the doctor-patient relationship (More, 1994). Yet Peabody appealed to the empiricism of his listeners: neglecting personal factors, he argued, is as "unscientific" as not controlling for all the variables. Caring was important to Peabody because it was more effective and more scientific. By "personal" he seems to have meant that the doctor shows an interest in the patient's personal life. Peabody advised medical students:

> Make time to have little talks with [the patient]—and these talks need not always be about his symptoms. Remember that you want to know him as a man, and this means you must know about his family and friends, his work and his play. What kind of a person is he—cheerful, depressed, introspective, careless, conscientious, mentally keen or dull? Look out for all the little incidental things that you can do for his comfort. These, too, are a part of "the care of the patient." (1927, p. 881)

Peabody did not comment on how such encounters affect the doctor himself or herself. Though he stated that the personal bond with the patient is the deepest satisfaction in medicine, he implied that caring means finding out about the patient in detail and in this way showing that you care. This kind of caring is devoid of mutuality; it is separate caring.

Peabody was of two minds about caring. On the one hand, it was the effective scientific instrument of an elite professional. It required going out of your way to have little chats and make patients comfortable. It was vastly enhanced by house calls, which revealed the basic facts about a person's life. Inherent in these descriptions of caring is a sense of the enormous class difference between Peabody and the majority of his patients. With patients, Peabody always remained completely in charge.

On the other hand, Peabody himself was a patient as well as a physician. Perhaps his understanding of the need for a gentler, less masculinist view of care came from his vulnerability as a patient at the mercy of his disease. When he gave the lecture quoted earlier, he was already terminally ill with the cancer that would kill him within a few months. His father noted in his memoirs: "To those who listened to the address, the scene was particularly touching; for they knew, as he did, that he spoke from out of the shadow of disease, and that each allusion to the patient as a person, rather than as a 'case,' carried an unspoken and poignant reference" (quoted in Scannell, 1986–87, p. 47). It was clear to Peabody's father and to his physician friends that his understanding of the need for doctoring to be personal came from his own experience of being sick. Peabody had the good fortune to be friends with his physicians; they knew him well and visited him at home frequently. They joined him for tea in the garden with his family. Caring in that context did not require "little talks" for them to find out about him. Neither science nor effectiveness fueled the care of Peabody as patient. Rather, mutuality was characteristic of the care he received. He talked about caring as a personal relationship because he was a patient privileged to know and be known by his doctors. Powerless over his disease, he could identify with the more "feminine" vision of care that derived from an era when physicians had little they could do for patients. But as an influential physician himself, his recommendations on caring conveyed a clear and "masculine" demarcation between doctor and patient. His words on caring reflect this split in his own understanding of caring.

More recently, Edmund Pellegrino (1985) has pointed out that caring is "foundational" to medicine. He distinguishes four senses of care: (1) compassion, being touched by the caring person; (2) doing for others what they cannot do, *nursing* the sick; (3) taking care of the medical problem; and (4) taking care in the sense of doing it well, conscientiously and competently. Integrating these forms of care is a moral obligation arising "out of the special human relationship that binds one who is ill to one who offers to help" (p. 13). Caring is also a moral obligation because the patient is vulnerable and the doctor is powerful in an inherently unequal relationship. The vulnerability of the patient requires that the relationship not be based on mutual self-interest or contract but on "profession" and trust. By profession he means "the promise the healer makes when he or she enters into the relationship with the person who is ill" (p. 13). The "act of medicine" is the link between the patient who is ill and seeking help and the doctor's vow of profession. For Pellegrino, the act of medicine constitutes "the moment of clinical truth," the collaborative decision about what to do. That decision comprises both the "right" decision, the one that, following the cure model, is technically correct, and the good decision, the one that fits into the patient's way of life and self-definition as a person.

To Pellegrino, there are three components to the good of the patient: (1) what is biomedically good, or "medically indicated," (2) what the patient conceives of as good within the context of his or her own life, and (3) the good of the patient as a person who has the human freedom to make his or her own choice. The physician should act to preserve patients' capacity "to act in a fully human way—that is, to express and act on their perception of their own good. That good is owed all patients, simply because they are human" (1985, p. 24). But something is missing here. How does the doctor find out what fits into a patient's way of life or how they define themselves as a person? How does the doctor carry out the promise? We see here that caring must be moral because it deals with a power imbalance, but we do not see how the parties are in relation. Caring arises out of the moral obligation to be good, out of the physician's act of profession and attempts to tailor his or her acts to serve each unique patient. What is good, and therefore what is caring, derives from the patient's autonomy. This kind of good is predicated on human separateness, not on relatedness. Even though Pellegrino claims a "special human relationship" binding the one caring to the one who is sick, his doctor and patient are quite separate, even as separate as Peabody's medical student and patient.

Separateness underlies these medical views of caring and persists today despite the new respect for patients' experience. Paying attention to what the patient is experiencing is a crucial element in contemporary patient-centered medicine. This approach explores patients' belief systems to discover their explanatory models of illness. It investigates what the patient may be feeling: fear, shame, and loss as well as pain. Michael Balint (1961), who pioneered the investigation into the meaning of the symptoms of patients of general practitioners, stated that the main task of this "whole-person medicine" is "to understand the meaning for the person of the complaints and illness that he offers to his doctor. The aim of therapy will then be to enable the patient to understand himself, find a better solution for the problem facing him, and thus achieve the integration which has not developed or has broken down because of disturbed relationship of the individual with his environment" (p. 42). Balint never considered the idea that this process should promote the involvement of doctor with patient; rather, he believed that the doctor could gain therapeutic efficacy by recognizing his or her own emotional responses and the interplay between those responses and the patient's behavior. The doctor could then notice and control otherwise automatic reactions. The patient's patterns would emerge more clearly, "help[ing] the doctor to become *still less emotionally involved*, thereby opening more possibilities for planned therapeutic interventions" (p. 206, my emphasis). For Balint, the discovery of the meaning of the illness to the patient and of the clinician's own responses promotes distance and prevents emotional involvement. Separateness is essential to the pursuit of the therapeutic end.

Some physicians do identify separateness as a problem (Baron, 1981, 1985). Bemoaning the distance that has come to typify the relation between doctor and patient, Baron locates the separateness between the doctor's understanding and the patient's experience in "vocational distance" (1981, p. 14). Knowledge available to ordinary human beings is no longer available to doctors, since they have become "ignorant of knowledge they already possess" (p. 16). Baron suggests that inquiry into the phenomenological world of the patient transforms the doctor because it puts him or her back in touch with the reality of human suffering. His goal is to remedy the personal isolation that plagues him as a doctor. If physicians can come to recognize patients' experience and to "make this way of being our own," perhaps they can overcome the distance between themselves and others (p. 16). Although Baron longs to "bridge clinical distance" (1981), he views persons as separate atoms that, at best, can move closer together but are never connected. He seeks to recover his own humanity through the internal cognitive process of encountering the patient's reality, not through any kind of relationship.

This approach to the doctor's inquiry suggests only what questions a doctor might ask of a patient, not what might happen to the relationship when the doctor asks them, nor what happens when the doctor, in touch with this reality, cares about the patient whose reality it is. For instance, suppose I learn to ask the questions that allow me to find out that my patient is being battered by her husband. Should I really be transformed by getting in touch with the "reality" of her suffering? Or should I become activated to support her attempts to gain safety, thereby gaining respect for her strength and endurance?

In contemporary medicine, the focus on communication—specific elements of behavior that can be observed and counted—sidesteps the relationship. The focus on behavior may be useful in educational settings: it gives trainees a clear idea of how they should conduct interviews and how they should comport themselves with patients. It addresses both cognitive omissions (failure to see the patient's point of view), which result in one-sided and incoherent interaction (Baron, 1985), and technical omissions (failure to ask the right questions or to engage in the right proprieties), which result in inadequate information and nonempathic communication (Platt & McMath, 1979). Correction of these deficiencies through improved communication skills *can* improve patient care and enhance patient satisfaction. But communication skills do not constitute the doctor-patient relationship. As we saw in chapter 7, even empathy can be taught as a technique: the trainee is enjoined to *identify* the patient's feelings (not *identify with* the patient's feelings) with an expectation that such an approach will encourage the patient to be more open with the doctor. The expectation is that the doctor will thus acquire more and better information to guide the treatment plan. In this "separate" view of empathy, the doctor offers technique, not responsiveness. In fact, the focus on cognition and communication technique distracts both parties from more directly considering the relationship—that is, from exploring the tentative bonds between themselves as human beings, with all their strengths and frailties.

In a relational approach, caring is a form of joining or connectedness between persons. This connection changes how clinicians see themselves in the world and how they feel about patients. Nel Noddings, a philosopher of education, describes the "displacement of interest from my own reality to the reality of the other. . . . When I am in this sort of relationship with another, when the other's reality becomes a real possibility for me, I care" (1984, p. 14). Put another way, what the patient tells me affects me, at times even transforms me, and the transformed clinician I become is newly capable of deeper relationships with this patient and others. The one cared for is aware of that mutuality and of its centrality in the relationship. Caring creates a kind of self-knowledge that offers "the capacity to be moved, to be inspired or to receive strength from the qualities we discern in people with whom we are in relations" (Mullett, 1987, p. 320).

A TRANSFORMED UNDERSTANDING OF RESPECT

For medicine to adopt a relational understanding of caring, commonly used words and concepts must be reexamined and reinterpreted. We saw in chapter 7 how separateness governs the interpretation of empathy in medical thought and limits what we mean by "knowing." Respect, like empathy, is another presumed virtue or good in the doctor-patient relationship and is central to any understanding of caring. Respect has also been variously interpreted: as a hallmark of human separateness, and as a measure of human connection. Three philosophers, Robin Dillon (1992), Lorraine Code (1987), and Marilyn Friedman (1987a), have clarified these different understandings of respect. Friedman points out that the perspective of care generates a view of respect that contrasts with the view of respect from the justice perspective:[2]

> The insight that each person needs some others in her life who recognize, respect, and cherish her particularity with its richness and wholeness is the distinctive motivating vision of the "care" perspective. The sort of respect for person which grows out of this vision is not the abstract respect which is owed to all persons in virtue of their common humanity, but a respect for individual worth, merit, need, or even idiosyncracy. It is a form of respect which involves admiration and cherishing, when the distinctive qualities are valued intrinsically, and which, at the least, involves toleration when the distinctive qualities are not valued intrinsically. (1987a, p. 108)

Dillon calls these two kinds of respect "recognition respect" and "care respect." Recognition respect recognizes the equal worth of the other. It is the respect accorded to all persons, and it requires our acknowledgment that the personhood of the other puts certain moral constraints on our behavior. One exercise of recognition respect would be to leave a person alone to develop and use her own capacities, respecting her rights to live her own life. Recognition respect applies to any person, regardless of his or her particularities, and does not differ from person to person.

It is recognition respect that underlies exhortations to medical students to treat patients "with respect." Respect in this setting is shown in the concrete behaviors associated with basic politeness, such as ensuring that patients and family members are comfortable, ensuring patients' privacy, limiting interruptions, and, in interviews, offering time for questions. Patients list such examples of recognition respect when asked to describe what kind of treatment they prefer (Mathews & Feinstein, 1988). This respect derives from an appreciation of what is just in health care treatment and forms the basis of the patient bill of rights. It is the respect we would accord to any human being, not only to one human being in particular. What is startling is how often the basic elements of recognition respect are lost in medical settings, and how grateful patients are when they are accorded even this minimal kind of respect.

In contrast to recognition respect, care respect sees a person not as an abstract individual but as a particular person who has a unique way of looking at himself or herself and the world. Someone showing care respect knows about the other person's self-definition and tries to see the world from that viewpoint, "valuing an individual in her specificity, seeking to understand her in her own terms, and caring about and seeking to promote her well-being" (Dillon, 1992, p. 74). Whereas recognition respect aims to preserve autonomy and self-sufficiency, care respect goes beyond noninterference to seeing and supporting the other in her or his life, to caring about the other's projects and trying to promote her or his good. Recognition respect is shown by distancing from and leaving the other alone, whereas care respect appreciates the individuality of the other; it is not remote from the other. To someone exercising care respect, it makes a difference which person you show it toward because you treat each person you know differently. "Care respect has the resources to maintain a constructive tension between regarding each person as *just as valuable* as every other person and regarding this individual as *special*" (Dillon, 1992, pp. 74–75).

The distinction between "just as valuable" and "special" struck home recently when a visiting medical student commented that all my patients were "so interesting, so special." The patients she had seen with me were not particularly unusual; what she was noticing that was unusual to her was how well we knew each other. In the context of a caring relationship, each of my patients feels special, not just to me but also to an outside observer. Her observation supports the conclusion that if care respect is to be grounded in the particularity of the other, it must clearly involve *knowing* the person (Code, 1987). Edmund Pellegrino (1982, 1985) holds that this is true for medicine; Patricia Benner argues for it in nursing: "Knowing a patient is central to the ethics of care and responsibility" (1991, p. 3). Respect and empathy, crucial elements of a relational view of caring, require knowing, a kind of knowing based on human connection. To get specific about what this might mean, I want to examine a concept familiar to clinicians: reassurance.

REASSURANCE

Traditionally, the doctor offered reassurance to the patient by remaining unruffled. Osler called this imperturbability *Aequanimitas*, "coolness and presence of mind under all circumstances, calmness amid storm, clearness of judgment in moments of great peril, immobility, impassiveness, or, to use an old expressive word, *phlegm*" (1932, p. 4). Osler's male physician showed no indecision, worry, or emotion on his face. He was inscrutable. Osler admitted that the physician who practiced this stance could be accused of hardness, but he thought this attribute was essential "in the exercise of a calm judgment, and in carrying out delicate operations" (p. 5). This is indeed the portrait of the patriarchal doctor of old.

Today's clinicians, who can engage in appropriate communication skills to reassure patients, may eschew inscrutability. Reassurance therapy (for patients with benign diseases) breaks down neatly into an orderly sequence of six steps: (1) elicit a detailed description of the symptom, (2) elicit the affective meaning of the symptom, (3) examine the patient, (4) make a diagnosis, (5) explain the symptom, and finally, (6) reassure the patient (Sapira, 1972). It is in the step of eliciting the affective meaning of the symptom that we again see a communication skill replacing a relationship. "Tell me more about how this symptom worries you" is the recipe. Sapira acknowledges that long-term relationships offer more potential for "superior" reassurance, but he asserts that the steps outlined above lead to optimal reassurance even when doctor and patient are strangers.[3]

In contrast to the stranger model of medicine, the relational framework enables reassurance to draw its meaning from the context of a long-term and ongoing clinical relationship. Patients can be reassured as they need to be because they are known in the setting of their lives and in the history of their specific relationship with the clinician. I may know how the problem of keeping a sick child at home will change a family's daily routine—for instance, that the mother may have to lose a day's work. I may remember the last time the mother had allergies in the fall or sinusitis in the winter. We may be able to measure whether the problem this time is as bad or worse than the last time. I am acknowledging that the patient is special and unique at the same time that I am placing her illness in perspective. Or I may share my familiarity with community illness: "You have the flu that's going around." Or I may draw on my steadfastness and dependability to reassure: "I want to see you again if it's not better by Monday." In such a statement, I am giving the patient a timetable of expectations, showing a willingness to recheck my diagnosis at a later point, and making a personal commitment to stick with the patient through the illness.

Knowing the patient means knowing that he or she may feel judged by the clinician. Patients feel judged for both what they have done and what they have not done. Mothers feel that keeping children healthy is their duty, and that sickness in a child suggests they may have been negligent (Korsch, Freemon, & Negrete, 1971). Worrying about being judged may make patients feel defensive, guilty, or hostile. In an era when illness is increasingly blamed on patients for what they have done (smoking, drinking, drug use, unprotected intercourse, and so on) or not done (exercise, diet, avoiding stress, rest), reassurance certainly requires knowing how and whether a particular patient is likely to feel judged. Often the clinician will not be able to anticipate exactly what past experience explains the patient's choices and feelings of judgment.

I took the opportunity at a follow-up visit for a miscarriage to suggest a complete physical exam to Sheryl Sharmat. I knew from terse acknowledgments during encounters over the years that she had been physically and sexually abused by a relative during childhood and raped by an acquaintance in adolescence. She had always been overweight and probably reached sexual maturity at a young age. For as long as I had known her (fifteen years), she had avoided undressing for physical examinations and refused pelvic exams. At the end of her only previous pregnancy, she arrived at the hospital in labor having had no prenatal care. She was often critical of her child, hypercritical of herself, and defensive about her smoking, her weight, and her parenting. I knew that she was in a stable relationship with a man she cared for and that she had talked to him about her previous experiences. She had been excited about the new pregnancy and saddened by the miscarriage.

When she agreed to my suggestion of a complete exam, I was pleased. I took it as a measure of progress in her struggle to come to terms with her past abuse. Beginning, as usual, at the top, I noticed yet again her mutilated and decayed teeth. I knew she was unemployed, without insurance, with little likelihood of being able to pay for dental care. I thought money was the issue. But her teeth were far worse than most. She must have been in pain with all those broken pieces. Running the risk that she would take my question as a criticism, I asked, "Where are you at with dental care?" Despite what I did know, I was totally unprepared for her answer.

"I'm terrified of dentists. . . . I was sexually abused by a dentist when I was little."

"Oh, Sheryl, not that too," I lamented. "Can you tell me about it?"

"He would feel me up when I was in the chair."

"Did it happen once or a lot of times?"

"A lot of times."

"Did you tell your mother?"

"No. He told me he would pull out every tooth in my mouth if I told."

"Oh God. You never told me about this."

"No. I don't like to think about it. I don't want to talk about it any more."

"It was good you told me. I never knew why you never got your teeth fixed. . . . Would you see a female dentist?"

"Yeah. Are there any?"

I made her an appointment with a female dentist. She gave me permission to tell the dentist of her prior experience. We set a goal that she would at least keep the appointment, but that she did not have to sit in the chair or have any treatment. After a certain amount of rehearsing, she was able to keep the appointment and undergo a cleaning and evaluation.

With Sheryl, knowing the patient was not enough; I thought I knew her. But knowing meant being prepared to find out more. Suspending judgment (another element of care respect) about her dental care let me into another realm of her experience, one that had been previously sealed to me by virtue of her shame and my assumptions about routine health care.

In reconsidering the concept of reassurance, we can certainly agree that an essential step in reassurance is finding out what the patient is concerned about, including what the symptom means to the patient and what feelings it brings up. This step is integral to any patient-centered clinical method. But when we go to examine feelings, we must be prepared to encounter fear and shame, perhaps over abuse or mutilation. Just asking for the "affective meaning of the symptom" cannot itself create a safe enough environment (that is, a relationship) in which a patient can reveal to us the source of his or her shame. Fifteen years and dozens of encounters had not prepared me for Sheryl's fears. It was, I think, my knowledge of her as a survivor, and her entrenched way of defending herself, that let me know that I should approach the matter of her teeth with care.

In discussions of reassurance, no one talks much about how to address fear. Clinicians have various ploys. One standard technique to address the patient's fears is declaration: no, this is not scarlet fever. Our authority, our expertise, the power of our personality, are the forces that shore up this form of reassurance. It is true because we say so. The drawback to this method is the drawback to all forms of authoritarianism: authorities can be and often are wrong. A person distrustful of authorities is unlikely to find such declarations reassuring and more often than not may look elsewhere for evidence or support to disprove them.

Another method is to join our declaration to some information: for example, "This cough is not pneumonia because there is no fever and the sputum is not purulent." Here we let the patient in on our thought process, on how we arrived at our conclusion that we are not worried that the patient's symptoms indicate pneumonia. This method gives the patient more tools with which to sort out symptoms the next time, but it also has the potential negative side effect of implying that the patient is stupid: how silly of you to worry about pneumonia with no fever and no phlegm! Individual patients require different answers, different words, different information, td be reassured because they are worried about different things. They may be unaware of their worst fears or unable to state them if asked. Providing information is not a neutral, disconnected activity; for information to succeed in offering reassurance, the clinician must tailor it, through the relationship, to the needs of the patient.

Though not traditionally understood as a form of reassurance, patient education is a way of giving patients the tools to manage their own health and illness and thus to take better care and to reassure themselves.[4] Patients are especially appreciative of clinicians' efforts to provide information. In a meta-analysis of thousands of doctor-patient interactions, the amount of information given by clinicians was the best predictor of patient satisfaction (Hall et al., 1988). (Of course, how information is given is crucial. Is the clinician really trying to explain something, or is she or he handing out a pamphlet as a way to brush off the time-consuming patient?) In fact, doctors strongly underestimate the amount of information that patients want (Strull, Lo, & Charles, 1984). Providing information can show patients that we think they are smart people who can use it; they see us recognizing them as in charge of their own or their children's health care. Even though patients may not take in some or most of the information offered, the act of providing information is a demonstration of at least recognition respect.

For information-providing to show care respect, it must go further. It must be grounded in our knowing of the patient. I use "knowing" rather than "knowledge" because I mean the process of knowing rather than any set of facts about the person. It is one thing to know that a person reads at the fourth-grade level. It is another to understand that she or he is proud of knowing how to read and would appreciate receiving appropriate materials to read.[5] Patient education requires a knowing on the clinician's part that implies caring. One example that clarifies this connection between caring, knowing, and patient education comes from Dru Alvino (1986), a nurse in a neonatal intensive care unit. She describes "informing" as a process of caring—in contrast, for instance, to the duty of obtaining informed consent. She relates the story of a woman who had given permission for innumerable procedures on her premature brain-damaged baby. Over the course of many months, it became clear to Alvino that no one had ever clearly told the mother that her baby would never be normal, would never even be able to sit, hold a bottle, walk, or talk. The doctors had concluded that the woman was just unintelligent because so many doctors had talked to her. Alvino arranged a conference with the mother, social worker, and doctor for the ostensible purpose of obtaining her permission for yet another invasive procedure on the baby. During the meeting, Alvino detailed to the mother exactly how the baby would never be able to function, and for the first time the mother realized that her baby would never be normal. She was then able to decline any further procedures and allow the infant to die.

Alvino traces a sequence to this informing-caring: she first had to recognize the mother's need for care. She found herself thinking during her working hours and during her off hours about the woman's need for information. This kind of recognition reveals a taking-into-herself, a preoccupation with the other (Jordan, 1991b). Second, she recognized in herself her awareness of and respect for the other woman as different from herself, "identity-in-difference" (Mayeroff, 1965). This kind of internal inspection of self-with-other allowed Alvino to arrive at what had not been asked and what had not been said. Only after the recognition and the taking-in was she able to complete the task of informing by offering knowledge, with the intention of bringing about positive change for the sake of the patient. Alvino shows us in the very real world of the neonatal intensive care unit that the apparently cut-and-dried task of offering information for decision-making depends on relational knowing.

FIRST ENCOUNTERS

If we must know people before we can care for them, what does this mean for our relations with strangers? What is the meaning of relational caring if we have no experience with the other person when we greet them as a new patient in the office or as a sick person at the hospital? This situation calls upon the clinician to create a context in which caring can start and to initiate a relationship that nourishes the sense of caring and that may someday call forth all of the clinician's intellect and energy. Some of the elements necessary to create that context are:

Acting as if we consider the other worthy in the first place. The "as if" means that we perform the minimal activities of recognition respect: being courteous, ensuring privacy, and so on. It also means acknowledging that patients require recognition for the achievement of coming for health care. One way to show such recognition is to compliment the patient for what they have done well. With adult patients, a clinician might comment on their timeliness, their attention to detail in their medical care, the good questions they ask, or all that they are doing in their lives. With an adolescent, the clinician might note how well she dresses and grooms her baby—even if the baby's resulting appearance

conflicts with our own standards for gender stereotyping of children—
or how prompt she was for her appointment. There is no one who
comes into our office who does not need and deserve some recognition
of worth for how they are doing in their life; too often, despite our
acknowledgment that we are powerful figures in the lives of our
patients, we neglect to offer the approbation, the compliment that could
convey this positive regard.

Setting the stage. Another way I can prepare for relational caring is to
ask questions that show my interest and help me imagine the patient's
reality: What is your mother's name? (Often this helps me learn how it
is that a patient happened to come to our health center.) What street do
you live on? (This answer helps me imagine how she arrived and what
an office visit might entail.) These questions show her that, to me, she
is not just a person who is interchangeable with any other person and
worthy of impersonal respect, but a certain person, with specific experiences; I am recognizing her specifically.

Assuming growth. I assume that the person before me is in the process
of growing and developing and that even though I do not yet know
what his or her personal project for growth might be, the result of this
interaction with me should be a facilitation of that growth. "To help
another person grow is at least to help him care for something or someone apart from himself, and it involves encouraging and assisting him
to find and create areas of his own in which he is able to care. Also, it is
to help that other person to come to care for himself, and by becoming
responsive to his own need to care to become responsible for his own
life" (Margaret Lock, quoted in Mayeroff, 1971, pp. 10–11). It is neither
unreasonable nor unduly presumptuous to imagine that teenagers
hope to have friends, be liked, find work, be appreciated by parents,
and explore their sexuality. It is not unreasonable to think that a young
mother wishes to be a good mother and to raise a healthy child, nor that
a person recovering from an illness or operation hopes to resume his or
her usual activities. But does a patient need permission to stay home
longer and garner her strength before tackling her full workload, or
does she need to be pushed toward trying again after losing confidence
from being sick? What does growth mean to her? These are the questions that can be answered only by coming to know a person.

THE PATIENT PERSPECTIVE

Separate caring or connected caring—how do patients see it? Empirical
studies in medicine and nursing have approached this question assuming the dominant understanding of caring as a practice of separateness.
For instance, researchers at Yale–New Haven Hospital asked fifty adult
inpatients three questions:

"How do you feel about the doctors' care here?"

"What do you like or dislike about them and what they do for you?"

"What attitudes or behaviors toward you would you like the doctors to have?" (Mathews & Feinstein, 1988, p. 160)

These questions, and the answers they generated, reflect the authors' orientation toward caring as a set of skills—behaviors—that can be acquired.[6] "Responsiveness to patient's concerns" is subdivided into (1) eliciting expectations and desires, (2) inviting opinions, (3) answering questions, and (4) relieving worries (p. 166). "Demonstrating solicitude" toward the patient is composed of taking a personal interest in the patient and viewing him or her as special. Unasked is the question of how you relieve worries or view the patient as special when you do not *know* the person. Absent from a taxonomy of behaviors are ideas like knowing the patient, maintaining a relationship over time, or staying with the patient. "Care" in this setting seems to have nothing to do with relationships.

In a comparable study from nursing, fifty hospitalized patients described an experience in which they felt cared for by a nurse (Brown, 1986). The responses were ordered into themes that often combined into two patterns: first, a linkage between demonstration of professional knowledge and skill, surveillance, and reassuring presence (patients offering this description had usually perceived some kind of emergency in their care); and second, recognition of individual qualities and needs, promotion of autonomy, and spending time. In this pattern, the nurse's focus was not on needs for treatment but on patients' reaction to their condition and decisions. Once again the investigator's formulation of caring highlighted the importance of skills and attitudes.[7] The nurse-patient relationship, although present in the shadows, was secondary.

Patients' appreciation for caring-in-relation can emerge only from research that assumes the centrality of relationships. One study that approaches this understanding is a study of caring as it was perceived by ten women who had experienced a miscarriage. Swanson-Kauffman (1986) used extensive interviews to create five categories of caring in the event of miscarriage: knowing, being with, doing for, enabling, and maintaining belief. "Knowing" referred to seeing the miscarriage through the woman's eyes, to looking "for the personal meaning of the loss in her life" (p. 40), and not in preconceived terms (like "It was nature's way of cleaning up a mistake," and so on). "Being with" meant feeling with the patient and allowing a relationship to develop that felt personal rather than professional. "Doing for" was a matter of doing whatever the patient needed done, *as she would do it for herself* if she had the skills, energy, or health to do it. "Enabling" was the term Swanson-

Kauffman used to mean helping the woman to get through the loss and to grieve. It required understanding the meaning of the miscarriage to the patient. "Maintaining belief" referred to the clinician's trust in the woman's capacity to get through the loss and to choose whether or not to try getting pregnant again. In contrast to previous studies, Swanson-Kauffman approached a relational description of caring, or what I call caring-in-relation. Even Swanson-Kauffman's category that most clearly involves a set of behaviors—"doing for"—puts those actions in the context of the patient's relationship with her healthier self.

This glance at empirical studies of caring suggests that the methodology researchers use to frame patients' views of caring is subject to their assumptions about what constitutes care. Not surprisingly, since all of the researchers were clinicians also involved in the provision of care, their personal definitions were intrinsic to their research. Whether themes are identified that relate to separateness or to in-relation views of caring depends on the orientation of the researchers. Those who had no relationship with the patients they interviewed obtained answers with no relational themes. Swanson-Kauffman, who developed at least a short-term relationship with her subjects in the course of her interviews, discovered relational answers.

Fortunately, medical research is not our only source for understanding patients' longing for relational caring. Two especially articulate lay narratives offer insight into what patients construe "caring" to mean. In *Intoxicated by My Illness* (1992), Anatole Broyard tells us how much he wanted the urologist who took care of his prostate cancer to *see* him, to take him and his prostate seriously:

> I see no reason or need for my doctor to love me—nor would I expect him to suffer with me. I wouldn't demand a lot of my doctor's time: I just wish he would *brood* on my situation for perhaps five minutes, that he would give me his whole mind just once, be *bonded* with me for a brief space, survey my soul as well as my flesh, to get at my illness, for each man is ill in his own way. . . . Just as he orders blood tests and bone scans of my body, I'd like my doctor to scan *me*, to grope for my spirit as well as my prostate. Without some such recognition, I am nothing but my illness. (1992, pp. 44–45)

Broyard longs to be *known*, to be taken into the mind and eye and spirit of the doctor. He wants to be a unique person-in-relation, recognized and known by the other.

In *Heartsounds* (1980), Martha Lear writes passionately about her physician husband pleading with his cardiologists to listen to him. His helplessness had two elements. First, as a physician, he wanted to understand exactly what had happened to him. He kept trying, without success, to make sense of his symptoms—his worsening heart failure and his loss of short-term memory. Second, he wanted them to *hear* his anger and frustration about his postoperative brain damage. Even though he was a white male physician like his doctors, he never felt that they took him seriously as a person. For them, he had ceased to be a real person and had become instead a patient. His doctors, like many others, were unwilling to say, "Things went wrong," or, "You sustained brain damage from low blood pressure," or, "You had another heart attack during surgery." Instead, they took the defensive position of blaming his symptoms on the severity of his heart condition. They tried blithely to *reassure* him without ever hearing what was the matter or addressing the importance of his loss. Both the Broyard and Lear accounts show the desperation for being-in-relation that sickness evokes and medicine evades.

To sum up, medicine has traditionally taken a view of caring characterized by separateness. This view focuses on the behaviors, skills, and attitudes of clinicians in their approach to patients with whom they have little or no connection. A contrasting understanding of caring derives from a view of persons as fundamentally in-relation. Recognizing persons as in-relation compels us to reinterpret what we mean by knowing, empathy, and respect. Commonsense practices like reassurance and patient education take on different, relational meanings in the context of caring-in-relation.

How can we better understand the relational understanding of caring? Theorists in three related fields—mothering, nursing, and teaching—offer specific applications of a relational understanding of caring. Sara Ruddick (1983) considers mothering a "skilled practice" governed by three interests: preservation, growth, and acceptability. Each interest has its parallels in clinical caring. Fostering the growth and preservation of children strongly parallels the promotion of health and healing in patients. We encourage and cherish growth at all ages, from the infant's newest accomplishment to the resolution of a half-century of anger during a terminal illness. By preservation Ruddick means advocating for a child's safety as well as what she calls "holding": "an attitude governed by the priority of keeping over acquiring, of conserving the fragile, of maintaining whatever is at hand and necessary to the child's life" (p. 217). Holding is a particularly apt way of thinking about the need to conserve and garner resources for patients with limited time left to them or with limited energy, such as those with chronic and debilitating illness.

Acceptability, too, is a value in clinical work. Ruddick talks about mothers shaping an acceptable child: "They want the child they produce to be a person whom they themselves, and those closest to them, can appreciate" (1983, p. 220). Do clinicians feel this way about their patients? The answer is sometimes yes, particularly when one needs to share care of the patient with another clinician, nurse, therapist, or specialist. We want our patient to be someone other doctors and nurses will find interesting, worthwhile, and valuable. Sometimes it is necessary to cajole or even beg specialists to accept a patient who does not initially appear to be the sort of person they would like to see. The patient may not speak English, may not be able to pay, or may act in some way that doctors usually frown upon. As the person attached to the patient and trying to obtain the necessary care for her or him, I try to portray my patient in a way that reveals acceptable or good aspects: for instance, highlighting the patient's clinically puzzling illness, or the fact that he or she is particularly deserving. When a patient I know well comes into the hospital in labor and I realize that the staff may view her negatively, I find myself trying to convey enough about her to the nurses to enable them to find something to like about her. Clinicians, like mothers, want those they care for to be acceptable to others because they know that patients will do much better if the receiving practitioner comes to care about them.[8]

Ruddick's view of mothering as "skilled practice" contradicts essentialist notions that mothering is "natural," intuitive, and inherent in women. Likewise, caring in nursing exemplifies "expert human practice" (Benner & Wrubel, 1989, p. 4). Nurses' narrative accounts of real clinical moments reveal their self-reflection while engaged in highly complex interactions with patients. Nurses carry the insights from these paradigm cases as they move on to take care of other patients. "Skilled ethical comportment" includes not just words, beliefs, and values but also stance, touch, and orientation: "Thoughts and feelings fused with physical presence and action" (Benner, 1991, p. 2). The relevance of mothering and nursing to caring-in-relation lies in the understanding of skilled practice. Skilled practice means knowing what to do in relation to a particular person in a particular situation; it is not predictable and cannot be derived from protocols. Caring is not a set of behaviors and communication skills; it is not reducible to technique. It is grounded first in the relationship with the other. From this relationship emerges what skilled practice ought to be with or on behalf of that other.

From these excursions into mothering and nursing we can see that in clinical work caring-in-relation differs from "separate" caring. A focus on the separate and autonomous quality of the patient (and the clinician) turns caring into a matter of the skills and attitudes. When we place the relationship at the center of clinical work, caring takes on a different meaning because it emerges *from* the relationship. The principles of skilled practice in mothering and nursing likewise hold for medical practitioners, even though the exact nature of their skills may be different. With Benner, I would hold that knowing a patient precedes assessing a patient. With Sheryl Sharmat, for example, I found myself gingerly approaching the matter of her dental care from my prior knowledge of her painful identity as an incest survivor. While not expecting yet another disclosure of abuse, I was prepared to support her in her fears of dental care. I offer this as an example of skilled practice. Other more ordinary examples from my work include allowing a seventy-nine-year-old woman to cry about her younger brother dying rather than performing her annual physical exam, and accepting the shoulder and head pain of a woman formerly beaten by her husband without needing to medicate it or investigate it—and opening the possibility of translating the pain into a known and understandable part of her body that she can eventually recover. The skill lies in my relationships with these women; caring enabled me to learn what was problematic and shaped my response to it.

Noddings (1984) argues that caring serves as the foundation for a new kind of ethics. Stepping away from the traditional view of ethics as a matter of the rights and duties of separate individuals adhering to a variety of frameworks (utilitarian, deontological, and so on), Noddings takes the *relation* as ontologically basic, and the caring relation as ethically basic. "Taking *relation* as ontologically basic simply means that we recognize human encounter and affective response as a basic fact of human existence. . . . Both parties contribute to the relation; my caring must somehow be completed in the other if the relation is to be described as caring" (p. 4). Noddings believes that caring requires "engrossment," which may vary in intensity or at times be latent. The attitude of "one-caring" is "readiness to bestow and spend oneself, to make oneself available. . . . The one caring, in caring, is *present* in her acts of caring" (p. 19). She is reactive, responsive, engrossed in the other, receptive. Dispassion and detachment, the virtues of the autonomous individual, are not virtues in the caring ethic.

Noddings sees technique as destructive to caring. She argues that when caring is organized by rules or devolves into problem-solving, the focus shifts from the one cared for to the problem. The resulting pitfall is the "premature switching to a rational-objective mode" that tends toward the abstract (1984, p. 26). When the motivational displacement and engrossment in caring are missing, opportunities for self-interest arise.

> Those entrusted with caring may focus on satisfying the formulated requirements for caretaking and fail to be present in their interactions with the cared-for. Thus caring disappears and only its illusion remains. . . . [Caring must be] re-established and redirected from a fresh base of commitment. Otherwise, we find ourselves deeply, perhaps inextricably, enmeshed in procedures that somehow serve only themselves; our thoughts are separated, completely detached, from the original objects of caring. (p. 26)

This is the answer to Baron's (1981) sense of isolation in clinical distance described earlier—his clinician needs to reestablish caring from a "fresh base of commitment": engrossment in the patient.

This review of recent understandings of caring in mothering, nursing, and teaching points us toward the requirements of caring in clinical relationships. We can begin to elaborate a fuller account of caring and distinguish the essential elements. We can examine in what ways our clinical work already exemplifies those elements.

CARING IS RELATIONAL

Relations are primary; they define what it is to be a person. Caring is not a matter of contract. Making caring definitional changes how we think; the meanings of empathy and respect are transformed by the relational understanding of caring. Empathy comes to imply a mutually changing and reciprocal process, even though the parties are not equal. Clinicians show relational caring by making the patient feel *known*, by paying attention to *meaning*, by expressing real *feeling*, and by practicing *devotion*.

In making people feel *known*, the clinician recognizes them as who they are in their world. This is especially important during the conduct of ordinary care (which tends to become routinized), such as the treatment of upper respiratory infections, ear infections, and lacerations. We acknowledge this specialness by paying attention to individual particularities, by acknowledging the details we know about a patient's life: what floor she lives on, on what street, how it is to go to and come from her home. We do it by knowing enough of what a person's experience is to know that she or he may be reluctant to ask for a needed item ("Do you need any papers filled out?"). We do it by reviewing shared experience: recalling how long we have known each other; remembering family members with the same condition; recalling dates, such as the birth date of a baby relinquished for adoption or the anniversary of the death of a husband who hanged himself in a closet on Halloween.

In attending to *meaning*, we show relational caring by recognizing what the symptom or illness means in the patient's life—for instance, acknowledging that the parent of a croupy infant must have been up all night, or how scary a fall on the bath mat must have been for a seventy-nine-year-old woman who lives alone. We also pay attention to what the treatment will mean. We might ask the mother of a two-year-old who needs antibiotics whether she prefers chewable tablets or a liquid suspension for her child. We are recognizing that giving medicine to two-year-olds is a challenge and that sometimes one method is less of a sticky struggle than another. Or we might ask a pregnant teenager whether she prefers her prenatal vitamins as one big pill or two little ones. Again, we are acknowledging that taking pills is hard, and we want to make it as easy as possible. The patient certainly participates by making a choice, but more important, the patient is able to participate within the context of recognition of the meaning of each possibility to her or his experience.

Clinicians also show caring through the expression of real *feeling*: gladness, sadness, disappointment, or even scolding. This expression is different from the technique of reflecting back the patient's feeling. It is one thing to say, "You sound angry," or, "That sounds frustrating," or, "You seem pleased." It is another thing to say, "I am really sad for you." Courses that train us to be better listeners encourage us to identify the feeling the patient is expressing. But those courses do not tell us how to be in the relationship. Sharing the feeling is different: it says to people not just that we have heard them but that what they said has touched us as a person. Sending sympathy cards and attending funerals are tangible examples of showing feeling, as opposed to recognizing the feeling a patient must be having.

At times clinicians can show caring through open affection. This is easiest at the extremes of life—with infants, who respond to unambivalent caring, and with older patients, who cherish the contact and fear no ulterior motive on the part of the doctor. Touching and other nonverbal forms of affection are clear elements in caring (Gadow, 1985). Nevertheless, physical expressions of affection are hard with toddlers, adolescents, and those patients whose histories of inconsistency, deception, or loss in personal relationships do not permit them to trust. It is also crucial not to confuse our patients with touch that could be construed as sexually provocative or abusive. It is one thing for me to hug an eighty-year-old man; it would be another thing for me to embrace his forty-five-year-old son—although at his father's funeral I might do so. Thus, our caring for patients and our affection for them must contain a commitment to protect them from abuses of power.

Clinicians show caring through *devotion*. Patients may recognize that the clinician cares through the meticulous and detailed way she or he arranges things for the patient or because of the clinician's willingness to do something that takes extra time and effort: a night call or emergency room visit, a home visit, agreeing to admit a patient to a hospital convenient for the patient but inconvenient for the doctor, stopping by a patient's house on the way home from the office, sending a card commemorating an important event. Something "extra" may also include bending the rules: seeing a patient who arrives forty-five minutes late; squeezing in a visit for the person in the family who stayed home sick that day; writing a sick note for someone who needs to miss work. None of these acts are particularly efficient, and doing them daily for every patient could lead to chaos, yet in the individual instance a doctor's willingness to make an exception shows flexibility and caring for the patient (Ben-Sira, 1976, 1980).

CARING INVOLVES SKILLED PRACTICE

Caring is not a mindless matter of reflexes, hormones, and instincts. Nor is it a matter of detached problem-solving or dispassionate adherence to rules. Caring requires engaged thought, effort, and practice. Skilled practice means applying what I know about a person—from his or her past history and past relationship with me and from what I know about the community and health care setting—to his or her fears, symptoms, and medical findings. It means staying constantly aware of what I know and of what I do not know and can only imagine.

The ability to imagine the patient's experience is perhaps the greatest asset to skilled practice, and lack of imagination the surest cause of failure. As we carry out relational caring, our skilled practice in showing patients that they are known, exploring meaning, showing feeling, and demonstrating devotion must reflect imagination. How would I conduct a pelvic exam differently if I knew that the patient, a Vietnamese woman, watched as pirates raped her daughter and then threw her overboard? Perhaps I do not know what has happened to a patient, but when I am able to imagine the possibilities it changes my practice. Perhaps I can try to find out more; patients cannot always tell me. I need to imagine what a patient is unable or unwilling to say. Conversely, failure of imagination can be an act of destruction. A woman brings in her beautiful newborn and everyone admires the baby. The nurse weighing the baby gives her a cuddle and says, "Oooh, I could just take you home with me!" She does not know that as a teenager this mother was pressured into releasing her first child for adoption. In her unintentional comment, the nurse lacked the ability to imagine this possibility.

CLINICIANS MODEL CARING RELATIONSHIPS

How we conduct ourselves, live our lives, and work with patients offers a model of how to be a caring whole person in the world. Our experiences and our feelings are not removed from our work but rather contribute to it. Our capacity for bringing ourselves into our work emerges in our self-disclosures: we are revealed as genuine. Our genuineness sets the stage. It says, I hear you, your feelings have touched me, I will be direct with you as well. It delivers to the patient an expectation of, even an invitation to, further genuine disclosure. Our openness encourages patients to extend their openness to us. Our responsiveness says, This relationship is a joint project. We both come to it as full human beings.

THE ONE-CARING MUST BE CARED FOR IN TURN

A person caring must care for himself or herself and be adequately cared for by others in order to do the work of caring. Self-care is more than a matter of meeting one's basic needs for food, shelter, clothing, and sleep. Ones-caring—mothers, nurses, teachers, day-care providers—need time for themselves and time with others like themselves to think about the work they do and how to do it better. They need an opportunity to examine their own weaknesses in the work of caring and to find strategies to ameliorate those weaknesses. They need to find ways not to give up whole parts of themselves in order to keep caring; instead, they need the unity and commitment to define the work of caring in ways that are not subservient.

Likewise, caring in relation requires that clinicians take care of themselves to ensure that they become neither self-effacing nor self-destructive. The need for vacations, for sleep, for exercise, for care of ourselves in sickness, for care of our families, for grief when death strikes us personally, all show us caring for ourselves as worthwhile human beings. Clinicians must locate sources of personal and group sustenance to continue caring for patients; they must examine how their own unique histories create problems in caring for patients and must seek ways to address these problems. Rest, meditation, exercise, vacation, writing, reading, and music are forms of self-care; support groups, Balint groups, supervision, and psychotherapy offer more explicitly clinical forms of self-care.

Although the caring ethic is naturally "other-regarding," it is not self-sacrificing because caring is both self-serving and other-serving (Noddings, 1984).[9] As Noddings puts it, the one caring needs no special justification to care for herself; to continue caring, she must maintain herself as a person who is strong, courageous, and capable of joy. For nurses, storytelling is one way to recover caring; nurses' narratives about their work can be nourishing and liberatory, and by extrapolation, caring narratives could be liberatory for doctors and other clinicians (Benner, 1991). We might rephrase Peabody: the secret of the care of the patient lies in caring for oneself while caring for the patient.

CARING REQUIRES A REINTERPRETATION OF DEPENDENCY

In a view of persons as separate, any loss of independence or sacrifice of autonomy through dependence implies sickness, weakness, disability, or immaturity. Dependence posed as the opposite to independence often carries a negative connotation: growth and progress are equated with detachment, and "attachments appear as an obstacle to the growth of the autonomous self" (Gilligan, 1986, p. 248). In contrast, being-in-relation theory views dependence and interdependence as healthy, necessary features of human existence (Stiver, 1991c). For instance, Gilligan found that adolescent girls viewed dependence as being able to rely upon someone. They did not see dependence as clutching or clinging but rather as "attachments" that "arise from the human capacity to move others and to be moved by them. . . . In this active construction, dependence, rather than signifying a failure of individuation, denotes a decision on the part of the individual to enact a vision of love" (1986, p. 249). To them, being dependent did not mean being helpless, powerless, and without control but rather being able to have an effect on others. The interdependence of attachment empowers both the self and the other, not one at the other's expense. The activities of care—being there, listening, the willingness to help, and the ability to understand—take on a moral dimension, reflecting the injunction to pay attention and not turn away from need (p. 249).

FLEXIBILITY IS INHERENT IN CARING-IN-RELATION

This principle implies preparedness for the come-what-may, an acknowledgment that we cannot predict the future and that the relationship we are in will straddle whatever may happen. The flexibility of caring-in-relation is different from the duties spelled out in a contract relationship with a patient; caring-in-relation is more inclusive and sustains more uncertainty. Flexibility is an attribute of skilled practice: it conveys a quality of "staying with" or "presence."

I recall an encounter with a middle-class woman whose visits for her children's regular physical exams always bordered on the contentious. She made it clear that she did not want or need my advice on how much protein or how much weight gain was advisable and that she did not believe in fluoride. At one point I asked her point-blank what she did want from these visits, and she replied, "Shots." Her third pregnancy was uncomplicated, and she delivered on a weekend when I was away. The baby had a rare and potentially fatal condition at birth that was immediately obvious. On my return, we jointly arranged and dealt with the visits to a specialist, the potentially poor prognosis (most of the case reports in the literature stated that babies with this condition died in several months), and the sensation of being caught in the completely unknown. Quite miraculously to everyone, the condition literally disappeared. Our mutual relief and eventual acceptance that the child would be fine was also shared. The relationship has subsequently changed: she is less confrontational with me, and I am more accepting of her. We have a shared past. I was quite flattered when she called me at home on a weekend to ask where her mother should have a malignancy investigated, in our city or in Boston. I knew this call was an affirmation of her trust in me.

This woman could never have anticipated that she would need me to be present for a rare congenital occurrence. What I offered was a kind of fidelity, a promise of presence despite her reluctance, resistance, and prior lack of need. Her initial need for a hands-off approach to well-child care was followed by a desperate need for me to help her contain her fear over the possibility that her child would die. These events required my flexibility.

Like Ruddick's mothering, caring is based on an assumption of changing capabilities in the one cared for. A mother's stance must be continuously flexible to adapt to the needs and requirements of a child, who is never at a standstill. This flexibility in stance is essential for the doctor as well, not only because of the wide variation among patients in their needs for attention, help, and encouragement, but also because of the great swings between feelings of independence and dependence that individual patients experience as they journey through health and illness. Such flexibility is demonstrated in the care of a healthy thirty-five-year-old woman who develops aseptic meningitis and then recovers; a healthy thirty-five-year-old who suffers a stroke from a cerebral aneurysm and remains permanently disabled; and a healthy thirty-five-year-old who gradually develops rheumatoid arthritis. Each of these moments in clinical care calls upon the clinician to remain flexible enough to adapt to the changing needs in the person cared for: skilled practice.

CARING ENHANCES THE GROWTH OF THE CARER

Often, when tired, we think of caring as draining and exhausting. Being-in-relation theory helps us recover our sense of how pleasurable we find caring to be. Sharing something of ourselves is a gift to the patient when not offered out of need; it allows the patient a window through which she or he may care back. The clinical result is reciprocity—a type of responsiveness different from role reversal or a need to take care of the doctor. Reciprocity is a recognition by the one cared for of the one-caring as a person. Our patients' eagerness to care for us is readily demonstrated when we experience life changes: pregnancy, illness, death in the family (see chapter 8). Being-in-relation theory provides us with a richer understanding of the patient's responsive caring for the doctor, whose needs and capacities, as we well know, vary across time.

In relational theory, reciprocity implies mutual growth. Growth-fostering relationships are characterized by the development of empathy, the process of mutual empathy, and the emergence of mutual empowerment and self-knowledge (Surrey, 1991a). Miller (1986, p. 3) points out the mutual enhancement that takes place in relationships that foster growth:

- Each person feels greater vitality or "zest"
- Each person is more capable of action
- Each person has a clearer picture of herself and the other
- Each person feels a greater sense of worth
- Each person feels more connected to the other and more motivated to relate to others beyond the relationship

This sense of enrichment from relationship is the reward of caring-in-relation. My caring is "completed" in my long-term patients by their recognition and acceptance of who I am as I care for them, as well as how I care for them (Noddings, 1984).

CARING MUST BE GROUNDED IN THE SOCIAL CONTEXT

Placing the caring relation in a social context means grounding it within the specific situation—including the race, gender, family, and community—of the one cared for, as well as within the practices and values of the health care setting, where caring can be not only permitted but facilitated. Paying attention to the social context means acknowledging the intersection of all these features with the unique history of the one-caring as a person with the same complexity of context. In other words, I acknowledge what I can and do know about a person's situation in her family, but also what I cannot know about her experience—for instance, her world as a sixteen-year-old woman of color who is also the mother of two infants. Understanding the social context includes a commitment to learning about all kinds of factors outside the patient's medical and even psychological reality. For instance, knowing the history of medical experimentation on black and Puerto Rican people allows the clinician to understand why patients of color might be skeptical or resistant toward new treatments. Such broad contextual thinking is essential to morally situated clinical work (Friedman, 1987b).

POTENTIAL PROBLEMS WITH CARING AS AN IDEAL

While the meaning of caring and the nature of its skilled practice have achieved some consensus among the varied practitioners of caring, embracing caring as an ethical ideal creates some problems: caring for people at a distance, inequality of the ones-caring, and essentialism.

CARING FOR PEOPLE AT A DISTANCE

If we must know people to care for them, how can we practice caring for people whom we have never and will never meet? Relational caring as I have described it *is* limited to those persons with whom we have direct contact and accepts a lesser form of involvement with those who are distant yet may deserve caring as much or more than those nearby. Caring for those nearby (what Noddings [1984] calls "proximate caring") may benefit those who are close but does nothing for those at a distance who may be far more needy. If I care only for those people I know, my caring is likely to be biased in favor of people like me and against those who are distant or different.[10] For instance, I may more readily find myself caring for white working-class patients who are fearful of people of color than for people of color in another city who are afraid in their own neighborhoods. Such individually construed caring is potentially unfair, prejudicial, and racist, lacks a social focus, and allows me to close my eyes to the need for social change.

The problem of how to respond to those more needy at a distance is, of course, a constant dilemma in all clinical fields: no matter how much we may do here, there are always innumerable sick and hungry and suffering persons elsewhere. On a broader scale, caring only for those already receiving care is the major moral problem facing a medical care system characterized by exclusion, limited access, and high cost. Those in the system *do* get the care, such as it is, while those outside get none at all. This reality forces all of us to see that a care perspective is only part of the picture; justice and rights are indeed relevant, particularly in our connection to those with whom we have no direct contact. But in clinical work, proximal caring is central. We cannot talk about taking care of all patients, only specific patients. Nevertheless, relational caring is *not* an answer to failures of the just distribution of resources, including access to health care.[11]

THE PROBLEM OF THE INEQUALITY OF ONES-CARING

A preoccupation of those thinking about care, from the feminist perspective as well as others, is the inequality between the one-caring and others, often men, who do not share in the caring. This inequality occurs between individuals inside and outside of families, within institutions, and in society at large. Women do most of the care of the young, the old, the helpless, the sick, and the dying, as well as a disproportionate amount of the household work to support the lives of other family members. Likewise, at their paid work women are more likely to perform the support and maintenance functions that receive low recognition and reward. Class differences allow some privileged women to take advantage of this system: women of color and poor women do caring work that sets upper-class women, like Zoe Baird, free to pursue lucrative careers. At every level of our society, governmental pressures to reduce the costs of health and social programs depend upon the unpaid "informal care system" provided by women in the community to keep sick and elderly people at home, with limited support and respite. This work is reinforced by an ideology of caring that makes it synonymous with women's roles (Finch & Groves, 1983).

Given this pattern of inequality and often exploitation of ones-caring, it is not surprising that feminists are reluctant to build an "ethic" based on those relations in families and in society that have historically been used to oppress women. The link between caring and low status is firmly entrenched. Women are underpaid, lack social support, and have little or no control over the conditions under which they care. Day-care

providers, nursery school teachers, nurses' aides, nursing home atten-
dants, hospice workers, all are paid poorly and accorded little respect.
Even in relatively elite settings, such as universities, the work that
requires the most intense caring—advising, tutoring, writing and study
skills instruction—usually falls to those with the least status: part-
timers, adjuncts, women. An ethic of care appears to dictate that
women remain in caring relations to husbands, parents, children, sick
people, people in power or with money, even when those relations are
essentially oppressive to women.

In the health care system, women do the vast majority of the caring.
Medicine, which has historically delegated all caring functions to nursing—in other words, to women—is the exception. Female physicians,
male nurses, and "midlevel practitioners" (nurse practitioners and
physician's assistants) may have softened the strict gender distinctions
between men who doctor and women who nurse, but at political, practical, and metaphorical levels, the gendered nature of clinical activity is
still sharp. One need only walk onto any hospital floor to remember
that women nurses, social workers, aides, physical therapists, and respiratory therapists are still the ones who are carrying out doctors'
"orders."

In nursing in the United States, low status and low pay have historically been tied to the ideology of caring. Whenever in the history of
modern nursing nurses began to demand recognition in the form of
improved salary and working conditions, such moves have been coun-
tered by exhortations about the importance of caring (despite abysmal
wages and endless hours of work) and allegations of nurses' selfishness
and lack of caring (Reverby, 1987). Thus, the ideology of women caring
has been used to keep nurses underpaid and unrecognized. In
response, nursing faces tremendous pressures to turn away from relational definitions of clinical work in the pursuit of legitimacy and professionalism. Insofar as caring is connected to gender, and gender is
connected to lower status and less professional respect, nurses continue to face a choice between allegiance to the gender-associated relational definition of their work (caring) and the more prestigious pursuit
of a kind of professionalism detached from nursing's relational origins.[12] Clinical power stripped of personal caring, the masculine style of
rational doctoring, is oppressive to nurses and patients; personal caring
without power, the traditional condition for female nursing, perpetuates oppressed conditions and relations for nurses. Gender and power
suffuse caring in all health care relations.

Even within medicine itself, as a culture and as an institution, caring
is inevitably linked with lower status. Specialties that focus on relationships have lower status: family physicians, pediatricians, psychiatrists,
and primary care internists have lower incomes and less prestige than

subspecialists, surgeons, and those who emphasize procedures over relationships. Not surprisingly, women are far more strongly represented in the relational fields. And women practitioners in all specialties occupy less prestigious positions than their male colleagues. Thus, medicine itself recapitulates the linkage between gender, caring, and lower status. Despite the defined social need for more primary care practitioners, neither medicine nor society in general has figured out how to encourage more trainees to enter the less prestigious work of primary care. Not surprisingly, within medicine it is those in the relational disciplines who argue for the need for caring in clinical work; it is those less privileged in the system who recognize the social and emotional inadequacies and relational failures of a hierarchical, gender-stratified system.

With increasing numbers of women in medicine, and increasing recognition of the relational core of clinical practice, at least some quarters of medicine are likely to reclaim caring as central to their work. Not only do women physicians spend more time with each patient, they also use verbal styles that enable patients to speak more freely and they are less likely to interrupt patients (Roter, Lipkin, & Korsgaard, 1991; West, 1984). With chronically ill patients, women physicians do more information-sharing and more partnership-building. They spend more time collecting a medical history, compared with their male colleagues, and in the process they allow their patients to spend more time talking (Roter et al., 1991). This research suggests that women physicians' styles are characteristically more likely to be perceived as caring. As medicine seeks to portray itself as caring, educators are likely to identify women's caring as a set of specific skills that can be taught and learned.[13]

Yet caring in medicine will continue to encounter significant pitfalls. As with caring practices in other domains, caring in medicine needs to be disentangled from self-sacrifice. Despite the prestige and power of physicians, dedication to work at the expense of self-care has historically characterized how doctors go about their work. In response, patients have forgiven doctors' poor communication and poor manners as the understandable result of fatigue and overwork. Doctors have appeared entitled to the caring attention of secretaries, nurses, and spouses because of their hard work on behalf of others. Even doctors' high incomes have been excused as a compensation for the long years of self-sacrifice. Again, for doctors as well as mothers, self-sacrifice is linked to an expectation of later control. To make medicine less patriarchal, medical training must renounce self-sacrifice. Medical training, which often pits patients' needs against the self-care needs of the trainee, resulting in resentment and hostility, will need to be informed by a perspective on care for self and others. Thus, caring must include care for self if it is not to be corrupted into oppressive caring or to require that others (nurses, spouses, and so on) engage in oppressed caring to maintain the doctor's caring.

Caring in clinical work is, of course, different in some ways from caring for one's children, one's partner, one's parents, or one's friends. Clinical caring is paid work, and highly rewarded work compared with other caring work in our society (day care, child care, care for the infirm, aged, and retarded, and the ordinary work of caring for the children or elderly in one's family). Clinical caring has beginnings and ends, vacations and paychecks, and occasionally even sick leave. Family caring has none of these benefits. But clinical caring *is* contaminated by the ideology surrounding the social expectations of women caring: long hours, lower pay and less status (than technical or procedural work in health care), and expected selflessness. Efforts to limit the commitments of clinical caring through part-time work are construed as inadequate caring or, alternatively, insufficient dedication to one's profession (Wheeler, Candib, & Martin, 1990).

Being-in-relation theory recognizes that women's work and women's psychological suffering are framed by the subservient conditions under which they do their caring (Miller, 1976). Women are taught to serve the needs of others, to use all their abilities on behalf of others, "as if women did not have needs of their own, as if one could serve others without simultaneously attending to one's own interests and desires" (p. 61). The problem with women's abilities and desires for affiliation, as Miller points out, is that the main kinds of affiliation available to women have been subservient affiliations. Healthy relational caring does not and cannot occur under oppressed conditions. Respect for caring and for those doing the caring demands a recognition of the skill, intelligence, and effort involved. This recognition must go beyond token appreciation and find a place in governmental economic and political policies (Finch & Groves, 1983).

THE PROBLEM OF ESSENTIALISM

If we define women (and not men) in terms of relationships, women will be restricted to relational work and the *relationship* will be reified as women's domain. If caring is defined in terms of women, then women will be defined in terms of caring. Critics worry that Gilligan's depiction of women as motivated by caring within relationships can be all too easily extrapolated to social expectations that women *should* care, that women are in fact socially obligated to care, while men are not. Caring may have been ignored in traditional moral theory, which was developed by and applied to men, but caring is neither the prerogative of nor the only territory open to women.

The theme of the centrality of caring to women, as outlined by Gilligan and Noddings, though enormously popular, has provoked sharp disagreement from many critics (Card, 1990; Hoagland, 1990b;

Houston, 1990; Puka, 1990). Framing women's moral thought in terms of caring, feminists have argued, perpetuates women's restriction to their socialized caring roles as helpmeets and nurturers and compels them to keep on caring even within relationships that are damaging to them. Such expectations that women should be the ones-caring and not give up on relationships constrain them from leaving violent and abusive situations. Adherence to the ideology that women should do the caring often allows care for others to preclude self-care. Such situations may result in women being stifled, silenced; they may find themselves in physical danger. In short, caring is destructive for some women.

While feminists have been critical of caring as an ideal because of the subservient and oppressed conditions in which women care for others, caring has also been under attack in the self-help movement. Caring too often becomes "codependency." Raised in a dysfunctional family, the codependent adult (almost always a woman) continues to look after the feelings of others, to put others first, and to strive for perfection but never feel good enough.[14] She may live with an addict, an alcoholic, a batterer, a gambler, a workaholic, a so-called sex addict (or sexual offender), or a man who buries himself in sports. Her problem? She loves too much (Walters, 1990).

The codependency movement has stripped gender away from caring. Women's traditional socialization—to take care of the relationship, hold the marriage together, support the man through his problems, and look after the children, while working an additional eight hours a day in a caring role as a nurse, secretary, administrative assistant—was transformed into a form of pathology; the woman herself has the problem. The codependency movement is unwilling to address gendered inequality and oppression in the dysfunctional family or dysfunctional workplace. In Miller's terms, the problems of women who have been labeled "codependent" can be reframed as the problems that adhere to subservient affiliations. The problem is not caring or caring too much, but caring when you are not an equal.

Being-in-relation theory offers an alternative to the charge of essentialism—of defining women as relational and therefore unequal by definition. All persons start out as relational, but the pressures of male and female development push men to deny their attachments and separate from their relational identity in the name of autonomy. Women are encouraged to deny awareness of their own needs in favor of the needs of others, in the service of caring (Miller, 1976). Just as we need a new kind of autonomy that is based *in* relationships rather than outside of them, we also need a new kind of caring that is not based on subservience. Women would no longer be defined as relational, because both men and women would locate their identities within relation. We could then move beyond conventional understandings of autonomy (relinquishing relationships to become separate and self-directed) to a more complete vision: "a fuller not a lesser ability to encompass relationships to others, simultaneous with the fullest development of oneself" (Miller, 1976, p. 95).

In the 1990s, caring is in fashion. It has been used to market everything from airline tickets to dental appointments. It has been claimed by women finding their different voice and rejected by others because of its link to oppression. Caring-in-relation offers us a way through these contradictions. One final issue to be addressed is the asymmetry of the relation between the one-caring and the cared-for. Caring-in-relation accepts that asymmetry—exemplified, for instance, in the work of mothers and teachers, whose caring takes place in highly asymmetrical relations, at least for long periods of time. As I pointed out in chapter 6, clinical relationships parallel the relationship between mother and child because the definition of moral conduct in both is based on recognition of inequality between the parties. Caring-in-relation recognizes that "unequal meetings" (Noddings, 1984, p. 67) are an inevitable feature of human relations: between a well person and a sick one, a professional and a client, a parent and a child.

The power inequality cannot be wished away or denied—doctors, teachers, and mothers are inevitably more powerful than those they care for. While a partnership model asserts the equality of the parties, a contract cannot in fact resolve the real power differences. Instead, caring-in-relation offers another way of looking at power—power not as a force to coerce or control, but as an energy on behalf of the other. The dynamic is mutuality and reciprocity rather than contract and negotiation. As we see in chapter 10, the elements of caring-in-relation share the assumptions of the practice of empowerment.

CHAPTER 10

Power-in-Relation

A SELF-IN-RELATION VIEW of the doctor-patient relationship frees up *caring* to supplant *contract* as the central definition of the connection between doctor and patient. But if we make caring primary and forgo the contractual view of the doctor-patient relationship, are we open once again to the charge of paternalism, or worse, abuse of power? Gilligan argues that our two moral predispositions toward human connection—toward justice or toward care—derive from the experiences of inequality and attachment embedded in the parent-child relationship (1986, p. 245). A care-based theory of clinical work takes attachment into consideration but must also find a way to address the issue of inequality. Toward this end, we need a relational understanding of power in the doctor-patient connection.

The reigning understanding of power in medicine is "power-over." This view of power as domination limits our ability to appropriate any other kind of power for the clinical relationship. It allows for forms of remediation and strategies for negotiation but provides no opening for considering any kind of power other than domination. Medicine's response to the problem of domination—the strategies of contract and negotiation—begins after the power relations are already established; the legitimacy of power-over is never questioned.[1] The methods it offers to defuse the doctor's power-over usually take the form of more effective "communication strategies" to facilitate understanding between doctor and patient. While these recommendations may make both doctors and patients feel more effective, they do not question the basis of power in the relationship.[2] Many strategies are entirely cognitive and do not address the fundamental need for empathy if the relationship is going to play a role in healing. Other strategies call for empathy (Mishler et al., 1989) but do not clarify how the doctor might attain it. Thus, despite the increased attention paid to the doctor-patient interview over the past ten years (Lipkin et al., 1984; Smith & Hoppe, 1991), recommendations about communication designed to address the power imbalance in the relationship often do not make empathy central; conversely, recommendations concerned with empathy and caring usually do not address the problem of power-over. Although clinicians concerned about these issues have defined the hallmarks of a good interview (Mishler et al., 1989), deliberate empowerment of the patient is not a commonly accepted goal of medicine or of individual physicians.

If we turn from medicine and examine other endeavors characterized by unequal relationships, we discover that feminists have defined a legitimate form of power: the power to empower. Essential to the operation of the power to empower is a state of empathetic readiness consistent with caring-in-relation (see chapter 9). The feminist conduct of unequal relations in domains outside medicine—teaching, mothering, research, psychotherapy—centers on empowering the less powerful. Examination of this approach reveals the qualities integral to empowerment activities in clinical work.

Outside of medicine, the women's movement in general and feminist health activists in particular have made specific contributions to our understanding of the power imbalance in women's health care. The most direct and explicit contribution was reclaiming women's right to know about their bodies. Both a symbol and a force in its own right, the Boston Women's Health Book Collective's *Our Bodies, Our Selves* (1971) offers an example of women health activists acquiring and disseminating information about their bodies to women and making it available in a respectful and accurate form. By showing that ordinary women can learn about their bodies and explain what they understand to others, this book made an immeasurable difference in transforming power relations between doctors and women patients. I will return to the question of how patient education serves to empower.

In the 1970s activists in the women's health movement initiated self-help efforts ranging from an underground abortion service in Chicago to classes in self-examination of the cervix to menstrual extraction clinics. Education, peer counseling, diagnosis, and treatment were coupled with social and emotional support for women receiving care or learning about their bodies in these settings. Although physicians and nurses provided consultation, legal authority, or technical assistance in some self-help settings, professionals did not figure prominently in the self-help movement expressly because of its antiprofessional position. An explicit conflict emerged between the self-help movement and the growing number of women health activists who became health care professionals: the lay women who ran women's health clinics in the 1970s prevented physicians from occupying decision-making roles because of their distrust of the professional role (Ruzek, 1978; Walter, 1988). The self-help movement empowered women by keeping them away from professionals and later, after self-help groups had faded away, by rendering women watchful if not suspicious of what medicine had to offer them.

However, even as self-help activism waned, another social force for empowering women patients was growing: the increasing number of outspoken women physicians. Many women patients perceived women doctors in various specialties as offering an alternative to traditional power relationships. However, powerful forces work to make women physicians act like men: socialization into the male world of work, coupled with discrimination and harassment by men. (The resignation of Frances Conley, a prominent neurosurgeon at Stanford, brought such harassment to public attention in 1991.) Despite the appearance of success, women physicians remain excluded from the most powerful echelons of medicine (Lorber, 1984, 1991). From midlevel positions, they seem unlikely candidates for transforming medical institutions or building alternatives that challenge the male medical hierarchy. Nevertheless, women clinicians could indeed conduct relationships differently. Empowerment work can act as a force for change despite women's own and their patients' lack of power-over in the world outside the examining room.

Likewise in nursing, feminists have confronted the gender stereotypes held both by nurses themselves and by doctors and hospital hierarchies.[3] Primarily in the outpatient setting, nurse-practitioners have created a legitimate and authoritative role. While they may not explicitly articulate how they use power differently from physicians offering similar services to patients, nurse-practitioners and patients share a conviction that the care is different. Nurse-practitioners practice on their own license, with their own malpractice insurance, and in some states write their own prescriptions. They have established a separate, though sometimes overlapping, basis of authority with physicians.

Feminists and women health activists advocate clinical relationships that reduce the power imbalance or, perhaps implicitly, offer a different model of power altogether. When a woman chooses a nurse-practitioner or a midwife (almost exclusively women) over a physician, she is often consciously choosing a clinician *not* viewed as so powerful as a physician, a clinician whose conduct may not reflect such unequal power dynamics. More positively, the practice of nurse-practitioners and midwives may be more grounded in a belief in the normality of developmental and physiological processes, including pregnancy and birth, rather than preoccupied with a pathological model. A woman's choice of a female clinician may also reflect a preference for a clinician more like herself.

Feminist critiques of medicine have made it legitimate to choose a clinician as similar as possible to oneself: for instance, to minimize her experience of the homophobic aspects of medical practice, a lesbian patient may choose a lesbian physician. However, despite the increasing possibility for such matches of patients and doctors, distrust of even women physicians lingers among feminists. Moreover, a clinical relationship based on the choice of a practitioner like oneself, while apparently less open to abuse because of greater symmetry, contains its own unique potential for abuse.[4]

Feminist alternatives to traditional medicine—self-help, women clinicians, nurse-practitioners, matching values—all offer ways to sidestep, if sometimes only temporarily, the dominating relationships typical of medicine. Yet while patients may choose to avoid all contact with mainstream medicine, women practitioners inevitably deal with the institutional Goliath. For women clinicians whose work brings them into formal medical settings, medicine's power-over is so pervasively displayed that it raises the question of whether feminist practice can even survive in the medical environment. If the only kind of power in clinical relationships is power-over and the best one can hope for is to be less dominating and less abusive, then feminist clinical practice is impossible. Fortunately for medical practice, teachers and psychotherapists have been struggling with the same questions. In both these domains, heavily populated by women, feminists are exploring new ways of thinking about the power vested in them by virtue of their chosen work.

In the classroom, feminist teachers face a dilemma about the nature of power similar to that experienced by women doctors. They see power-over as inevitably connected to social oppression, yet they themselves also use power in positive ways when they are being effective teachers. Nevertheless, gender-linked visions of power—power seen as masculine—leave no room for women to be powerful teachers except by imitating men. Because of the association of power with male power, it is difficult for women in the classroom to discover an "authentic voice not based on tyranny" (Friedman, 1985, p. 207). Women need to develop a pedagogy that validates intellect and authority based on knowledge and experience but does not look to male-associated bases of power for that legitimacy. Since teaching is universal in medical settings and essential between clinician and patient, the need for a nonoppressive form of power in teaching is felt in medicine as well.

How we construe ideas of power is tied to gender. Men are likely to conceive of power in terms of domination, whereas women see power in terms of relationship and nurturance (Gilligan & Pollak, 1988). The philosopher Nancy Hartsock reflects: "Against power as domination over others, feminist thinking and organizational practices express the possibility of power as the provision of energy to others as well as self, and of reciprocal empowerment" (quoted in Harding, 1986, p. 149). Jean Baker Miller describes this kind of power in psychotherapy as a way to "be powerful in ways that simultaneously enhance, rather than diminish the power of others" (1991, p. 205). The term "power to empower" describes the appropriate, legitimate, even necessary power of the feminist clinician.[5] The power to empower "simultaneously enhances the power of the other and one's own power." The resulting mutuality serves to give power to the relationship itself, "to create, sustain, and deepen the connections that empower" (Surrey, 1991a, p. 164). Thus, empowerment is both mutually empathic and mutually empowering. Empowerment arises within the context of relationships that promote growth, whether in the classroom, the workplace, the therapist's office, or the medical setting.

The medical setting is the last place most feminists might look for empowerment, yet it is clearly as essential there as in any other location. It is always fashionable to condemn medicine as an arena impervious to feminist reinterpretation. The fact that most doctors are not feminists should be no more paralyzing than the fact that most sociologists, anthropologists, philosophers, psychologists, and specialists in every other academic field are not feminists; yet feminists are actively and visibly engaged in redefining the tasks and territory of each of these disciplines. Medicine is unique in that the feminist critique comes entirely from outside the discipline. Nonclinicians rail against medical abuses of power without offering an alternative basis for reconsidering the field. While graduate students in, say, sociology or psychology study feminist critiques of their chosen fields, medical education goes on largely unchanged despite the increasing number of women students. Within medical education, parallel feminist critiques are unknown and phrases like "patriarchal power" are alien. The feminist project in medicine has not yet even been defined.

To arrive at a feminist understanding of power in clinical relationships, we can study unequal relationships in some other areas in which feminists have redefined the practice of power: mothering, teaching, research, and psychotherapy. Each of these activities, like the practice of medicine, is at risk of fostering the abuses that result from power-over; in fact, the abuses of each area have been well documented. But all of these activities have been reconsidered by feminists and reinformed and transformed by the desire to use power to strengthen and empower the less powerful rather than maintain or amplify the power of the more powerful in unequal relationships.

Each of these areas also shares some specific features with medical practice. Medicine shares with mothering the goal of helping a healthy child develop into a healthy and productive adult; the necessity for patience while growth and healing take place; the constant awareness that unpredictable catastrophes are a permanent hazard; the conflict between care for others and self-care, expressed as exhaustion and self-sacrifice; the need for moment-to-moment responsiveness; the long-term and evolving nature of the relationship; and the unpredictability at the outset of what kind of person and what kind of relationship will develop. Doctors, particularly women doctors, because of the very similarity of their caring role to that of mothers, may also be on the receiving end of the strong feelings some patients have toward their mothers, sometimes occasioning reactions and outbursts that initially seem inappropriate.

Doctors share with teachers a belief in the value of learning for human growth and a willingness to contribute a part of themselves to the learning process. Doctors teach younger doctors, doctors from other specialties, medical students, nurses, and other health care workers about the specifics of medicine, and every clinician is involved in some way in patient education. Doctors and teachers pursue long years of training in preparation for their "unequal meetings" (Noddings, 1984, p. 67) with those who will be in their charge. Doctors also teach by example: their visibility makes them perennial models of human conduct. It is perhaps for this reason that their failings are so disappointing and make people so angry.

Doctors share with therapists the responsibilities of the clinical role; an awareness that the relationship is the medium in which healing takes place; an acknowledgment of the interconnection of symptoms perceived as either mental or physical, and the relation of these symptoms to the larger arenas of family, work, and society; the privilege of having private and intimate knowledge of other human beings; the risks and burdens of bearing the secrets of other human beings; the onus of serving as the focus for the patient's unpredictable, inchoate, and sometimes overwhelming feelings; and the formality of clinical relationships, with all the trappings of offices, appointments, and billing systems.

Doctors share with researchers a curiosity about the natural world and an energy for finding out about it; a belief that many things can be found out (a respect for empirical investigation); an appreciation for the complexity of the scientific endeavor; and an awareness that empirical generalizations do not necessarily apply to the individual case, yet an appreciation of the importance of findings from individual cases. Doctors are aware that each individual living through an illness or taking a medicine is a kind of scientific experiment in which $N = 1$ (N is the statistician's symbol for the number of subjects in the experiment). Finally, doctors and researchers must both wrestle with the conflict between the status of neutral observer mandated by ordinary science and their complicated relatedness to those they learn from or study.

These areas of overlap between doctors and mothers, teachers, therapists, and researchers pertain to the work of any practitioner, not only women or feminists. Unequal meetings are inevitable features of the work. An adult may choose to avoid relationships with parents or children, going to the doctor, pursuing formal education, seeing a therapist, or doing formal research. However, it is impossible to avoid all experiences of sickness and healing, of teaching and learning, of caring and being cared for, of inquiring about, or being regarded as a resource for inquiry about, the world. Insofar as these unequal experiences are part of human relations, feminist contributions to mothering, teaching, therapy, and research are relevant to all of us.

THE REQUIREMENTS OF EMPOWERMENT

Given the reality of the domination of patients by doctors, how would we set out to construct an alternative practice? What would *empowerment* of patients mean? Acknowledging that patients themselves will be variously aware of, and comfortable or uncomfortable with, the traditional power-over in the relationship, what does the practice of empowerment entail?

RECOGNITION OF OPPRESSION

Empowerment first of all requires a "commitment to understanding the world from the perspective of the socially subjugated" (Harding, 1986, p. 149). The practitioner must accept and assume all of the realities of domination in a person's life and dedicate the doctor-patient relationship to recognizing it, not perpetuating it. The commitment to empowerment sharply distinguishes a feminist approach from enhancing communication skills and other patient-centered methods that genuinely seek to identify the patient's perspective (Brown et al., 1986; Lazare & Eisenthal, 1979; Levenstein et al., 1986; Smith & Hoppe, 1991). These approaches operate comfortably within conventional medicine, which does not make the central connection between the personal experience of illness and the social structure. "The noncritical nature of medical discourse encourages clients' continued functioning in a social system that is often a major source of their personal problems" (Waitzkin, 1984b, p. 344). In contrast, an empowerment approach *requires* recognizing a person's context, particularly the sources of inequality and oppression she may experience—her family, her work, her race, her poverty, her chronic disease. This recognition does not assume that the doctor has the power to fix the patient's contextual problems; rather, it acknowledges the contribution of context to the patient's health status and clarifies the unfairness or immorality of her oppression. The ethical commitment of the feminist practitioner must be to oppose that oppression.

I am not urging, as some critics might argue, that we make inquiries into nonmedical areas in order to help patients cope, thereby "medicalizing" social problems. Rather, I see naming social forms of oppression, like battering and racism, as an essential step for a doctor and patient to make together in order to recognize where the patient's symptoms come from and what sustains them. Doctors who accept and use language that acknowledges the oppression people experience are supporting the reality of their patients' experience of that oppression. (Such discussion changes the doctor as well, as I discuss later.) For instance, questions like, "How did they treat you there?" or, "What is it like for black people (or Puerto Rican, or Vietnamese) to go there?" can encourage patients to discuss their experiences of racism in medical care facilities; if the patient wishes, such discussion can lead to further exploration of the issue of racism. When I asked a black patient about her experience of racism as an employee at an all-white medical center, the resulting discussion at that visit and many subsequent ones explored the patient's sense that her supervisor singled her out for criticism. By bringing up racism as a concern, I was acknowledging that racism was an ever-present fact in her life. My finding is not unique: any clinician working with women of color hears from patients about their daily encounters with racism from representatives of various bureaucracies.[6] Of course, asking the question is not enough. Clinicians must listen to the answers and allow themselves to be affected by what they hear.

The recognition of a patient's feeling of disempowerment, or oppression, means acknowledging in conversation with him or her that the economic system brutalizes people, that women and children are physically and sexually victimized, and that sickness disrupts the fragile economic and psychological balance in which most people live.

A twenty-one-year-old Puerto Rican mother of three children under the age of four came in seeking to sign papers to obtain a surgical sterilization. She had used Norplant (implanted progesterone capsules) as contraception for the last year, with resultant weight gain, but she was starting to lose weight. She could not stand the thought of having another child, and she wanted to attend classes to become a home health aide. Her husband was unemployed. There was no work for him. She acknowledged that someday perhaps, when her children were all in school, she might want to have another, but that time seemed very far away. I raised the awful possibility that something might happen to one of her children or to her husband, changing her life completely. Or what if her husband started something with another woman, and she threw him out? Ten or even five years later she might regret having had a sterilization. I also reminded her that many people think that women of color on welfare, like herself, should not be allowed to have more children. She needed to think out whether those people would have any influence on her decision. My explicit mention of racism gave us both pause. She decided to stick with the Norplant. I made a mental note to reflect back on this discussion at the time of her annual visits.

In this example, I am not derogating the importance of patient choice; rather, I hope to reinforce the importance of the context in which that choice takes place. I did not neutrally lay out alternatives and then appeal to this young woman's right, as a patient, to decide. Instead, inquiry that made relevant the effects of racism, poverty, and sexism on her life, as well as sexist and derogatory experiences she may have had in medical institutions, helped her situate her decision within the real power relations that determine her world. One of these power relations is the doctor-patient relationship. By placing sterilization in the social context, I encouraged her to see even our relationship as subject to the same restrictive forces. Neither clinicians nor patients customarily make the link between symptoms and social conditions; from an empowerment perspective, the responsibility to call attention to it lies with the clinician. What features of context are most salient to a given woman at a given time is up to her to define when an empathetic clinician offers her the opportunity.

In corresponding ways, feminist researchers make the fact of women's oppression central to their investigations and direct their work toward active struggle against that oppression and toward emancipation (Mies, 1983). Mies proposes methodological guidelines that replace the "view from above" with a "view from below" (p. 123); research, formerly an instrument of dominance, must be made to serve the interests of the oppressed and dominated. The feminist researcher engages in "conscious partiality," which goes beyond empathy: it corrects distortions and widens perceptions. Mies's perspective on research places the researcher herself within the investigation.

Like women researchers and women patients, women clinicians work within institutional and social frameworks shaped by gender. As in women's studies, in which "gendered subjects teach gendered subjects," women clinicians heal in gendered contexts where they also are "embedded in the work they produce and are similarly inscribed in the practices in which they participate" (Rothfield, 1987, p. 526). This awareness of the embeddedness of both parties is basic to an understanding of oppression and empowerment and partly underlies patients' preference for clinicians like themselves.

EMPATHY

Empathy is an essential element in empowerment. Recognition of oppression informs the empowering clinician's stance toward the world; empathy informs her stance toward the patient. Empathy requires *being with* and *being open to*. It is a readiness to feel the other's feelings as one's own and to use that experience for the benefit of the other. For Noddings, the one-caring experiences a "readiness to bestow and spend oneself, to make oneself available" (1984, p. 19), and a "displacement of interest from my own reality to the reality of the other" (p. 14). Empathy is a prerequisite for empowerment because it is through empathy that a person knows she has been heard, felt, or touched. Empathy validates her experience and forges a connection with another human being.

Empathy requires *inclusion*, the capacity to see from both one's own and the other's perspective. Inclusion allows the one-caring to practice confirmation—that is, seeing the one cared for as she or he both is and might be, as she or he envisions his or her best self (Noddings, 1984, p. 67). Empathy—incorporating "being with," "being open to," and inclusion—leads to confirmation of the other and a commitment to act on his or her behalf. Thus, empathy leads to empowerment because it confirms the *worthiness* of the other. In the psychotherapy setting, the experience of receiving empathy, perhaps for the first time, can lead to the growth of much needed self-empathy in the patient (Jordan, 1991a).

Clinicians will argue that empathy as described by Jordan and Noddings cannot be practiced by a doctor or nurse-practitioner with every single person in a session of fifteen or twenty patients. I would argue that even brief interactions can be empowering. What would they entail? The ability to tune into each person where he or she is at the moment: a man with a sore throat, a woman in for an annual physical, a teenager with a colicky baby, a five-year-old in for a kindergarten physical, a teenage brother and sister whose parents have HIV infection. Noddings makes the parallel to teaching: "I do not need to establish a deep, lasting, time-consuming personal relationship with every student. What I must do is to be totally and nonselectively present to the student—to each student—as he addresses me. The time interval may be brief but the encounter is total" (1984, p. 180).

Empathy is an element of long-term relationships, but it need not be active at every moment. What needs to be active is an openness to another person's experience at the moment of encounter. This openness is amplified by a clinician's rich imagination and familiarity with the wide range of experiences and interpretations that a person might bring to the clinical encounter. The clinician uses his or her imagination to offer an understanding of the patient's experience, without trying to limit the patient's experience to a category that the doctor has preconceived. Empathy enables the clinician to hear what the patient is not saying, what the patient is perhaps embarrassed about or afraid to say.[7] For instance, it is axiomatic that pregnant women worry about their babies being normal, but the specific content of that worry varies. If I say, "Everyone worries about whether their baby will be okay, but sometimes people have a particular thing they worry about; is there anything you worry about especially with this baby?" I accomplish several tasks: I am saying that worrying is normal, I am acknowledging her uniqueness, and I am making it easier for her to share her concern. Questions that arise from the empathetic imagination can diminish fear, isolation, and sometimes guilt. Empathy also enables the clinician to look for signs that she or he might have misunderstood the patient and to hear clearly when patients say that they do not feel understood.

RESPECT FOR THE PERSON AS A PERSON

Lorraine Code (1987) distinguishes treating a person "as a person" from treating him or her "like an object," by which she means stereotyping the person. I use the phrase "respect for the person as a person" as a way to extend our consideration of personhood to persons who may be treated as less than full persons—who may be senile, retarded, or otherwise disabled. Empathy toward such persons seems more difficult, perhaps irrelevant. It is easier to be empathetic toward members of their families. Code draws on an example from May Sarton's novel *As We Are Now* (1973) about a nursing home's denigrating care for an elderly woman of fluctuating mental abilities. Despite her ups and downs, the woman had an idea of herself and a sense of who she was, what she wanted, and how she wanted to be treated. Code calls for clinicians to invoke the "moral imagination" to treat a person as a person with an idea of her own selfhood despite fluctuations in abilities (Code, 1987). Her vision of a person's idea of selfhood reverberates with Noddings's vision of the person "as he envisions his best self" (1984, p. 67). When a clinician holds on to this "vision" of the other, sometimes against formidable odds, he or she is acting powerfully on the patient's behalf.

Let me offer a striking example. Some years ago our health center agreed to provide physical examinations for disabled adults entering an independent living center. My first patient from the center was a nineteen-year-old woman with severe cerebral palsy. She was in a motorized wheelchair that she controlled with her only usable finger. I could not understand her guttural speech or her facial contortions. She could not consistently hold her head up or control her drooling. After a few desperate moments, I asked her if she knew how to use a typewriter. She managed to make me understand a "yes" answer, and I ran out of the room to locate a typewriter on a mobile stand. Pleased with my ingenuity, I stood next to her as she typed, expecting some limited request. My smugness gave way to sheer awe as she painstakingly, letter by letter, tapped out with her left fourth finger the question, "What are the risks for me of taking the birth control pill?" Perhaps more than any other person, that one young woman taught me what it means to respect a person as a person.

Responding to the Changing Abilities of the Other

The requirement that the more powerful person be able to adapt to the other's changing abilities is a prominent theme in feminist discussions of mothering, teaching, and therapy. It is particularly apt for medicine. Jean Baker Miller observes:

> The one who exerts such power recognizes that she or he cannot possibly have total influence or control but has to find ways to interact with the other person's constantly changing forces or powers. And all must be done with appropriate timing, phasing, and shifting of skills so that one helps to advance the movement of the less powerful person in a positive stronger direction. (1991, p. 199)

Ruddick describes the quality in mothering that fosters growth and welcomes change; in response to change, she must be "a changing mother. . . . Change requires a kind of learning in which what one learns cannot be applied exactly, often not even by analogy, to a new situation" (1983, p. 218). Thus, unlike scientific practice, which depends on repeatability, maternal thinking is based on flexibility and adaptiveness. "It is not only children who change, grow, and need help in growing; those who care for children must also change in response to changing reality" (p. 219).

The implication of Ruddick's understanding for the doctor-patient relationship is that the doctor, like the mother, needs to develop a capacity to make constant changes in his or her stance, both from patient to patient and in caring for the same patient over time. In doctoring, a flexible stance is essential in work with children, whose abilities change and grow so rapidly, and also in the care of people who are sick and whose ability to handle information and events fluctuates during the course of illness, sometimes leading to recovery and resumption of previous abilities, and sometimes not. For instance, over the course of two weeks a competent woman in her eighties can become acutely ill with an infected gallbladder, undergo surgery, become paranoid and delusional in the surgical intensive care unit, and then resume normal functioning in her own apartment. Such wide variation over time and across clinical conditions requires a flexibility on the clinician's part that includes a tolerance for uncertainty about the outcome.

A patient's changing powers require that the doctor pay scrupulous attention to her as she sees herself (Code, 1987) and also maintain a fidelity to her as she has been in the past and to the values that the physician herself espouses, and for which the patient may have chosen her in the first place. My allegiance to the feisty independence of the woman in the surgical ICU allowed me to weather the period of her altered mental ability without denying her personhood. The physician's flexible stance must transcend not only the fluctuations of illness but also life transitions. Doctors who treat patients over many years see their abilities change remarkably—for instance, the transformation over ten years of a thirteen-year-old girl growing up into a twenty-three-year-old woman. Being her doctor when she was thirteen required one kind of attention; what she needs and expects is very different ten years later. I need to be able to change in response to her changes, yet the element of respect must persist. If I took her seriously and treated her with respect at thirteen, I am far more likely to remain her doctor at twenty-three. Being-in-relation requires that the clinician change as the relationship changes.[8]

Lorraine Code (1987) warns against getting stuck in old definitions of a person, practicing a futile kind of fidelity to a historical person who no longer exists. Just as it would be constricting and limiting for a parent to treat a twelve-year-old like the ten-year-old she used to be, it is disempowering to patients to hold them to what they used to be, to anticipate no growth or change in them. For example, a patient switches from being cared for by me to one of my partners because she feels that I always treat her the way she used to be when she was "crazy." Now she is different, but she feels that I do not treat her in a way that recognizes her difference. I may have an alternative interpretation of her need to switch doctors, but I must address the criticism of my failure to recognize her change. Similarly, a robust elderly man may reject the idea of life support systems, but when he suffers a sudden massive coronary and is successfully resuscitated by the ambulance crew, he gains a new appreciation for life. When he begins a progressive deterioration and suffers more and more breathing trouble and fatigue, he accepts, indeed chooses, to be intubated and ventilated because, at that moment, he wants to continue to live. He is not ready to die. Fidelity at that moment to his previously stated rejection of life support must be supplanted by a new understanding of how desperate it feels not to be able to breathe and a new appreciation of his desire to live. Fidelity to another aspect of who he was as a person, a man who saved every nut and bolt and bit of old machinery for its potential usefulness in repairing something someday, a man who would work all day to rebuild a machine to avoid spending a quarter on a new part, that man wanted to keep his old body going a little longer if some way could be found to rig it up. Fidelity must be coupled with a flexible stance to "accommodate the unexpected turns personhood can take" (Code, 1987, p. 156).

LANGUAGE

The deliberate choice of empowerment as a goal is new to medicine. Given that language, in both form and content, is a medium through which domination is achieved and maintained, any consideration of empowerment must address how the language of doctor-patient interaction would need to change. Specifically, we need to examine what kind of language—or questions, since doctors' primary speech mode is questioning—might best convey empathetic readiness and thus empower patients. Following the method of a Norwegian feminist general practitioner, Kirsti Malterud, the doctor can initiate this sequence of empathy-to-empowerment by changing the kind of questions he or she poses to patients (Malterud, 1987a, 1987b, 1990, 1994). Once again, the doctor must initiate this transformation in the unequal relationship.

Malterud's work merits detailed description because it is an explicit application of feminist principles to medical practice and it is not widely available to North American clinicians. She begins with the assumption that language reflects the power relations between doctor and patient: the person in charge can define the legitimacy of knowledge and how language is perceived. The doctor (often a man) will define the "context of communication" and thereby "reject or lose the patient's knowledge and considerations" (1990, p. 233). "Traditionally, the patient's subjective experience of her symptoms, their consequences in her social life, and the expression given by her in her own language (illness) is not included in the valid medical concept of disease" (p. 234). Malterud proposes a method of communication "based upon the deliberate medical use of the conversation between doctor and patient": "The intention of the method is to influence the social relation and interaction in the consultation by (1) strengthening the position and power of the female patient, and (2) promoting the ability of the female patient to share with the doctor her knowledge about her health complaints and illnesses" (p. 234).

Other analysts of medical communication have proposed changes in doctor's language skills to enhance communication, but Malterud is unique in defining her goal as *strengthening the power of the female patient*. Using questions that enhance the patient's power contrasts with models of the medical interview that identify specific language skills to improve patient satisfaction. Qualities such as attentiveness, facilitation, and collaboration certainly render an interview more "humanistic," but the goal of patient satisfaction is not the same as the goal of empowerment (Mishler et al., 1989). Likewise, the goal of mutual collaboration—recognizing and supporting patients as partners with physicians (Szasz & Hollender, 1956)—sounds desirable, but the grounds for the partnership are unclear. Everything in the context, structure, and language of doctor-patient interaction makes doctors more powerful and patients less so. How can doctors, at the point of making a diagnostic or treatment plan, suddenly dismiss the power relations in favor of a partnership model? When doctors talk about partnership, they want a willing, informed, and agreeable junior partner. Wanting patients to be powerful is not how most doctors view collaboration. Thus, the intent of Malterud's feminist model differs from the humanistic goal of improved patient satisfaction, even though some of the methods are similar.

Malterud uses four key questions in her work with patients. First, she asks for the patient's definition of her problem: "What would you really most of all want me to do for you today?" (1987b, p. 211). On the surface, this question appears neither profound nor transformative; it is very similar to the question "How do you hope that I can help you?" advocated for interviews with psychiatric patients (Lazare & Eisenthal, 1979). Once again, however, the intent is different. Lazare and Eisenthal see their question as providing the jumping-off place for negotiation between doctor and patient. Malterud locates in the answer to her question the distress women feel in their life situations that leads them to develop symptoms. Her question allows a patient to bring up the conflict between feeling overwhelmed by the work of caring and the centrality of caring to her self-definition: "I feel dizzy when I stand up—seeing zigzags before my eyes. I wonder if there is something wrong with my brain. It might be nerves—I have been living under an enormous pressure because of health problems in my children the last twenty years. You know, that is why I exist—to take care of my children" (1987b, p. 213).

In interviews in which I have felt flummoxed by the diffuse and overwhelming nature of the patient's presenting concerns, I have found that using Malterud's question cuts through vagueness and sharpens the focus. Patients' answers are often completely unexpected: "I'd like to try some Seldane to see if it would help the mucous," or, "Just get me out of here in time to get my laundry from the laundromat before it closes." Physician reluctance to ask the question stems from fear—fear that the answer will be so overwhelming that she or he cannot possibly respond. Noddings calls this "the legitimate dread of the proximate stranger" (1984, p. 85)—someone who requests more than one can conceivably give.

Malterud's second question asks for the woman's view of causality: "What do you yourself think is the reason for x?" (the health complaints described in her own words). When necessary, she adds: "Yes, we'll certainly find out about that—but I am sure you have been thinking about what might be the causes of x." This statement might be complemented with, "Since you have suffered from x for y days, you must have been thinking of its possible causes." Implicit in Malterud's repeated effort to elicit the patient's explanation is the awareness that patients' assumption of powerlessness makes them reluctant to suggest an explanation. Patients commonly use responses like, "You're the doctor," and, "That's what I came here for," to deflect the question. Persistent efforts to elicit the patient's idea of causality are well worth the trouble: the answer offers an entry into her understanding of what makes her sick and opens a window onto her experience of worry. The patient is unlikely to give a scientific explanation of what has made her ill, but scientifically verifiable causes are only a small portion of any explanation. "The patient's so-called model of illness differs most significantly from the clinician's not in terms of exotic symbolization but in terms of the anxiety to locate the social and moral meaning of the disease" (Taussig, 1980, pp. 12–13). The kinds of explanations patients make—being run down, under pressure, overworked, in constant fear—are valid at a different level from biological explanations and tell the clinician a great deal about what changes will be necessary for recovery.

Malterud's third question seeks to elicit the woman's expectations of the doctor: "What do you think I should do with x? I'm sure you thought of that before you came here?" As with the first question, doctors' resistance to asking this question stems from their fear of the answer. They do not want to find out what the patient wants them to do because it might be too much work or because they might disagree with what the patient proposes. It might be against medical principles, or too expensive. Sometimes patients want administrative actions (referrals and certifications) that doctors would rather deny. Finding out the answer to this question early in an interaction allows the doctor either to situate her or his response within the patient's expectation or, if the doctor's response disappoints the patient's expectation, to open the disagreement up for discussion.

Malterud's fourth question elicits the woman's actual experiences of handling her health complaints: "What have you so far found to be the best way of managing the illness?" The question conveys the doctor's respect for the woman, and the answer validates her as an authority on her own health issues. Malterud's questions use language to strengthen the patient's position. By asking for the patient's opinion in an open-ended way and getting her definition of the problem, these questions remind her of her problem-solving resources and support her as a source of knowledge by acknowledging her experiences. The systematic return to her own words legitimates her use of medical language and confirms her as the expert. These steps challenge the usual conduct of the medical encounter because they imply "the existence of multiple response alternatives outside the imagination of the doctor" (1990, p. 236). They support and empower the patient by legitimating her explanations, her experience, and her language, "verifying the competence claimed by her own words" (p. 236). Malterud's method points the way toward enabling patients to reflect on their own understanding of causality and to offer their desire for clarification and naming of their symptoms, not necessarily for treatment or cure.

Laying out such an approach as a list of questions makes it appear to be a set of moves; it would be better thought of as a kind of openness or imaginative inquiry, an empathetic readiness to learn. On the other hand, a set of specific questions is helpful because it parallels the medical model of inquiry, which is typically based on questions (Frankel, 1990): both the doctor and the patient expect that the doctor will ask questions to explore a certain set of symptoms. In this model, doctor's questions that recognize the patient's experiences of both her body and her context, that verify her use of language, that acknowledge her explanations of her symptoms, and that draw on her personal resources for problem-solving—such questions are first steps in making the doctor-patient relationship a source of empowerment.[9]

TAKING THE OTHER PERSON SERIOUSLY

I distinguish this quality from treating the person as a person, from empathetic readiness, and from considering the patient in her context. Taking a person seriously incorporates paying attention to where she is at the moment, respecting her fears, listening beneath her jokes, and not making light of or trivializing her concerns. Patients are concerned about how doctors think of them; as a doctor, taking the patient seriously means taking into consideration what he or she might be afraid you will think. Malterud gives the example of the patient who presents her symptoms as overwhelming because she is afraid the doctor will blame her for her symptoms. I am reminded of the patient who dramatically swamped me with her symptoms: she had sinusitis, a cough, premenstrual syndrome, itchy feet, and she was overweight. When I asked her Malterud's key question, "What would you really most of all hope that I could do for you today?" she replied, "Oh, I wish you could put me in the hospital for four days so I could quit smoking." She herself saw smoking as central to her problem but did not want me to lecture her or blame her, as she already was hypercritical of herself.

Malterud suggests that a doctor take two steps to show that he or she recognizes the patient's situation: invite mutuality humorously, thereby averting the threat of embarrassment; and allow a dignified retreat so that the patient can be in charge of her own position. These steps, avoidance of embarrassment and dignified retreat, reverberate with the awareness among feminist researchers that what a woman says at the moment may be what she *can* say. For example, in a German project on violence against women, it emerged that the battered women had initially not told the truth about their past. "Faking" is part of women's survival—researchers (and doctors) need to accept it and take it seriously. The researchers' initial conviction that honesty was the highest priority needed to be replaced by the understanding that the subjects were saying what they could (Klein, 1983). As Maria Mies puts it, "The truth of a person cannot be asked for, is not static, but grows and develops during the course of a life time" (quoted in Klein, 1983, p. 95)—or, I would argue, during a relationship.

Clinicians need to remember that patients say what they can say as they listen to women trying to explain their symptoms. Perhaps the patient cannot accomplish the physical or emotional work of caring but cannot resign from it either. For some women, being part of a hopeless relationship may cause symptoms, especially "if the woman feels responsible for maintaining the relationship while at the same time she has no influence or power, and is hit by the reflections of the conflicts" (Malterud, 1990, p. 237). This pattern may reflect the presentation of women in abusive relationships. Indeed, health complaints may develop in situations that require a woman to "hide her feelings out of concern for others or herself" (p. 237). Cultural standards of suitable sick behavior also influence how a woman suffering from overload presents herself to the doctor: a woman worrying about unlikely serious disease may be vague so as not to come across as a hypochondriac, while another woman may hide her health beliefs in order not to be blamed for something she thinks is her own fault. The excessive detail of the presentation may be an attempt to hide shame for not preventing the problem and to ward off the doctor's "unrealistic recommendations to reduce stress and strain" (Malterud, 1990, p. 238).[10]

Averting embarrassment and ensuring a dignified retreat are acts that allow a woman to mobilize her survival strategies. I learned this when a Vietnamese woman brought her child in for follow-up after hospitalization for asthma. She had a sore hand. When I examined it, it was so tender that I suspected a fracture. She stated that it happened when she fainted, and that she had been fainting frequently. It did not look to me like an injury from fainting, but I did not challenge her account. She went for an X ray, which showed a fracture. She then confided in the translator that her husband had been beating her and had forced her hand against a wall. Later she told me that she had been embarrassed to tell me that her husband was beating her again. It was more tolerable for her to confide in the translator—knowing full well that the translator would pass the information along to me—than to tell me directly about the beating. I learned that sometimes a woman needs to tell a story that is not entirely true, not because she is a liar but because the reality is too painful to acknowledge consciously at the moment or in front of a particular person.

CHOICE AND CONTROL

Empowerment is tied to a patient's sense of control over her life; it includes accepting her priorities, legitimating her choices, and allowing her control over as much of the circumstances of medical and health care as possible. Nurses committed to combating powerlessness can offer measures of control even to patients who are totally dependent (paralyzed and intubated) (Boeing & Mongera, 1989). Legitimating a patient's choices and putting her in control when she is terminally ill may mean accepting and supporting her choices about when, where, and how to die (Quill, 1991).[11] Paradoxically, empowerment can also mean supporting patients' choices in relinquishing responsibilities. For instance, an eighty-two-year-old woman who had nursed her husband for five years until his death chose to sell her house of forty years and move into a small apartment in a condominium complex for the elderly. She garnered the energy she had previously used taking care of her husband and cleaning and managing the old house and yard for her new priorities of traveling and visiting friends. Similarly, a young cancer patient decided to request that the hospice worker pick up her son at school and bring him home. Although she was openly angry about no longer being able to meet him at school and jealous of the worker's health and ability to do the task, her empowerment lay not in talking about the loss but more in her deliberate choice to have some energy to be with her son when he got home. Thus, the acceptance and legitimation of choices to cut back or reduce activity can empower people of diminishing resources to use their energy to their own best perceived interest.

Just as caring-in-relation requires a reinterpretation of dependency (chapter 9), so too with empowerment. In ordinary parlance, dependence and empowerment seem to be contradictory. This problem resolves when dependency is redefined as:

> a process of counting on other people to provide help in coping physically and emotionally with the experiences and tasks encountered in the world, when one has not sufficient skill, confidence, energy and/or time. . . . What each of us requires emotionally from others is to feel affirmed and validated in one's feelings and perceptions. This notion of dependency would allow for experiencing one's self as being enhanced and empowered through the very process of counting on others for help. In these terms, dependency would be seen as normal and growth-promoting. (Stiver, 1991c, p. 160)

The implication of this reformulation of dependency for the doctor-patient relationship is that the recognition of emotional needs (dependency) can be viewed as empowering the patient; recognizing those needs does not need to be seen as taking power away. This framework contrasts with the patriarchal understanding of dependency: the one cared for is either deprived of something or terrifyingly helpless. When autonomy is upheld as the ideal of human development, dependency is translated into a pathological helplessness. (Infancy, old age, and illness offer examples of this dreaded dependency.) The view of human beings as in-relation, in contrast, sees the connection between counting on, relying on, and trusting others in the fabric of a full and healthy life.

Taking the patient seriously means supporting the patient's priorities for physical integrity over medical arguments for intervention. Examples include the refusal of an incest survivor to have a pelvic exam because it would rock her precarious sense of control over her body; a Jamaican man's refusal of amputation because he cannot accept the idea of surgery on his leg to prevent gangrene of his toe; the refusal by an unlettered alcoholic man of a laryngectomy and likely cure because he prefers to retain his ability to speak for the short time before his cancer inevitably spreads. Empowering such patients consists in accepting their priorities as legitimate despite the inconsistency between them and the medical model.

Taking the woman patient seriously means accepting that *health* per se may not be her first priority (Raymond, 1982). Women may choose to live "self-defined lives" in which health is not "the final statement, the conclusive and comprehensive category for female existence" (p. 213). While it is important, it is not the central question in the creation of woman-defined living. I have this discussion regularly with a patient who is an intellectual woman and weighs 260 pounds. She succeeded in losing 100 pounds on a starvation diet ten years ago, only to regain it over the following two years. We both understand that her weight is genetically controlled and that it is not good for her health. We both know that she eats neither too much nor unwisely. Yet at this time in her life, knowing what she knows, she does not see weight loss as a priority. Although I know her weight may harm her health and shorten her life span, I support her choice about how she wants to lead her life now. A strategy of empowerment for women in the medical setting supports woman-defined living as the central task and makes health an element but not the only goal of clinical work.

Childbirth is one moment when a woman's priorities for a self-defined life can be examined. Empowering a woman during birth begins with finding out her expectations and aspirations for the birth and learning what kind of outcome would promote her sense of mastery. The clinician must engage in this process before labor because the responses should come from the woman's competent adult perspective; she can give her best sense of who she is and who she wants to be as a mother when she is not in pain. The story of the birth is hers, and she will be the one to live with it and integrate it into her story of herself. Familiarity, comfort, and participation in this narrative becomes the clinician's role.

For childbirth to promote a woman's sense of mastery, the meaning of mastery unique to her must emerge. Fidelity to her values is most likely to promote a woman's sense of mastery (Laslie, 1982). For some women, the goal of no medication and no intervention is paramount; others want a pain-free birth, perhaps like the one a sister or a friend had. Some fear the loss of composure, being out of control, or what others will think of them if they scream or swear. Others fear the pain but fear the foreign medical territory and English-speaking professionals even more. And many adolescents are caught in the middle, uncertain what messages to believe. Of course, not every woman can put her image of mastery into words (especially if no one ever bothered to ask her before), but the role of the empowering clinician is to elicit her fears and preferences and create an atmosphere that strengthens her on her own terms.[12] A woman-centered childbirth experience needs to be distinguished from family-centered maternity care in settings where hospital staffs make it clear that they are most comfortable with the nuclear family "as the normal social context for birth" (Laslie, 1982, p. 187; Midmer, 1992).

Empowerment during childbirth is more than a matter of offering patients a choice: "You could have this or you could have that; here are the advantages and disadvantages." Instead, it is a continuous process of sizing up the situation, figuring out what could put the woman more in control, more in charge, and enable her to be less passive. Empowering a woman during labor often takes the form of suggesting a change in position: standing, walking, or taking a shower. Apart from the merits of the sitting and standing positions as they affect labor itself, encouraging the woman to resume the upright position reminds everyone present that she is a full person, not a sick and helpless patient. Often empowering strategies cannot come from the woman in labor herself because she is unaware of the possibilities or does not remember them at the time. The clinician's active listening is central. Just as empowerment in teaching requires listening to the changes that students undergo, a birth attendant who would empower a woman in labor must ask about and listen to her reports of what is happening in her body: what she feels, where it hurts, how her breathing and speech change. The clinician must pay attention to what is helpful and what is not helpful and be constantly prepared to change; what is comforting at one point may become noxious and objectionable a few minutes later.

Promoting mastery in the childbirth experience includes helping the patient define her own expectations and aspirations as a woman prior to labor, showing respect for those expectations, eliciting her fears, and identifying sources of support. Attending the process of labor requires adherence to the values of the family and the woman; attention to her experience on a moment-to-moment basis; respect for her decisions; and constant reexamination of the setting to recover sources of empowerment for her. The birth attendant has the responsibility to clarify what is optional in hospital practice and to maximize the woman's potential for freedom within the fewest possible constraints.[13]

NARRATIVE

Each woman is the keeper of her own history, the narrator of her own story. Empowerment means shaping the medical care to fit her personal narrative—for instance, finding out that the patient with the fractured hip who feels inept and weak in physical therapy is the same woman who taught her daughter to walk again following polio (Taussig, 1980). A woman's emotions and intentions are not just momentary; her personal narrative has been long under way and will keep on going. If we are to understand others in a "morally adequate way," we need to attend "to how their beliefs, feelings, modes of expression, circumstances and more, arranged in characteristic ways and often spread out in time, configure into a recognizable kind of story" (Walker, 1989, p. 18). Doing so requires paying minute and specific attention to "individual embroideries and idiosyncracies."

Eliciting women's own narratives of their lives is a central feature of feminist work in anthropology, sociology, and history. Taken as individuals and in groups, women's accounts of their experiences make unique interpretations of historical and psychological events (Blaxter, 1983;

Robinson, 1990). Medical practitioners rarely use narrative and life history work to elicit people's experience and understanding of illness—partly because it is time-consuming, but more important, because medical discourse tends to dominate. The creation of the narrative in the presence of a doctor allows a woman to put her experience in its historical and social context and to move beyond the individual or psychological framework to the level of myth and metaphor. The clinician can be one of the co-creators of the story, searching beneath the surface for unstated themes related to healing myths and refigured narratives that might promote healing (Shapiro, 1993). The clinician must never forget, however, that the empowerment approach takes the woman's own interpretation of her story as primary.[14]

EMPOWERMENT AND EDUCATION

Giving patients information about their bodies, their illnesses, and their medications is certainly basic to medical care, regardless of the doctor's goals about patient empowerment. Studies show a direct link between the amount of information physicians provide and the degree of patient satisfaction (Blanchard, Labrecque, Ruckdeschel, & Blanchard, 1990; Hall et al., 1988). Patient education usually means providing information understandable to patients about their health care, illness, treatment, and outlook. The doctor commonly uses the process to support his or her plan of management, and it is not often a source of controversy. Sometimes doctors relegate "patient education" to others; often such education consists in giving clear instructions and making sure the patient understands them. This kind of teaching and learning depends on what Freire (1970) calls the "banking" concept of education: material is "deposited" to be "withdrawn" later. A far different kind of patient education may occur with the educated or professional patient whose ability to read the medical literature and sort out the statistics of experimental protocols may be as good as the doctor's. Such patients can make their own assessment of the evidence rather than having to rely on the doctor to interpret scientific studies (DiGiacomo, 1987). However, outside of university settings, such patients are uncommon. Lack of familiarity with scientific material and limited reading ability prevent most patients from collaborating with the physician to gain sophisticated and technical information.

More commonly, patients' limited reading abilities compromise their health status and disempower them in health care settings (Weiss et al., 1992). The growing realization that many patients cannot read, or can barely read, patient information, medicine labels, and instruction sheets has led some educators to focus on patient literacy (Davis et al., 1990; Davis et al., 1993). Alternatively, doctors may conclude that using written materials for patient education is a waste of precious time. The difficulty that many patients have with consent forms for treatment, surgery, and participation in research protocols, most of which are written in legalistic language accessible only to those with postgraduate education (LoVerde et al., 1989), leads many doctors and nurses to be dubious if not cynical about the role of written materials. However, focusing on illiteracy once again raises the issue of power-over versus power to empower: a patient's illiteracy can be used to exacerbate the power discrepancy between clinician and patient, or it can serve as the opening wedge in a strategy of empowerment. Paulo Freire's work teaching unlettered Brazilian peasants showed that even those who cannot read possess a critical consciousness about themselves and the world they live in. Finding out what patients already know, asking them what they want and need to know, encouraging them to ask questions (Greenfield, Kaplan, & Ware, 1985; Greenfield, Kaplan, Ware, Yano, & Frank, 1988), and enhancing their skills at managing their illnesses are tasks that emanate from a very different concept of education.

Education that assumes the patient's preexisting critical consciousness requires an openness on the part of physicians about the whole medical endeavor; they must recognize patients for their special knowledge and allow patients into the uncertainty of medical knowledge and teaching (Lindemann & Oliver, 1982).[15] If a measure of doctors' power over patients is the control over uncertainty (Waitzkin & Stoeckle, 1972), then empowerment includes letting patients in on how little may be known with certainty about their problem. This uncertainty is not equivalent to therapeutic nihilism; rather, it is sharing the task of medical care with the patient in the most profound sense. For instance, patients now know that the radiation given to children in the 1930s and 1940s caused later thyroid cancer, and that the DES given to pregnant women in the early 1950s caused genital abnormalities and cancer in their offspring. Although those treatments were given with scientific confidence but now are in disrepute, doctors do not present today's treatments as questionable, even though we are often uncertain of their long-term effects. My own experience includes prescribing, in the 1970s, antihypertensive treatment with thiazide diuretics in doses that now have been shown to be associated with excess mortality (Wikstrand et al., 1991).[16] I remember encouraging patients to take their medicines and reminding them of the importance of blood pressure control for their long-term health. Now I am humbled to realize that the treatment I (and thousands of other clinicians) tried so hard to promote was harmful. I wonder, was I cautious enough? Did I tell patients often enough that "we don't know" the long-term effects?

In some ways, drug treatment is the most rapidly changing and uncertain aspect of medical practice, but it is also one in which patients can actively participate as their own individual control. Even placebo treatment can be assessed by patients who are fully aware of the placebo effect.[17] Only patients can tell what the effect of the medicine is; they have to be the final arbiter of whether it is useful or not. Patients, of course, do not and cannot know that a given drug has been or may in the future be statistically associated with increased mortality, but they do know if it does not feel right. When a patient tells me now that a drug is not right for her, I need to respect that judgment, not because she has any mystical or intuitive knowledge about the drug's effects, but because her knowledge of the drug's side effects on her is as useful a criterion as large-scale statistical studies in deciding about drug treatment for her. Her assessment is as valid a measure *in her direct care* as any other measure available to me, and may be better.

Understanding patients' potential for critical consciousness enables us to reconsider the whole notion of patient "compliance." Patient choices to adjust or stop medications may reflect their effort to control, regulate, or manage their own illnesses rather than a flaunting of authority (Conrad, 1987). Within their understanding of their illnesses and their medications, patients seek the best way to manage their lives, control their symptoms, and live as well as possible. For patients on long-term drug therapy, increasing, decreasing, and stopping medication are ways to gain control over symptoms and over the disease itself. For patients with epilepsy, who usually require at least one chronic medication, self-regulation of their drug treatment represents a way to take control over a disorder that at times seems to control their lives (Conrad, 1987). Clinicians can empower patients on long-term medication by expecting that they will self-regulate and inquiring into patient discoveries about their symptoms when they have done so. Knowing that medication doses are arbitrarily determined (Herxheimer, 1991), that human beings vary greatly in their metabolism of drugs of all classes, and that individuals have idiosyncratic reactions to even common drugs, clinicians should take a humble approach to patients' self-knowledge about their medications.

Or take the area of diagnosis. A forty-year-old man has experienced numbness on the outer aspect of his leg for two months. A sensory nerve serving that area has probably been pinched or traumatized. It is unlikely that there is any specific medical or surgical treatment for the problem. The numbness could be an unusual early sign of diabetes, which he is worried about. I could send him for nerve conduction studies of the nerves in his leg, or I could wait and explain that there is probably no determinable cause and no specific treatment. If I tell him exactly what the nerve conduction studies entail (twenty to forty electric shocks of an intensity harsh enough to make his leg jump off the table), he has a much better idea of whether he thinks the symptom warrants the evaluation. I can also let him know that he himself will know, long before any such test is repeated, whether the numbness is improving or getting worse. In contrast, the discomfort of the diabetes testing is far more congruent with his level of worry about that condition. He can easily weigh the inconvenience and the pain of that testing against the benefit of relatively certain information about his blood sugar level.

The joint participation of ordinary, technically unsophisticated patients must be made possible by legitimating their status as the experts about their own health care and their own bodies. Modern medicine denies that a patient has a "knowledge of a different kind but equally important as his or her own for the medical encounter" (Lindemann & Oliver, 1982, p. 140). Medicine implicitly denies this form of expertise by continually reminding patients of all the ways they cannot know when something is wrong—that they may have high blood pressure, or an abnormal pap smear, or breast masses too small to feel but large enough to be detected by mammography. All too few practitioners and patients are aware that the utility of screening for asymptomatic disease is actually limited to a relatively small number of conditions (Oboler & LaForce, 1989). By far the most useful indicators of problems doctors could and should address are those symptoms of which patients are aware. Yet except among clinicians who treat a large proportion of patients with chronic diseases (for instance, rheumatologists), the importance of patients' assessments of their own disability or level of symptoms is limited, ignored, or even denigrated. The patient as expert is not a common understanding among physicians.

Patient education also means informing people about real risk. People bring their healthy child to the doctor for a yearly physical examination. They believe that the doctor might find something that they themselves were unaware of about their child's health. The unstated hope is that the visit will prevent some dreadful disease from overtaking their child. Occasionally I do discover minor problems unknown to the parents and the child; more often I find that they watch too much television, get too little exercise, and eat poorly. My ability to influence these practices is limited. Statistically, the greatest cause of death and disability among healthy school-age children is trauma: car accidents, bike accidents, fire, drowning, and so on. All the medical visits in the world will not prevent these catastrophes; systematic use of seatbelts, bike helmets, and smoke detectors and adherence to swimming safety rules would make some difference. Parents need to know about these risks in order to make choices based on them; their annual visit with me might be better spent talking about these risks than doing physical exams to ward off cancer fears.

Patient education for empowerment teaches people to care for their own health needs as much as possible; it means giving them the tools and information to make decisions. Patients allowed to review their own charts ask more questions and become more active in interviews with doctors (Greenfield et al., 1985). Patients want far more information about their diagnoses, their prognosis, and their medications than doctors usually provide (Strull et al., 1984; Waitzkin, 1984a). However, patients are more dissatisfied when doctors do more talking than patients and dominate the tone of encounters (Bertakis, Roter, & Putnam, 1991). An empowerment approach can resolve this apparent contradiction. Patients want more information but do not want doctors to exert more power-over. If doctors begin from the position of readiness to learn about the patient's view of the world (empathic readiness), then it is far more likely that the information she or he provides will suit what the patient wants and needs.

Let me offer two examples. First, when doctors initially ask parents of developmentally delayed children about their sense of what is going on with the child, the parents are likely to accept diagnostic information from the doctor. When doctors attempt to give information about disabilities without going through this step, patients reject the doctors' diagnosis (Maynard, 1989, 1991). This finding reminds us of the importance of finding out where a person is at before trying to initiate a course of action. A second example comes from a study of the communication between doctors and patients about the treatment for abnormal pap smears. The doctor who initially asked each patient about her understanding of her problem performed fewer hysterectomies. He was open to hearing her perspective and fitting his treatment into it (Fisher, 1983). This finding suggests that even though questioning is a linguistic form that can reinforce doctors' power-over, questions that seek to elicit the patient's understanding and desire for information serve a different purpose. They enable the patient to talk about her own reality. The power of these questions is the power to empower, as opposed to power-over. Patients' strong preference for information, even when they do not wish to make medical decisions themselves (Ende et al., 1989), supports the importance of information itself as a source of power for patients.

Collaborative health models like the Peckham Experiment have attempted to give patients the tools and information to maintain their own health in the setting of an entire community committed to a healthy lifestyle (Ransom, 1983, 1985). But care of the "activated patient"—one who wants to understand her medical problem and the options in the management of her illness and to become able to take care of herself further into the course of illness—is problematic for physicians who do not embrace empowerment as a goal.

The vision of empowerment I have described is not free of problems. First, critics may argue that empowerment as I portray it is no more than technique. It is reducing empowerment to verbal strategies that turn it into technique, and technique does not serve empowerment because it keeps the doctor in control. Such a criticism is valid then if the clinician implementing this vision of empowerment regards it as no more than technique. Jordan points out that domination interferes with mutuality and contradicts it: "If one is primarily concerned with the establishment of a position of dominance vis-a-vis another, that motive eliminates the possibility of a real interest in the subjective experience of the other. Rather, one's own interests are felt as uppermost. Manipulation of others to achieve ends that are unilaterally defined becomes the focus of the interaction" (1991b, p. 93). In other words, interest in another in order to control him or her is not real interest but self-interest.[18] The power model is based on inequality, disconnection, and "a prevailing sense of competing subjectivities"; in contrast, mutuality requires capacity for empathy, interaction, and "reciprocally enhancing subjectivity" (p. 93). Jordan finds the two models totally at odds. Clearly, one who views empathy as a set of strategic maneuvers is functioning from a position of instrumentality and power maintenance, not one of empowerment.

More problematically, the use of an empowerment "strategy" might further potentiate doctors' power over patients, to "seize on the implicit with the instruments of modern social science so to all the better control it" (Taussig, 1980, p. 13). Doctors taking such an instrumental approach might use the language of empathy and support to lend human- and spontaneous-looking features to the doctor-patient relationship when they are actually only using linguistic devices to maintain and enhance their control. When such a technique is used from a position of dominance, it will only perpetuate the position of dominance. An extension of this argument is that empowerment-as-strategy is a counterfeit activity, that it is not genuine. Adopting a verbal strategy of empowerment when one is not truly interested in empowering the patient is an act of falsehood: the doctor is a phony.

This is a telling criticism. Clearly any improvement in clinicians' ability to communicate could be used in the service of abuse and domination. However, unlike the introduction of new technologies, which fortify the technical project in medicine, doctor-initiated changes in communication can change the entire form of the communication process. When a doctor makes overt his or her respect for the patient's opinion, the positions of the patient and the doctor are changed. Of course, that respect must be genuine, not merely a linguistic maneuver. Conversely, a doctor not truly committed to empowering the patient could not genuinely engage in a linguistic process of empowerment—that is, the doctor's underlying disrespect would emerge in nonverbal or verbal strategies that would be evident to patients regardless of how "skillfully" the doctor used such maneuvers. If, in fact, a clinician adopts language changes without sincere respect for the patient, she or he will be unable to convey verbal and nonverbal sincerity to the patient. A strategy of empowerment cannot prevent phoniness, but it remains a quality that patients are able to judge from a position of less power—perhaps even better from that position.

A second objection is that empowerment is merely another example of paternalism. From this point of view, all therapeutic relationships foster power-over or power as control (Hoagland, 1990a). Professionals take seriously their position as "responsible decision-makers" and thus accept the legitimacy of "'benevolent' control" (p. 141). Paternalism is *always* a potential problem when one human being sets out to help another. The doctor who tries to empower the patient may merely be satisfying his or her own desire to be important, to be seen as helpful, to do good for others. White people who wish to "help" black people, men who wish to "help" women, developed countries that wish to "help" Third World countries, and doctors who wish to "help" patients would do best to step back and listen to what the recipients of their help have to say. In medicine, listening to the patient's presentation of herself, exploring her context, and respecting her experience are the prerequisites to any strategy of empowerment. The clinician who disregards them is running the real risk of acting paternalistically.

On the bright side, however, empowerment of patients transforms clinicians. The process of eliciting the stories sometimes changes the doctor himself or herself. Doctors who may be dubious about the frequency of marital battering, childhood sexual abuse, or date rape yet are willing to ask patients questions about the violence in their lives, are profoundly affected by their growing realization of the universality of such abuse. Similarly, doctors may find that after following an instruction to adopt a new form—say, not to interrupt the patient's opening statement and to provide linguistic forms of continuation ("Mm-hmm," or, "Go on") until the opener is completed—they are more satisfied with the new form of inquiry than the old. A small change in behavior (or technique) may actually change for the better what happens between doctors and patients (Frankel, Morse, Suchman, & Beckman, 1991).

Empowerment of the patient requires that the clinician change as well. Because clinicians can live through no more than a fraction of life events similar to those that all their patients experience, we must be open to learn from patients, insofar as we are able, what it means to have epilepsy, to live with cancer, to survive a battering marriage, to pack three small children onto a city bus for an early morning appointment. The passage of time and the clinician's growing experience are essential to deepening this understanding of other people's social reality. (Not that beginning clinicians cannot engage in empowerment; sometimes the novice has more time, more energy, and more openness to engagement.) Life experience and clinical work provide the context for thoughtful self-criticism—recognizing our mistaken application of assumptions from our own values or training or past histories to the patient's experience. When self-scrutiny is lacking, when we think we know what is wanted or needed from us without asking, then we are indeed guilty of the charge of paternalism.

A third objection to empowerment as I have described it is that it expands the already extensive invasion of medicine into people's lives, that bringing the psychosocial dimension of a patient's life into the medical encounter extends medicine's hegemony over human activities by medicalizing social problems (Arney, 1982; Illich, 1976; Stimson, 1977; Waitzkin, 1989). The patient appears sicker in more dimensions, and the doctor is rendered more powerful as a result. Such expansion puts more and more of modern life under medical purview (diet, exercise, weight, sex, recreation, work, sleep, family life) and further reduces personal privacy and agency. This argument is the tough challenge that Foucault's work presents to anyone who chooses to be a clinician nowadays. The answer may in fact be a matter of faith: if the medical relationship has anything to offer that can outweigh this kind of ideological control, it must lie in the resiliency of the human spirit and the depth of connection that individuals in relation can make to each other. Clearly medicine can condemn a person's way of life, invade her privacy, assault her body, render her powerless in the face of technology, while at the same time enjoining her to participate in the process. Empowerment as I have defined it, however, begins at the point of respect for the patient and for her right to reclaim her life and create her own understanding of illness or health. It requires the engagement of one human being with another in a mutual project. Empowerment is an act of resistance to medicine as a totalitarian agent of social control because the doctor and patient are not engaged in medicine's project but rather in the patient's own empowerment as a woman.

Lastly, some critics will argue that individual empowerment does not create social change. Of course, they are right. The empowerment of individuals is only a small step. And medicine is only one arena of people's experience of disenfranchisement and powerlessness. Nevertheless, I can imagine the strength and resourcefulness that respectful and empathic relationships could elicit from people who have never been recognized. I can imagine the power and energy of people coming together to make social change after each had felt the surge of personal empowerment. I can imagine relationships with patients, with children, with students, as the steps toward a world where people can claim, together, their power. Likewise, empowerment strategies offer clinicians the opportunity to engage, in small ways, in social change through relationships that engage, transform, and empower.

If, given these arguments, clinicians decide that empowerment makes sense as a way to approach their work, what would empowerment in a feminist practice of medicine look like? I will offer two examples from families I know well.

Dolores Rodriguez,[19] a forty-six-year-old Puerto Rican woman, slumped to the floor from her chair while waiting at the social security office. Bystanders told her later she had been unconscious. She went home and later came to the hospital complaining of dizziness and pains in her chest. The emergency room staff admitted her to be sure she had not had a heart attack, even though the history of her symptoms did not sound typical of a cardiac event.

Mrs. Rodriguez takes care of her two adult retarded daughters, both of whom are deaf; one is more deaf and more limited than the other. Her husband, who alternates between being unemployed and under-employed, also has many physical complaints and is somewhat hard of hearing. He does not share in any of the housework or care of the daughters. Both parents have long-standing anger at each other dating back to the time of their marriage, but they have been unwilling to con-sider either individual or joint psychotherapy. Over the years both par-ents have appeared to be chronically depressed, and at times they seem to compete with each other in the intensity of their physical complaints. Almost twenty years ago Mrs. Rodriguez had lumbar disc surgery, and she has had low back pain ever since. Although she has heard about overnight respite care for people like her daughters, she does not want them staying somewhere else overnight.

After admission to the hospital, Mrs. Rodriguez underwent a series of tests to detect any heart injury and to check on her heart's rhythms and contraction. She also underwent studies of the circulation to her brain to find any vascular explanation for her dizziness. Thirty-six hours after admission, when all her tests were negative, she still com-plained of feeling dizzy; she did not feel ready to go home from the hos-pital. Her sister came up from New York to look after the daughters. The next day she still felt dizzy and said that the social worker who talked to her about a day program would be in to see her on Monday; she wanted to wait to talk to her. Also, her husband had gone off to Boston to visit his sick aunt, so she had no way to get home. She went home Monday, a little better, half-believing that she might have a dizzi-ness problem but still wondering if there was something the matter with her heart. Why, if nothing was wrong, did she get the flutterings and poundings? She came back to the office the next week feeling some-what better.

We talked about the long-term care of her daughters "should any-thing happen" to her. She said that her husband claimed he would look after them, even though he had never taken any care of them since infancy. Her sister in Puerto Rico would be willing to have them, but they had never been to Puerto Rico. I asked her about the possibility of taking a trip with the girls to Puerto Rico. She told me then that she had been approved for social security disability. When her checks started to come, she was thinking about such a trip. (She could receive social secu-rity disability payments in Puerto Rico whereas welfare payments had required her to remain in Massachusetts.) Her husband did not want her to go, but she was serious about it. She had told him that "the days of slavery are over." Thinking about Puerto Rico, she thought that things would be easier there, with the exception of the medical care. She was not pleased about the kind of medical care she could get there. I reminded her that, however good we were, our health center could not provide the day-to-day care her daughters would need if she were unable to provide it.

In the setting of enormous family burdens, an uncommunicative and unsupportive husband, and a bureaucracy unresponsive to the needs of Spanish-speaking retarded people, empowerment of Mrs. Rodriguez has been a formidable challenge. However, her personal dignity, her forbearance, and her substantial skills in handling the state bureaucracy for the retarded have been consistent strengths. She is also considered a wise and intelligent woman in her church. Within her world, physical illness and body pain have been the only acceptable paths to support and respite. Now with the option of geographic mobility, she can consider breaking out of the entrenched gender conflict of her marriage. Empowerment here means helping her to think about the choices and supporting her decision.

In the two years that have passed since I first wrote this account, Mrs. Rodriguez has grown more determined to return to Puerto Rico with her daughters. She is not talking to anyone about her plans, however. She says that one day she will just leave, and everyone in her world will be surprised. In the meantime, she has decided to write down everything that has ever happened to her. She has asked me to read it when it is done. I like to think that seeing my written accounts of some of her life events encouraged her to tell her own story.

I have known thirty-two-year-old Josefina Santana Perez since her daughter Jessica, now fourteen, was an infant. Josefina is a fully bilingual Dominican woman who works as a teacher's aide in a bilingal classroom. She is an assertive woman who can be very demanding with the on-call doctor when she wants treatment for her problem with urinary tract infections. In retrospect, her demands usually appear appropriate. Jessica is the oldest of her three children; the other two are boys. The father of all three is currently in jail, due to get out soon. The mother has a new relationship and is newly pregnant.

Josefina brought her daughter in for a checkup; Jessica sat on the examining table with her head hung down, long hair around her face. Her mother immediately asked me if I wanted a baby-sitter, told me I could have her, I could keep her. I asked Jessica why she was there, and she said, disgustedly, "for a physical."

"You don't like physicals?"

"I hate going to clinics."

"I don't blame you. And you've been to a lot of them, I bet."

Recently I had received a request for information about Jessica from a counselor at a local family service agency. I asked her about the counseling. Jessica had gone four or five times but still did not know the "lady's" name. Josefina told me that her daughter argued with every single thing she said. I laughingly reminded her that her mother said the same about her, that she still hadn't stopped arguing. "She sounds just like you!" Josefina jokingly accepted the analogy. Jessica smiled for the first time to see her mother repositioned as the argumentative one. I continued to deflect Josefina's criticisms of her daughter and established that Jessica was not in trouble with the law, had not skipped school, and was not pregnant. Josefina told me that Jessica had had a period around the time of her own last period; Jessica acted embarrassed. I shooed Josefina out to do the physical.

Alone with Jessica, I asked her what she would most of all like for me to do that day. She said, "Get me off punishment." I asked her what she was being punished for. It turned out that she got detention and missed a therapy session. Her mother had punished her by grounding her for a week, with no TV and no phone calls. She was three days into it. She didn't like the therapist, who "asks too many questions." A seventh-grader, Jessica was in the college track at her junior high school. She found schoolwork easy and sometimes didn't do her homework. She had had detention three times, once for tying another girl's sleeves behind her back, once for putting a boy's books on the window sill where they fell out after the boy had been bothering her, and once for being late for class. She did not smoke, drink, do or sell drugs, or miss school; she was not having sex and was not close to doing so. She described the constant bickering with her younger brothers. She liked to stay over at her traditional grandmother's because it was quiet, but recently her mother and stepfather had stopped her from staying on week nights because they said it was bad for her schoolwork. She said that she liked her stepfather and felt okay about her mother's pregnancy. We didn't talk about her father much at that visit.

On the physical side, Jessica wanted to know if I had anything for pimples. Her exam was normal. She was not particularly uncomfortable or awkward about her body. Afterwards, I went over several issues: the confidentiality of our talk, my openness to birth control when she was ready for it, and my support for her situation. I reminded her that she was not a bad kid and had not done bad stuff. I told her that I thought rewards work better than punishment when parents want kids to do things, and that I would tell her mother that. I asked her what kinds of rewards she might like, and she said, "New jeans." I asked her to suggest something that didn't cost money, and she replied, "Being allowed to go someplace."

When Josefina came back in, I reminded her of all the good things Jessica was doing—going to school every day, eating breakfast every day, unlike most of her peers, and not drinking a lot of soda. Josefina acknowledged all this to be true. I also reminded her that three detentions was not the worst thing in the world, and that Jessica didn't like the therapist. Josefina agreed that the therapist was not working out. Then came the crucial part. Jessica was a Hispanic kid in a mixed junior high school. She didn't fit in with the Spanish-speaking Puerto Rican kids, who were likely to drop out of school, but neither did she fit in with the white middle-class kids, who saw her as a Puerto Rican kid. I reminded Josefina that Jessica had to take "shit" from both sides, and also from any boy who tried to tease her. I also reminded Josefina that she herself didn't believe women should take "shit" from men, that she wouldn't want her daughter to take it either, and that sometimes it was more important to defend yourself and keep your self-respect than it was to be good. Sometimes the kid who defends herself gets caught when the kid who provoked it does not. I redefined Jessica in terms of racial and gender issues as a teenager who was carving out a solid and self-respecting peer position for herself. Josefina acknowledged the truth of all that I was saying. She knew how it was to work as a Hispanic person in a mostly white school system.

After that it was easy to talk about rewards and to reconsider the punishment strategy. At the end, Jessica threw her arms around her mother's neck and pleaded to come off punishment. I sensed Josefina had softened a lot. I reminded her that I was no better with my eight-year-old and that it's a lot easier to do this kind of talking with other people's kids than with your own. I suggested to Jessica that her mother had forgotten a little about what it's like to be fourteen. The next week, at her first prenatal appointment, Josefina told me that things were better. They had gone to their last therapy appointment, and she had agreed to let Jessica "go somewhere with her friends" once a week if she had no detentions.

Both mother and daughter felt confirmed after this half-hour appointment. The daughter's behavior became legitimated, even lauded, when interpreted in the setting of gender and race, and both were supported in the quality of stubbornness they shared. Other common ground was confirmed as well: Josefina and I share the problem of how best to raise daughters.

Individual efforts to reconstruct the doctor-patient relationship to be empowering can seem tenuous in a world where people are constantly being disempowered. Both clinicians and patients are subject to being treated as objects and to being humiliated and oppressed outside the clinical setting. This one relationship cannot fix all the oppression in the patient's life that stems from causes far greater than the doctor-patient relationship. Likewise, one doctor alone cannot stem the tide of authority, hierarchy, greed, racism, and sexist treatment that patients experience.

Still, each of us must start where we find ourselves. If the project is worth doing, it is worth doing in whatever form of work we take up— or else that work must be rejected as corrupt or bankrupt. We must dream of better possibilities. Just as we hope to raise our child to be a peacemaker in a world that rejects war, and we teach our student with the hope that she will become one who loves learning and can pass along that love to others, just so we hope that an empowering relationship with our patient will free her to discover her own potential and to empower others in her life. As long as people seek medical help, in health or sickness, some of us will be called upon to care for them. In the seeking and the caring a bond forms between the healer and the patient wherein lies the potential for empowerment. In an era when the forces against personal and community empowerment are so organized and the pathway toward social change so uncertain, joining another person in the task of empowerment is one of the few things worth doing. Medicine-in-relation offers us a way to renew our vision of clinical practice in the service of that empowerment.

NOTES

CHAPTER 1

1. The emphasis on separateness in late infancy and toddlerhood in the textbook examples draws heavily on the psychoanalytic construction of infancy. The modern theorist who made infant separation and individuation the centerpiece of her work was Margaret Mahler (Mahler, Pine, & Bergman, 1975). According to Mahler, the successful negotiation of the phases of infant separation and individuation depend on proper maternal conduct during this stage. Mahler identifies the transition from "symbiosis" to the onset of infant differentiation at about age four to five months, when the infant begins to distinguish his or her own body from that of the mother. This timing is rather "late," compared with Stern's findings.

CHAPTER 2

1. For discussions of a relational perspective on men's development, see Osherson (1986); "Men Nurturing Men," *Family Therapy Networker* 14 (1990), is an entire issue devoted to men's developmental issues. For a fuller discussion of a self-in-relation perspective on persons, see Schmitt (1995).

2. Work in men's development usually means "meaningful" work and career development. This emphasis has excluded consideration of the adult development of the many minority men whose work opportunities are constricted by racism to tedious, dangerous, or despised jobs and who are more subject to chronic under- and unemployment.

The Grant study offered enormous detail on a large group of privileged men across their adult lives in the midtwentieth century; it contains important conclusions about work, marriage, and mental and physical health for this group of men. Women make an appearance primarily as wives in marriages that are happy, conflicted, or miserable. Vaillant (1977), a psychiatrist, sees the study as supporting Erikson's views of the stages of adulthood. He outlines the falling away over time in the "healthy" subjects of immature psychological defenses like fantasy and acting out and the increasing use of mature psychological defenses like suppression, sublimation, altruism, and humor. Development appears to be a psychological process largely internal to the individual.

In the Grant study, "working and loving" turn out to be key criteria for long-term mental health, but Vaillant's operating definition of "loving" describes male experience. He measures loving by the accomplishment of six tasks: getting married without later divorce; spending ten years of marriage "that neither partner perceived as outright painful" (1977, p. 305); fathering or adopting children; believing that he had one or more close friends; appearing to others to have one or more close friends; and enjoying regular recreation with people outside his family. Vaillant recognizes that this score provides a "less real but more believable" way to measure love, but he accepts the scoring method for the sake of science (p. 305). He does not acknowledge that his measurement of loving may not pertain to women. Men who scored highly in the study turned out to feel closer to their parents and their children and to suffer less physical and mental illness in adulthood, while men with lower scores admitted more fear of sex, avoided competitive sports, took fewer vacations, and used more alcohol and tranquilizers. The scoring system distinguished two groups of men: those who were successful at maintaining marriage, friendship, and recreation (the conventional relationships outside of work for men) and those who were not. But relationships are not central in Vaillant's view of development or adulthood; they are markers for successful "adaptation." The contribution of the Grant study to an understanding of women's adulthood is questionable.

3.　Lerman (1986) makes this criterion a requirement of an acceptable feminist theory of personality as well.

4.　Sociological constructions of the relation between the domestic world and the world of employment are affected by economic conditions as well as by changing attitudes about women's employment: the ideology of dual spheres has given way to the concept of spillover between home and work. The spillover formulation tends to view the workforce role as primary for men and secondary for women. Research based in this model emphasizes the negative effects of women's employment. An emerging view of the interdependence between employment and family roles for both men and women permits examination of the constructive or detrimental effects of diverse roles (see Chow & Berheide, 1988; Forrest & Mikolaitis, 1986).

CHAPTER 3

1.   The Peckham Experiment was a large-scale project to integrate families into a healthy lifestyle through a social club, called the Pioneer Health Centre. The club contained a swimming pool, game and music facilities, a dance floor and theater, cafeteria, pub, store, and cooperative farm; it also sold milk and organic vegetables. Opened in southeast London in 1926, the club grew to 1,400 families, all of whom lived within walking distance. Entire families enrolled in the program, which emphasized the value of exercise, recreation, healthy diet, premarital and prenatal education, and an annual physical exam and health assessment for all family members. The club did not provide health care as we think of it today, but rather an environment that encouraged healthy activities and health awareness for families at various stages of development. Implicitly based on an understanding of the family life cycle, the Peckham Experiment maintained a self-conscious vision of the family as an organism that can grow and flourish in a community setting dedicated to healthy values (Ransom, 1983, 1985).

The Family Health Project was an interdisciplinary project that combined the fields of internal medicine, psychiatry, social work, nursing, and anthropology and was dedicated to understanding the role of illness in families. The Josiah Macy, Jr., Foundation supported the two-year project through a grant to Cornell University Medical College. Professionals from the various disciplines met weekly during the two years to discuss in detail the relationship between illness and family life in the fourteen study families. From an interview with Margaret Mead in 1978, Don Ransom learned that the concept of family equilibrium was introduced into the project by Gregory Bateson, who was Mead's husband at the time. The project was written up by the internist Henry B. Richardson in his book *Patients Have Families* (1945), which is now out of print (Ransom, 1985). *Family Systems Medicine* reprinted the fourth chapter, on the family equilibrium, in 1983.

2.   The study of the family came into vogue after the field of child development was well established and after Erikson's vision of adult development had captured the American imagination (1963). In her reflections on the family life cycle, Evelyn Duvall (1988) writes that it was her training in child development, linked with Reuben Hill's training as a family sociologist, that resulted in the formal statement of the family life cycle concept at the White House Conference on the Family in 1948. For clinicians, however, the family life cycle concept was a logical extension of placing the template of development theory over the structure of the family: individuals proceed through developmental stages; so must families. In

actuality, by the 1930s economic historians were already applying the family life cycle schema to describe transitions in family economics.

At the turn of the twentieth century, the British economist Benjamin Seebohm Rowntree identified the family life cycle as a useful concept for understanding the fluctuating economic conditions of families. He noted that family fortunes decline with increasing numbers of mouths to feed, improve as older children became workers, then decline again for the elderly. American sociologists applied this insight to American farm families in the 1930s, noting that for many families living on the margin of poverty, one child more or less could make the difference in subsistence. Regional variation in availability of land as well as ethnic and class aspirations for education and goods contributed to economic welfare. Even the contrasting effect on women's labor was noted: "The farm owner's wife does not work outside the house as much after children are born as before.... Because the tenant family is poorer, the tenant's wife works about the same number of hours outside in all stages, except that in the last stage, the amount of work done is restricted by age" (Loomis, 1936, p. 187). This awareness of the vulnerability of family economic well-being to the changing shape of the family was rooted in an acknowledgment of the hardships of families both rural and urban. Unfortunately, the family life cycle concept preserved in clinical work today is stripped of these early economic insights. For other references to the history of the family life cycle concept, see Loomis (1936), Hareven (1974), and Hill and Mattessich (1979).

3.　Such is our vision, however, that white history is history, and white family history is family history: Demos does not consider the "family life" of the native Americans, the Quinneboag Indians, whose communities and social structure were irretrievably altered and mostly destroyed by the white colonists.

4.　We have little trouble recognizing that the vision of the family as refuge, insofar as it described any portion of American society, pertained only to the middle class (Glenn, 1987) and had little relevance to the lives of the laboring immigrant multitudes of women and children as well as men who toiled in factories and mills; nor to black families before and after the Civil War; nor to rural families everywhere who struggled to eke out a living from the soil. Nevertheless, this vision of the family, with its prescribed roles for women and men, its vision of morality residing at home and vice in the economic world, served a function: it held up an image of what everyone should be struggling for. Thus, the ideology of the family in the nineteenth century served to separate the spheres of men and women in the service of an economy recognized as cruel and immoral.

5.　Married people have been found to be healthier in much research, but closer examination has revealed that women's health is associated with living with any proximate adult, not necessarily a husband (Anson, 1989). This finding suggests that it is a context of relatedness that affects health status, not being married. Infants of teen mothers suffer higher infant mortality than the infants of older mothers, but infants of *unmarried* teen mothers (black and white) die consistently less often than the infants of *married* teens, showing that it is not marital status but social and economic support that affects this key indicator (Centers for Disease Control, 1990). Coresidence with the maternal grandmother is associated with completion of immunization for the infants of teen mothers and with better cognitive ability and health outcomes for their low-birth-weight infants (Bates, Fitzgerald, Dittus, & Wolinsky, 1994; Pope et al., 1993). Maternal isolation, not father absence, was associated with adverse effects on inner-city schoolchildren's psychological and social functioning; children of mother-grandmother families did as well as those from mother-father families in terms of social and psychological functioning (Kellam, Ensminger, & Turner, 1977). The presence of another adult in a female-headed household improves adolescent conduct and maternal control (Dornbusch et al., 1985).

6. The construction of the family life cycle as separate from women's work shows a flagrant disrespect for history. The paid work available to women depends on the community economic structure. Local historical conditions combine with the particulars of the local economy to determine the location and type of work available to women and the resultant family structure prevalent in that community. For instance, in Newfoundland fishing communities "gangs" of women ran between their homes and the beaches where they dried the fish while the men were at sea for months at a time. Women took care of their families, took on paid employment, and managed the family income with only periodic entry of men into family life. Women were the central players in family and community life (Porter, 1988).

The New England mill communities also maintained a long tradition of working-class women's employment outside the home. Women tended to work before marriage, marry later, and return to mill work when necessary after they had children. Women had access to income and were able to be more independent in community and work life. Whole families were involved in the textile industry, and family life was interwoven with work life (Hareven, 1981). In mining and steel communities like Pittsburgh, in contrast, the excess of young men, coupled with the lack of employment for women, promoted early marriage for women and big families. The high rate of work-related injury and disability among men workers resulted in many women having to raise large families with few resources. Such an economy promoted more economic dependence for women (Elder, 1981).

Women's paid work is neither new nor fashionable for working-class women. Some have worked in their own homes, taking in washing, offering lodging to boarders, minding other women's children, doing piecework sewing. Others have gone out to work in mills or factories. Why is this historical understanding not central to the prevailing image of the family life cycle? Part of the answer lies in the post–World War II suburban dream of the happy housewife who was fortunate not to have to work outside the home. The family with a male breadwinner, a 1950s image promoted to move women out of the workforce and to open up employment for men returning from war, turns out to be the historical aberration. It was during the 1950s, of course, that the family life cycle concept began to take hold—and American women had more children in faster succession than in the fifty years before or the thirty years since (Glick, 1977, 1988).

7.   Further stigma may accrue to infertile women in the 1990s as feminist critiques of reproductive technology make infertile women seeking technological solutions to their problem appear misguided, oppressed, and potentially exploitative of other women (Sandelowski, 1990).

8.   Family caregiving extends beyond the family to include caring for other women's small children and looking after unrelated elders. Women also do most of the care of children in day-care centers and family day-care settings. When women in the family are not the ones providing care for the elderly and disabled, those who do—the staffs of nursing homes and home health agencies, as well as helpful neighbors—are mostly women. The status accorded to tending the elderly—who are perhaps disabled, incontinent, or demented—is equivalent to that given to looking after small children, and the pay is just as poor. Society views family caregiving and its extension, caregiving outside the family, however necessary, as not worth paying for.

9.   Keeping women in the role of family caregiver serves a long-term function in preserving gender inequalities in two ways. First, women who leave the workforce for a long time to look after a disabled child or elderly parent face decreased income, decreased social status, and reduced employability should they try to return to the workforce. Second, since poor women, women of color, older women, and women in poor health are more likely to leave employment when it conflicts with caregiving, and since younger, more educated white women are more likely to accommodate their jobs to caregiving, control over the working world is left to men (and some women) who have no caregiving responsibilities. Although some men engage in family caregiving, they are less likely than their wives or sisters to compromise their work schedules to look after a parent. The result is that women's income and status is compromised both inside and outside the workforce. Moreover, the values and attitudes that family caregivers could bring to the workplace are lost.

10.   There are various responses a woman can make to the care requirements for a disabled or demented mother: she can immerse herself in her mother's care; she can attempt to balance her mother's care against her family and work responsibilities; or she can try to integrate care for her mother into the rest of her life (Lewis & Meredith, 1988). The history of the caregiving relationship clarifies how the pattern evolves as her mother's incapacity progresses. This flexible biographical approach contrasts with the rigidity of a life cycle schema, which depicts some women caregivers as overinvolved with their aging parents. In life cycle thinking, "overresponsibility"

is interpreted to mean that a woman has failed to separate adequately from her parents (McCullough, 1980); having never forged a "separate identity," she finds family caregiving stressful and has difficulty balancing her needs with those of others (Gluck, Dannefer, & Milea, 1980). This interpretation suggests that caregivers need more separateness, yet the literature on the burden of caregiving suggests that family caregivers already suffer isolation and loneliness. Upbraiding women for failure to establish a separate identity and failure to individuate derives from the masculine interpretation of adult development. It begs the question, who will do the work if women do not? Thus, the social problems of inadequate services for the elderly and work overload for family caregivers disappear within the criticism of individual women as overresponsible and underdifferentiated.

11. The only two allusions to homosexuality in family life cycle texts addressed to family medicine readers are telling. One is a bare mention of homosexuality in a paragraph about the risk of AIDS among gay men. Inappropriately, it appears in a section about rape and sexual abuse in a chapter on legal issues in family practice (Henao & Grose, 1985, p. 401). The second reference is to the difficulty of grieving the loss of a partner in a relationship that was secret or disapproved of by family and the resulting distancing and lack of family and social supports for AIDS "victims" (Falicov, 1988, p. 329). The texts examined were Christie-Seely (1984), Crouch and Roberts (1987), Ramsey (1989), Henao and Grose (1985), and Falicov (1988).

12. Clinicians who do not deliberately support lesbian and gay relationships are unlikely to recognize such families in their practices; if they do, these families are likely to seem deficient or troubled to them. According social and legal legitimacy only to heterosexual relationships creates unique problems for gay and lesbian families: for instance, the potential loss of relationships with children or grandchildren when a lover dies or the relationship dissolves; the fear of state scrutiny or intrusion into parenting because of homosexuality; lack of legal authority over a partner's or child's health care if no durable power of attorney has been previously arranged. Gay men and lesbians, however, are actively challenging the strictly heterosexual definition of family by arguing for the legalization of their unions as family relationships and redefining the meaning of family in several legal areas, including housing rights, rights as next-of-kin, and rights as parents. I am indebted to Irving Zola for pointing out to me the sharp challenge to the definition of family coming from gay and lesbian legal struggles.

13. For ethnic families, the task of assimilation is one that family therapists identify as a source of conflict and problems between spouses and generations. Assimilation, however, is not a choice for African-American families. Portrayals of African-American families in family life textbooks fall into three categories: "deviant," "cultural equivalent" (for instance, in the middle class), and "cultural variant," a stance of respect for the strengths and cultural traditions of black families (Bryant & Coleman,

1988). In the last category falls McGoldrick, Anderson, and Walsh's text *Women in Families* (1989), which discusses black women and black families in a chapter on ethnicity and women. Although the chapter's discussion of the harsh historical and contemporary conditions of racism experienced by black people is very strong, the authors do not discuss the implication for people of color of subsuming race under ethnicity or viewing racism as a form of ethnocentrism.

Race itself is a socially constructed concept. Since social rather than biological attributes define race, some authors argue that it is more appropriate to regard black people as members of distinct ethnic groups rather than as members of a homogeneous biological category called the black race (Mullings, 1990). The Centers for Disease Control and the Agency for Toxic Substances and Disease Registry sponsored a workshop in 1993 to discuss the use of race and ethnicity as concepts in public health surveillance. No clear agreement was reached about the use of these terms, although a variety of recommendations were offered (Centers for Disease Control, 1993). Nevertheless, race is assumed as an objective category in social science and medical writings. Higginbotham (1992) points out that white speakers use the language of race to define difference, but that people of color adapt the same language to celebrate cultural identity and to strive toward liberation from oppression. However, since these arguments are not widely discussed by family scholars or medical educators, the more pressing problem remains the failure to identify the enduring oppression that people of color experience precisely because of their color (Rothenberg, 1990).

CHAPTER 4

1. Among refugee women, a past experience of rape during escape or internment often results in devaluation and later battering by their husbands (Friedman, 1992). Although the husband was not the rapist, the woman undergoes further abuse from him as a result of having been victimized by other men.

2. Malamuth, Sockloskie, Koss, and Tanaka (1991) attempted to develop a theoretical model to explain aggression against women. They studied several thousand male college students along a variety of variables, including childhood experiences of violence, delinquency, promiscuity, attitudes toward aggression, "hostile masculinity," social isolation, and coerciveness. They suggest that physical and sexual aggression against women result from interactions in two different dimensions: hostile masculinity and promiscuity. Men high on both scales engaged in both physical and sexual aggression; men high on hostile masculinity but low on promiscuity engaged primarily in physical aggression; and those low on hostile masculinity but high on promiscuity engaged primarily in sexual aggression. Interestingly, when they tested their model on student data, both the group

high on sexual aggression and low on physical aggression and the group high on physical aggression and low on sexual aggression showed high levels of hostile masculinity and sexual promiscuity. These data show that at the highest levels of hostility, physical and sexual aggression against women cannot be disentangled.

3.   Child abuse is often the last straw for a woman in a battering relationship. While she may not be able to act on her own behalf, her realization that her children are at risk may be the stimulus that enables her to act. Battered women try to protect their children even though they know that seeking help from social service agencies puts them at risk of having their children taken away from them (Gordon, 1992). In marriages in which the batterers abuse the children, women are more likely to look for help (Bowker et al., 1988).

4.   Women often begin their use of street drugs in the context of a heterosexual relationship; often a woman's male partner is dealing drugs and supplying her with daily narcotics (Anglin, Hser, & McGlothlin, 1987). Sometimes the addicted male partner takes advantage of the woman's addiction to use her as a source of income by forcing her to engage in sex work, supplying her with just enough drugs for her habit. Her powerlessness as an addict makes her less able to require that her customers use condoms. Here again, drug abuse reinforces the power discrepancy between men and women.

5.   In Campbell's study of marital homicides in Dayton, Ohio (1981), cited in her nursing text on family violence (1984), at least 64 percent of women killed by their partners (18 of 28) had been previously abused by them. Of the 29 men killed by their women partners in the same study, only 2 men acted in self-defense; 23 had precipitated the murder either by flashing a weapon or striking blows. Of the women homicide victims in Campbell's study, 30 percent had already separated from or divorced the men who later killed them; in other words, the women had recognized the hopeless collapse of the marital relationship. The men subsequently pursued and attacked them. These data show that behind the numerical similarity between the violent deaths of marital partners lies the profound asymmetry of violence in the family.

6.   Rosen and Stith (1993) suggest that, in working with a young woman in a violent dating relationship, the clinician take a strong stand against the violence while remaining neutral about the relationship itself. Many women come into therapy trying to save a relationship and need an opportunity to gain perspective before they can consider leaving it.

CHAPTER 5

1.   I will discuss primarily sexual abuse of girls. Sexual abuse of boys seems to have different long-term effects: because of male socialization,

boys are more likely to repeat their victimization and to become perpetrators themselves (Lew, 1988). I have chosen to use the pronoun *he* to refer to the perpetrator of sexual abuse because the vast majority of perpetrators are male (95 percent). I do not, however, mean to minimize the devastating impact of the far less common sexual abuse by mothers or other female caretakers, or of joint sexual abuse by male and female caretakers. Such abuse may in fact have worse consequences because of the loss of a potentially protective maternal figure.

2.   I refer to women who have experienced child sexual abuse or incest as *survivors* because the consistent use of this word, rather than *victims*, may enable clinicians to view these women as strong rather than weak; also, when abused women themselves adopt the word, they gain a tone of empowerment. I use the word *incest* to refer to the particular form of child sexual abuse that occurs within families. I do not accept any of the intimations of mutual consent or symmetry that have been associated with the word. Also, although the word conveys no particular relationship between perpetrator and victim, incest characteristically involves forced sexual exploitation by an older and stronger male of a younger and physically weaker girl.

3.   College samples differ from community samples in that they may represent a younger cohort; they are biased away from poor and lower-income groups; and respondents are preselected by virtue of their completion of high school and their commitment to achieving further education. College surveys also gather data through self-administered questionnaires rather than interviews; as a result, the relatively lower rate of reported abuse may reflect the different methodology.

4.   Some researchers suggest that, rather than sexual abuse being the cause of later symptoms, the symptoms result from a chaotic or unsupportive family background in which sexual abuse was only one element (Fromuth, 1986; Harter, Alexander, & Neimeyer, 1988). This suggestion does not account for the fact that women whose abuse occurred outside the family also carry an excess of symptoms. Bagley and Ramsay (1986) found that only half of sexual abuse occurred to women whose families were marked by coldness, lack of support, or parental separation. Fully half of the sexually abused women in their sample came from intact families. Their findings support the conclusion that incest and sexual abuse occur in inconspicuous families. Although survivors of intrafamilial abuse are more symptomatic than survivors of extrafamilial abuse, the persistence of symptoms in both groups serves as an argument that sexual abuse itself plays an etiological role in the later development of symptoms.

5.   The fourth edition of the *Diagnostic and Statistical Manual of Mental Disorders* (American Psychiatric Association, 1994), the technical handbook for the classification of psychiatric disorders (known as *DSM-IV*), defines somatization disorder as a condition in a person who by the age of thirty considers himself or herself sickly and has multiple clinically significant

symptoms (at least four pain symptoms, two gastrointestinal symptoms, one sexual symptom, and one pseudoneurological symptom), all occurring over several years, requiring medical treatment, and having no medical explanation. Such a description, based solely on the number of body symptoms or feelings, groups people with similar presentations but does not identify etiology. This descriptive, composite way of making a diagnosis—all it tells us is that these patients suffer a miserable bodily existence—typifies the current psychiatric approach to all diagnosis: eschew the search for causes and instead adhere to a classification schema based on purely descriptive findings.

6.   Fifty-five percent of sixty women with somatization disorder in a psychiatric group practice, when interviewed directly, gave a history of incest or sexual abuse before age eighteen, compared with 16 percent among a control group of women with primary affective disorders in the same practice (Morrison, 1989).

7.   This study also found that sexually abused women were more likely to have histories of depression (56 percent versus 25 percent for the control group) and of drug abuse (57 percent versus 22 percent). Moreover, among women with pelvic pain, those who had been sexually abused had more adult sexual problems (dyspareunia or inhibited desire, excitement, or orgasm) compared with women who had not experienced sexual abuse as children (74 percent versus 34 percent) (Walker et al., 1988).

8.   The argument about sexual abuse in psychoanalytic circles was recapitulated in the controversy that surrounded Jeffrey Masson's recovery and publication (*Assault on Truth* [1984]) of Freud's and Ferenczi's papers about the reality of childhood sexual trauma. See Janet Malcolm's book *In the Freud Archives* (1984) for this history. See Westerlund (1986) for an exegesis of Freud's blaming women caretakers for sexual abuse while discounting patients' accounts of sexual abuse by men as fantasy.

9.   Social service referral is not benign; historically, girl victims of incest or sexual abuse were labeled sexually deviant and were far more likely to be removed to foster care or to be institutionalized than the perpetrator was to be prosecuted or convicted (Gordon, 1988). Today it is still usually the victim who is removed, not the perpetrator. Thus, however sympathetic the verbal messages to child abuse victims, the social treatment they receive conveys the message that they were at fault.

10.   In Gordon's study of families reported for incest and sexual abuse to Massachusetts social service agencies over the course of eighty years, if the physician deemed that penetration had not taken place, the girl's allegations, regardless of the clinical history, were likely to be dismissed. If penetration had occurred, the girl herself was viewed as polluted and, what is more, contagious to other girls (1988, pp. 216–17).

11.   Physicians' suspicion of child sexual abuse is associated with certain characteristics of physicians: younger physicians, those who worry about underdiagnosis of sexual abuse, and those who think social service agen-

cies are effective are more likely to suspect child abuse. Those who think that the investigative process is harmful to children and that children are likely to be removed from the household are less likely to suspect child abuse. Those who think that they will be required to testify in court are less likely to report such suspicions to the child protective system (Willis & Horner, 1987).

12.   Russell (1986) found that 17 percent of women sexually abused as children told someone at the time of the first incident or soon afterward, 10 percent told someone later, and 19 percent said that someone else knew about it. Of forty incest survivors studied by Herman (1981), seventeen (42.5 percent) disclosed to someone while still at home, but only three (7.5 percent) came to the attention of any helping services during childhood.

13.   Masson (1984) reviews the history in nineteenth-century Europe of the argument over whether children falsify their experiences of sexual abuse. He reports a German tradition of considering children liars who accuse others for their own gain, and two French trends—one of considering rape to be commonly imagined, and a forensic tradition of believing children's accounts of assaults. Masson shows that Freud was familiar with these lines of argument before he outlined and then recanted his seduction theory. Echoes of this argument reverberate today in the form of disputes over children's accuracy and concern about the effects of allegations of child abuse on families.

14.   In two recent divorce and child custody cases, sexual abuse of the daughter by the father was the central issue. In one case, Dr. Elizabeth Morgan went to jail for two years because she would not reveal to the court the whereabouts of her daughter Hilary because she believed the child's statements that her father, Eric Foretich (Morgan's ex-husband), had sexually abused her. She was finally freed through a special law passed by Congress. During her imprisonment, it emerged that Foretich's previous wife had also brought charges against him of sexual abuse of her daughter. Foretich continued to attempt to get access to his daughter and subsequently followed Morgan to New Zealand, where her daughter was living, and demanded her return to the United States (Farber, 1990; *Newsweek*, 1990). In another divorce case, a New Hampshire mother disputed child custody with her husband on the basis of his sexual abuse of their child. On the eve of the judge's decision to allow visitation by the father, two other adults in the community came forward with the declaration that the father had sexually abused them as children. Their declaration was important in the custody decision (Baker, 1989).

15.   See, for instance, Bass and Thornton, *I Never Told Anyone: Writings by Women Survivors of Child Sexual Abuse* (1983); Wisechild, *The Obsidian Mirror: An Adult Healing from Incest* (1988); Morris, *If I Should Die before I Wake* (1982); Petersen, *Dancing with Daddy* (1991); Fraser, *My Father's House* (1987); Angelou, *I Know Why the Caged Bird Sings* (1969); Brady, *Father's Days: A True Story of Incest* (1979); Armstrong, *Kiss Daddy Goodnight: A*

Speak-out on Incest (1978); Allen, *Daddy's Girl* (1980); McNaron and Yarrow, *Voices in the Night: Women Speaking about Incest* (1982); and, more recently, Smiley, *A Thousand Acres* (1991).

16. A historical example demonstrates the transhistorical features of sexual abuse in patriarchal families. (While a historical case does not give us access to the participants, it does afford us a window on the abuses resulting from patriarchy in another era. The specifics are different, but the dynamics are unchanged.) One sexual abuse perpetrator who achieved notoriety in his day was James Henry Hammond, governor of South Carolina from 1842 to 1844 and a U.S. senator from 1857 until 1860, when he resigned on the eve of South Carolina's secession. Hammond was known as a particularly authoritarian man, even for his time; as a slave owner, husband, and father he was despotic. To demonstrate his physical and psychological domination, he frequently ordered severe beatings of his slaves, disbanded slave churches, and outlawed slave assemblies. Child mortality before age five among the slaves on his plantation in the first ten years of his ownership was 72 percent, far higher than averages anywhere else in the slaveholding South. He maintained physical and intellectual superiority over his wife, whom he had married for her wealth; she had six children during the first seven years of their marriage, reflecting an avoidance of the birth control measures that were known to and practiced by upper-class couples of the time. After the seventh child, a long-awaited daughter, was born, she had no more pregnancies for nine years. During this hiatus, Hammond began a sexual relationship with one of his slaves and had children by both her and her daughter. During this same period, Hammond also began molesting his four nieces. After two years, the oldest, by then twenty, refused his advances and six months later informed her father of her uncle's activities (Bleser, 1988; Faust, 1982).

In a diary entry of January 31, 1844, Hammond revealed that he had had sexual contacts with all four girls, then ages twenty, nineteen, seventeen, and fifteen, over the preceding two years. Hammond blamed the girls:

> All of them rushing on every occasion into my arms & covering me with kisses—lolling in my lap—pressing their bodies almost into mine wreathing their limbs with mine, encountering warmly every part of my frame & permitting my hands to stray unchecked over every part of theirs & to rest without the slightest shrinking from it, on the most secret and sacred regions—and all this for a period of more than two years continuously. Is it in flesh and blood to withstand this? (quoted in Faust, 1982, p. 242)

Hammond admitted in his diary to "every thing short of direct sexual intercourse" (quoted in Faust, 1982, p. 242). His brother-in-law, an extremely wealthy and influential politician, attempted to destroy Hammond's political career in revenge. What in fact transpired was that Hammond went on to become a U.S. senator after the scandal subsided while his nieces lived in ignominy, destined never to marry (despite their considerable fortunes) because he had publicly tainted their virtue. "No man who valued his standing could marry one of the Hammond girls" (Bleser, 1988, p. 180; Faust, 1982).

Most perpetrators, of course, have neither the wealth nor the power of a James Henry Hammond, yet the example demonstrates that the features of incestuous abuse 150 years ago persist as the central characteristics of abuse today: the perpetrator was a controlling and sometimes violent patriarch; his wife was rendered powerless by multiple consecutive pregnancies, less education, and social if not financial dependency; he had unlimited and unsupervised contact with the children he abused, his nieces; the abuse occurred over a period of years, involved consecutive sisters, and would have continued indefinitely had the oldest daughter not made her disclosure; the girls had lost the protection of their mother, who had died seven years before the abuse began; the perpetrator's version of the story was preserved for public view while the girls' account disappeared; and the perpetrator underwent little or no punishment and in fact maintained his power and station, while as far as is known the incest damaged the girls' lives as long as they lived.

17. Knowledge about prior sexual abuse may release abusive tendencies in men. Perhaps they find the taboo exciting, or they regard the girl or woman as already damaged, or they convince themselves that she was responsible for the abuse in the first place (Russell, 1986). Some perpetrators may be especially good at identifying whatever psychological vulnerability may make a woman less able to resist, escape, or report another event (Briere, 1989).

18. On a personal level, medical practitioners are heavily invested in the belief in their own responsibility toward patients. They feel that they work hard and do more than their share, and that patients, in turn, should hold up their end of the bargain. Practitioners may overextend themselves in an effort to "save" a patient only to find out that the patient cannot come through "for them." Prepared to work hard on behalf of others and to give unstintingly of themselves, physicians are likely to feel personally betrayed when the beneficiaries of their efforts do not act in a worthy—meaning responsible—fashion: for instance, using medicines given trustingly to overdose, breaking appointments, and failing to come through on practitioner-based expectations to begin therapy, attend twelve-step meetings, stop smoking, or lose weight.

Within this ideological context, patients who, even after they seem to know the risk, experience revictimization, are unable to leave abusive relationships, or expose themselves or their children to assault and sexual abuse or rape, evoke the disappointment and then the anger of the medical practitioner, whose work revolves around the spindle of responsibility. The obverse of responsibility is fault or blame ("I told her not to do that," "If only she had tried," "She didn't act responsibly," "She brought it on herself"). Health care professionals who have not examined their own attitudes about responsibility are the most likely to view revictimization experiences as the patient's fault.

19. Some trauma survivors recognize urges to reexperience the mental and physical excitement (mediated biochemically) that they first felt at the time of their original trauma. This mechanism may explain the "repetition compulsion" of some kinds of trauma survivors (Herman, 1992). However, the vast majority of women who have survived physical and sexual abuse are terrified by the internal reexperiences of flashbacks and find no addicting thrill or exhilaration in reliving the arousal and fear of their original trauma (see van der Kolk, 1989, for an opposing view).

CHAPTER 6

1. Some authors argue that patients cooperate in this process, that the conversation is a joint venture (Frankel, 1984; Treichler, Frankel, Kramarae, Zoppi, & Beckman, 1984). In this view, patients collaborate by taking up the subservient role. For instance, doctors may legitimately ask patients many questions, but patients hesitate and stammer when they try to ask the doctor a question (West, 1983). They match the doctor's linguistic assertions of dominance with responses of submission, much like a dog rolling onto its back. This view of collaboration implies that patients' collusion in the process of subordination somehow makes the resulting domination less the doctor's responsibility.

The idea of doctor-patient conversation as a joint project is confounded by confusion over the word *negotiation*. Sociolinguists use the word technically to describe the alternation in speaker turns in conversation. While ordinary conversations may indeed involve negotiation over specific linguistic forms, such as length of each speaker's turn to talk, doctor-patient conversations are unique in that the doctor has almost complete control over the discourse through questions (Frankel, 1990). Nevertheless, the sociolinguistic approach to medical communication incorporates the term "negotiation" in its sense of alternation to refer to the entire structure of medical conversation. Drass (1982), who studied the patterns of speech in medical interviews between patients and either nurse-practitioners or physician's assistants, defines the word: "A negotiation is the organization of acts, turns, sequences and phases through which a mid-level provider and patient accomplish the goals of assessing and managing a particular medical problem " (p. 325). Despite Drass's own findings of clinicians' tight constraint over patients' speech in every phase of their conversation, she nevertheless adheres to the use of the egalitarian-sounding term "negotiation" to refer to their exchange. Sliding from the technical use of the term into the commonsense meaning of "bargaining" gives the illusion that speech, behavior, and even diagnosis are under joint control: "Negotiation takes the form of an emergent interplay of two perspectives embedded in the discourse of the interactants" (p. 339). The use of the term "negotiation" (with its implication of shared participation) obscures the fact that one party controls the conversation, as well as any bargaining that may occur.

2.   Because of the presumption of self-interest, altruism poses a logical problem when persons are construed as separate and autonomous. I do something for someone else only if it benefits me. Acts that benefit only others do not make sense. In contrast, if we assume that from the beginning persons develop and survive in relation to others, altruism makes sense as a form of responsiveness. Altruism begins not with a rational decision to help the other but rather as an empathetic understanding of the other's experience (see Code, 1987, for further discussion of this point). Conversely, women who engage in supportive relations with children, students, or patients do so not out of a spirit of altruism or self-sacrifice but because they view such relationships as self-affirming and mutually enhancing (Stiver, 1991b).

3.   Patient autonomy can be understood to mean the patient's right to choose among available treatments. The ability of autonomous patients to compete for resources has major implications for the distribution of medical care: if each patient is entitled to choose what she or he wants, including the maximum in intensive care, regardless of the cost or likelihood of a good outcome, then the costs will be enormous. Patients already in the system will be privileged, and those without medical care will have access to even less. Scarcity of resources then becomes the argument against patient autonomy in this sense of the ability to choose among treatments. Medical ethicists argue that good citizens who are responsible members of the community would not demand the full use of costly resources at the end of their lives (Callahan, 1984; Danis & Churchill, 1991). Thus, the idea of community is beginning to challenge the primacy of patient autonomy in medical ethics. (Notions of community are, of course, subject to abuse: prejudice against minorities, the aged, or homosexuals can be interpreted as "a community value" and used to restrict care to these groups.)

Scarcity of medical resources poses a real world challenge to the assumption of the legitimacy of competition between autonomous patients. The fact that scarcity derives from an economy centered on weaponry remains uncontested. Certainly we could afford to maintain anyone who so wished it on mechanical ventilation and full life support if we were not so committed to unchallengeable deadliness as our strategy of national defense. Or put another way, invoking a social context of scarcity to constrain patient autonomy fails to situate scarcity within the even larger social context of militarism.

4.   The Society for General Internal Medicine offers a yearly training in the medical interview, a weeklong course in which participants spend two hours each day in a small group setting discussing personal issues. This

focus on the person in the course is a recognition that the doctor's thoughts and feelings are central ingredients in relationships with patients. However, interview training still focuses on what the doctor does and says and neglects the issue of what transpires *between* the two people.

5.   Nowadays health care relations are indeed bought and sold by employers seeking to minimize their costs by making contracts with the cheapest health maintenance organizations. Similarly, shifting economic forces often require patients and families to choose the cheapest available plan, thus forcing them to change doctors. The enormously destructive effect on clinical relationships of these market forces has gone largely undocumented, but for increasing numbers of people, a visit to the doctor has become a transaction between strangers.

6.   One valuable exception is the work of Michael Glenn (1984), who uses the term "contract" to describe the process by which doctor and patient come to an agreement about diagnosis. Schon (1983) also proposes a "reflective contract" as the conversation between professional and client when they have joined together in an inquiry into the client's situation. The client and professional recognize that they have different languages and different sets of meanings and understandings. However, this understanding of contract is not common in medical parlance.

7.   Mediation—negotiation in another context—is a process currently heralded as an informal means to reconcile differences. However, informal mediation between unequal parties serves to uphold the power arrangement. For instance, if I feel that my boss is sexually harassing me, a mediated solution implies that we will both make compromises when, in fact, I want him to stop altogether. In cases of sexual abuse and battering, mediated solutions often leave women and children vulnerable while the perpetrator retains his access to them (Scutt, 1988).

8.   Although one could argue that using operant conditioning to control behavior protects patient autonomy in the traditional sense more than, say, drug treatment, straitjackets, or isolation (see Dworkin, 1976, for elaboration of this point), the fact remains that contracting so employed is a deliberate means of control.

9.   Jose Bayona used this metaphor at a workshop ("Re-Inventing Lives: Toward Inclusivity in Collaborative Health Practice Models," Family in Family Medicine Conference, March 6, 1994, Amelia Island, Florida) to point out how reigning assumptions are invisible to the people holding them.

CHAPTER 7

1.   The polarizing effect of dichotomous thinking can be problematic: it poses two opposing realities, when many may exist, and forces us to choose between them. Forced choices narrow and rigidify the parameters of

thought. Dichotomies tend to be used by practitioners of the dominant mode of thought to define what is inside and outside the dominant schema. The promotion of dichotomous thinking in the scientific method, for instance, legitimates some methods and defines others (usually qualitative or experiential ones) as less valuable, unworthy of science, and invalid. Feminists have been particularly critical of the use of dichotomous thought in the characterization of male and female as opposites. Nevertheless, those out of power may claim and elaborate one end of the dichotomy: for instance, Reinharz (1983), noting the contrast between experiential and mainstream research in sociology, claims the former as appropriate to feminist work.

The construction of the categories themselves is also at issue. For instance, Harding (1987) argues that the categories of "woman" and "African" are categories *created* by the dominant oppressor group. Although we have no historical access to the time when the category "woman" was created in opposition to the category "man," we do know that the category "African" was created by white European men in the last few hundred years. Prior to Western imperialism, persons were not primarily identified in terms of race. African people were not defined as "other." Opposing male and female, white and black, serves those in power by allowing them to define all qualities deemed negative as belonging to the other. A culture that claims rationality and individualism as the hallmarks of masculinity relegates women to the condition of emotionality and dependency. Harding proposes that the dominant group (white European males) needed to create the category of the other as a repository for all the characteristics they did not possess themselves. Those out of power may claim as their own the particular characteristics that they see lacking in the worldview of the dominant group. The marginal oppressed group claims for itself values like a sense of community, connectedness with nature, and relatedness over individualism—hence, the overlap in values claimed by black philosophy and feminist philosophy (Harding, 1987; Tronto, 1987). See Patricia Hill Collins (1989) for the grounding of a black feminist standpoint.

The recognition of culturally drawn dichotomies leads to research on difference—male versus female, black versus white. But the focus on difference tends to entrench the differences rather than investigate the sources of the opposition. For instance, research on racial differences takes race as a fundamental category of difference and does not recognize that race is a socially created category. Such research reifies differences into mutually exclusive categories. Sameness, similarities, and overlaps disappear. Similarly, research on differences between males and females tends to emphasize difference and obscure similarities. Males and females who share characteristics become less visible. Differences are ascribed to gender itself, not to the crucial social and cultural factors that surround gender.

2.   Examinations of the diagnostic process in the clinician's mind inevitably describe the hypothetico-deductive model and its variations. For

instance, the diagnostician may construct a "map" rather than follow an algorithm in trying to solve a problem (Campbell, 1987). Contemporary descriptions of "clinical problem-solving" adhere to a strictly biomedical view of causation (Moskowitz, Kuipers, & Kassirer, 1988; Pauker & Kopelman, 1992). What is strikingly missing from such descriptions of the "diagnosing mind" is any consideration for the person and reactions of the mind's owner or for the fact that, at least in primary care, the vast majority of patient complaints do not fit a specific diagnosis. Moreover, diagnostic categories as they exist omit whole realms of human experience from consideration (Malterud, 1987a): for example, women's confinement to sex role activities and racist treatment of some patients may explain many symptoms but are nowhere acknowledged in diagnosis.

3. An objective approach to the patient's history would presumably examine the facts; a subjective interpretation would revolve around the speculations and intuitions of the clinician. This dichotomy occurs whenever interpretation is the main activity. Take the example of reading: as readers, we can take the text as objective fact, or we can accept the special nature of our own subjectivity in making our interpretation. Schweickart (1990) points out that when the author of a text is a student and the reader is a teacher, more is at stake than the reader's right to interpret the text. Schweickart argues that the ethic of care for the author must infuse such readings. The parallel between the teacher reading the student's text and the doctor hearing the patient's story is evident (see Mukand, 1990, and Charon, Greene, & Adelman, 1994, for further consideration of the doctor as parallel to the reader of a text).

4. In philosophy, the term "naturalist epistemology" has a specific meaning that is different from Kuzel's and closer to his use of the term "rationalistic" (see D. R. Gordon, 1988). His use of the term "naturalistic" derives not from epistemology but from the methodology of research, which can be conducted in the "natural" environment, removing or distorting the context as little as possible, but recognizing the entry of the researcher into the context as an element of the research itself. Kuzel, following Lincoln and Guba (1985), contrasts the positivist paradigm with the naturalistic paradigm. Naturalistic inquiry, in this sense, locates the knower and the known as interactive and inseparable; their very relatedness and effect on each other are central to the knowing.

5. By the mid-1960s, one-third of Puerto Rican women of childbearing age, living on the island, had been sterilized (Mass, 1976; Presser, 1980). Estimates of sterilization rates for Puerto Rican women in mainland cities ran as high as 51.6 percent (Schensul, Borrero, Barrera, Backstrand, & Guarnaccia, 1982).

6. For example, 100 women taking an oral contraceptive for 10 months yields 1,000 woman-cycles of experience with the drug. If 10 women take the drug for 100 months, a much smaller number with a much longer exposure, the number of woman-cycles is identical, but the kind of information

is very different. The difference between these two kinds of information is lost in a method of measurement that discounts time span in favor of time units. Most drug research favors short-term exposure with large numbers of subjects for the rapidity of results and resultant speed in marketing. This approach discounts the fact that many drugs are taken for years. Clinical experience with the long-term use of new drugs often does not occur until drugs are marketed. The "experiment" is conducted on real patients who are unaware that long-term studies have never been carried out.

7.   The effort to sever any connection between empathy and feelings in medicine is further evidenced in a recent study. Nightingale, Yarnold, and Greenberg (1991) attempted to divide physicians into two groups: the empathetic and the sympathetic. To do this, they asked doctors to respond to the following forced-choice scenario: A patient enters the office, sits down, and says, "Doctor, my husband/wife just died, and I feel terrible!" The English language gives you two ways to respond to this patient: (a) "I understand how you feel," or words to that effect, and (b) "I feel sorry for you," or words to that effect. Which do you use? (p. 420). Interestingly, some of their respondents felt that it was presumptuous to state that they understood feelings about experiences they had never had; others felt that the "I feel sorry" statement was demeaning. Despite these objections, the authors of this study hypothesized that "sympathetically sharing the emotional experience of a sick and frightened patients would . . . impair a physician's ability to make objective medical judgments on the patient's behalf" (p. 420). They contrast the emotionality of sympathy with the "more *objective* empathetic analysis," which, they hypothesize, would "facilitate a more adaptive problem-solving orientation" (p. 420, my emphasis). This passage shows how medicine has appropriated empathy as a tool of science and rescinded its emotional or relational meanings.

Nightingale et al. found that physicians who chose the "empathetic" statement ordered fewer lab tests on outpatients, stopped real-world cardiopulmonary resuscitation sooner, and were less predisposed to intubate a patient with chronic lung disease in a hypothetical management problem. They use these findings to support the idea that "sympathy," as defined by choosing the statement above, leads to less "objective" and therefore less cost-effective medical practice. The implication that empathy—defined by the physician's claim to know how the patient feels—is cost-effective fulfills Code's worst expectation about empathy's potential for abuse: "The location of empathetic knowing in a professional setting produces power asymmetries that can turn this ideally reciprocal, mutually affirming skill into an imperialistic, coercive practice" (1994, p. 89).

8.   The intense dysphoria, intrusive imagery, and loss of sexual interest experienced by therapists who work with survivors of sexual abuse reveals that "joining" the patient's feelings also means experiencing some of their symptoms (Briere, 1989). The reappearance of symptoms in the therapist

constitutes a kind of secondary post-traumatic stress syndrome, variously called traumatic countertransference or vicarious traumatization (Herman, 1992).

9. In addressing this same issue, Noddings (1984) makes a distinction between projection—taking the other person's viewpoint—and internalization—taking the other's view and making it part of self. Internalization makes it possible to move beyond separateness to a relational approach.

10. Noddings locates the imperative to action in an apprehension of the other's reality. Once one feels what the other feels as closely as possible, then one feels called upon to act. "The commitment to act in behalf of the cared-for, a continued interest in his reality throughout the appropriate time span, and the continual renewal of commitment over this span of time are the essential elements of caring from the inner view" (1984, p. 16). These words strike a chord with clinicians, who are often called upon to act on behalf of their patients, even though Noddings was primarily describing the relationship between teacher and student.

11. Nonetheless, some patients do obtain all their care in one institution, despite changes in doctors. Careful review of old medical records can sometimes offer a life-span perspective: the fifty-year-old diabetic of today can be seen with a fresh eye after reading a social worker's description of her difficulties as a single mother twenty years before.

12. Much discussion went on in family medicine circles about the definition of the word *family* in the early years of the formation of the field. I am still most happy with Ransom and Vandervoort's phrase: "a significant group of intimates with a history and a future" (1973, p. 1099).

13. This pattern of "circular" questioning situates the question and its possible answers in the larger family setting (Feinberg, 1990). It is a strategy familiar to family therapists but rarely used by physicians, even ones who regularly work with families.

14. The recommendation of Rosen and Stith (1993) to take a firm stand against abuse while remaining neutral about the relationship itself may be helpful to women clinicians working with women in oppressive relationships.

15. Separate and connected knowing cannot be reduced into each other, like adding discordant fractions. One example of such a reduction is the attempt to construe the narrative or naturalistic forms of research as forms of observation and therefore preliminary steps in science-making (McWhinney, 1977; Stephens, 1980). This stance implies that narrative/naturalistic forms are a more primitive version of scientific observation, as it is classically understood, and therefore are reducible to steps in scientific method. I disagree; the narrative/naturalistic form is not reducible to observation, because of the crucial role of the connected self in understanding the world through this mode. The transformation of the connected knower through his or her involvement with the other person removes this form of knowing from a step on the ladder of scientific method.

CHAPTER 8

1.   Of course, practitioners make contributions all the time by unintentionally displaying their negative attitudes. In words and gestures, in acts omitted and committed, doctors often reveal themselves to be authoritarian, condescending, sexist, racist, or homophobic. However, I do not focus in this chapter on the ways doctors distance themselves from patients. For a review of the copious evidence of doctors' practice of power over patients, see chapter 6.

2.   I use the term *self*-disclosure with some hesitation. It implies that we are inherently separate and isolated individuals who have a right to a personal privacy that we may choose to suspend by revealing personal information. It also implies that privacy, rather than openness, is the human condition, that self-containment rather than mutuality represents the ideal (see Friedlander, 1982, for an argument about the connection between autonomy and privacy). Nevertheless, for brevity I will use the term self-disclosure in this chapter, with the caveat that I do not intend to idealize either privacy or self-containment in human relations.

3.   The freedom of heterosexual women doctors to talk about their personal lives is an example of heterosexual privilege. Lesbian physicians may not feel safe or comfortable discussing the life context of their pregnancies or using examples from their personal lives in their work with patients who are not lesbians.

4.   In very oppressive relationships, those with less power (for instance, slaves, captives, and abused women) decipher a great deal about the more powerful. This knowledge, often dismissed as intuitive, is essential for survival. Patients with a strong history of abuse may be particularly adept at discerning the feelings and state of mind of their doctors—they are practicing a well-honed skill that has been essential to their survival in previous relationships with other powerful figures. I distinguish this kind of "gleaned" knowledge of the other's state of mind from what the less powerful person might learn from the explicit sharing of personal information by the more powerful.

5.   Mutuality would not be a characteristic of feminist research on those who abuse power—for instance, batterers and rapists. See, for example, Diane Scully's book on convicted rapists, *Understanding Sexual Violence* (1990).

6.   The participants in this discussion examined the role of talking about themselves in their classes, referring to the adage "The personal is political." The discussion took place on the Women's Studies List (WMST-L)—an electronic discussion forum maintained by Joan Korenman, director of women's studies at the University of Maryland at Baltimore (Baltimore, MD 21228–5398 [korenman@umbc2.umbc.edu]) on March 15, 16, 17, 18, and 23, 1992.

7. Lynn Schlesinger, Department of Sociology, State University of New York at Plattsburgh, personal communication, June 6, 1992.

8. Walker et al. (1988) identified six principles to assess the adherence to feminist principles of social service programs for families: (1) recognition of cultural context, (2) responsiveness to the vulnerable, (3) participation and equality, (4) celebration of diversity, (5) privileging of clients' perspectives on problems and solutions, and (6) empowerment of clients. They found that only a minority of programs (five of sixty-one) described in *Family Relations* over a ten-year period met any of these criteria; none met all of them. The authors attributed this finding to the difficulty of attempting to implement feminist principles in a hierarchical society in which inequality is considered a fact of life, not a problem to be confronted.

9. The connection between caring for others, suffering, and liberation has been identified as part of the Christian tradition for black women, who have historically cared for their own families and other families in the face of great adversity. Toinette M. Eugene points out that, in contrast to white feminists, black women consider the menial nature of much caring uplifting rather than debasing, because of the theology of servanthood linked to the suffering of Jesus. "This biblical model of feminist liberation theology is principally focused on human solidarity with those who suffer or who are marginalized in any way" (1989, p. 590). This tie between caring and suffering may be foreign if not objectionable to clinicians whose commitment to patients is grounded in other ethical or religious sources. Nevertheless, assumptions derived from the Christian tradition suffuse the thinking of the many practitioners who view their own service and suffering in the context of the suffering of others.

CHAPTER 9

1. In addition, the outcomes of encounters with new versus known patients differ. With new patients, Rost, Roter, Bertakis, and Quill (1990) found a negative association between physician control over the interaction and patient recall (what patients remembered about their instructions). They also found that, compared with new patients, established patients, when given more information about medications, were more likely to remember their medication changes.

2. Carol Gilligan argues in *In a Different Voice* (1982) and later writings that men are more likely to defend their decisions based on rights, using the justice framework, and women are more likely to frame their judgments from the perspective of care, for relationships and the feelings of others. Though empirical proof of the gender difference in perspective has been contested, the concept of contrasting frameworks for moral judgment has been the source of much philosophical and psychological discussion.

3.   In a review of medical reassurance in modern literature from Shaw to Drabble, Kessel (1979) divides reassurance into content and skills. In terms of content, patients want to know, he concludes, "that their illness will not prove serious or disabling or disfiguring or unduly painful or catching, that it will not prevent them from working, that they will not have to go away and that it will not take long to get better" (p. 1130). In terms of skills, Kessel includes a personal relationship with the patient and an appreciation of the patient as an individual. Here we come to the point of connection. What is comforting for one patient may be devastating to another. Some might need to hear that they are sick and need rest; others want to hear that it is nothing serious and they can go on about their business. One must know the patient for reassurance to take effect. Kessel does not say how this knowing takes place.

4.   Of course, not all information reassures the patient that the problem is trivial or self-limited. Common problems have rare complications and chronic illnesses have defined morbidity and mortality. Nevertheless, whatever the problem, patients find it reassuring to understand better what is known about it and what they can do about it.

5.   Despite the importance of reading and writing in medical education, thinking about patients as *readers* who have a variety of ranges of abilities is a foreign concept to most clinicians (see Davis et al., 1991, 1993, for an exception). The fact that patients' health status corresponds to their literacy level suggests that clinicians could benefit from paying more attention to literacy as an issue in improving patients' health (Weiss, Hart, McGee, & D'Estelle, 1992).

6.   Mathews and Feinstein (1988) arranged the responses into an extensive taxonomy divided into three groupings: (1) the personal style or amenities of the physician, (2) the emphasis on the patient's uniqueness, and (3) the performance of clinical activities. Even at this level, a relationship or connection between patient and clinician is absent.

7.   Brown (1986) isolated eight themes in patients' responses: (1) recognition of individual qualities and needs, (2) reassuring presence, (3) provision of information, (4) demonstration of professional knowledge and skill, (5) assistance with pain, (6) taking more time, (7) promotion of the patient as an active, decision-making participant in treatment, and (8) keeping watch or surveillance.

8.   Ruddick (1983) points out that the desire for acceptability contains the potential for inauthenticity, which she describes as: "to accept the uses to which others put one's children; and second, a willingness to remain blind to the implications of those uses for the actual lives of women and children" (p. 221). The mother who accepts that her son beats his wife, or who refuses to believe a daughter who tells her about sexual abuse, is functioning inauthentically. The mother's inauthenticity and obedience to "the values of the dominant culture" (p. 221) maintain the status quo, and her

position within it, at the cost of another person. Inauthenticity includes "training her daughters for powerlessness, her sons for war" (p. 221). Ruddick sees such obedience as a function of social powerlessness. The same can be true for clinicians, especially those of lower status, who may find themselves "selling out" the patient to protect their own acceptability at a hospital. For instance, a physician may describe a patient's problems as the result of "noncompliance" instead of allying with the patient, who is struggling to manage his or her sickness in a complicated world. I have at times found myself wanting the patient to be "good" while in the hospital so that hospital staff will like him or her and not be annoyed with me for bringing a "difficult" patient into the hospital world.

9. The connection between caring and self-sacrifice is complex. Our religious or racial allegiances may influence the meaning for us of self-sacrifice. For instance, Toinette Eugene (1989) argues that caring is liberatory for black women exactly because of its link to the sufferings of Jesus (see chap. 8, n. 9). In contrast, the psychologically minded would argue that it is precisely the carer's self-sacrifice that makes caring oppressive to the one cared for. The woman who forces her child to eat, compels her child to compete and perform, and lives off her child's accomplishments—this mother is seeking to squeeze from her child's life and existence the meaning missing from her own life. Clearly context is central to understanding the connection between self-sacrifice and caring.

10. Again, imagination is central to taking an ethical position. Code argues for the need to educate the imagination to "bring about right perception in those cases that stand outside the boundaries of one's own experience." She elaborates: "The fact that one cannot know everyone intimately indicates the cognitive and moral importance of an educated imagination so that one can be in a position to move empathetically beyond instances one has taken the trouble to know well to other, apparently related, instances. Such responsible cognitive endeavour seems to be essential to a moral life in which engagement with other people as the people that they are is a serious concern" (1987, p. 150).

11. Gilligan divides moral concerns into two preoccupations: justice and care. She argues that these concerns "arise from the experience of inequality and of attachment embedded in the relationship between child and parent" (1986, p. 238). For Gilligan, inequality and attachment characterize all forms of human relation. Each has its particular form of abuse: the abuse of inequality is oppression, and the abuse of attachment is abandonment. From these experiences arise the two moral predispositions that result in two distinct views of responsibility: the vision of justice promotes a commitment to obligations; the vision of care would have us commit to responsiveness in relationships. Certainly for clinicians, inequality and attachment are persistent features of their ongoing relationships with patients. Nevertheless, medical ethics, with its emphasis on patient auton-

omy and patient rights, has been preoccupied with justice and protection against the abuse of inequality; the predisposition for care and the importance of attachment have been neglected as anchors of both ethical and clinical work.

12. Nursing is still the primary clinical field preoccupied with an understanding of caring. Although the nurses who study caring do not consciously make gender an element in their study, the fact that it is women nurses who write and research about caring for other nurses means that the discussion takes place in a highly gendered context. Partially because of parochialism, but perhaps even more because of gender bias, the nursing literature on caring is completely unknown outside nursing. Any integrated understanding of caring will need to recognize the gendered insights about caring derived from nursing practice and to place these insights within the power relationships in health care.

13. Small modifications in the medical interview may make a significant difference in how patients perceive their care, even though no relational change has occurred (Debra L. Roter, personal communication, November 1992).

14. Although as many men as women were no doubt raised in dysfunctional families, women are the target of codependency workshops and make up 85 percent of the market for codependency books and groups (Kaminer, 1990). "Experts" estimate that between 75 and 90 percent of nurses are codependent (Snow & Willard, 1989).

CHAPTER 10

1. Likewise, studies of power in marriage focus on the outcomes of decision-making, failing to examine the underlying inequalities between men and women and the role expectations that predate and prefigure the decision under discussion (Komter, 1989).

2. One well-respected such strategy is the use of the patient-centered interview, a way of sticking to patients' agendas in order to recognize and address their concerns more promptly (Brown, Stewart, McCracken, McWhinney, & Levenstein, 1986; Levenstein et al., 1986; Smith & Hoppe, 1991). Improved patient satisfaction and patient "compliance" are the stated goals. Others call for a language-centered method (Ventres & Gordon, 1990), or "language competence," to enable doctors to become competent in patient language (Shuy, 1983). And some try to define the patient's explanatory model of illness in order to delve into the patient's meaning, at the expense of awareness of the interaction itself (Lazarus, 1988).

3. Nurses have revitalized the concept of in-hospital nursing through a claim for their primacy in patient-centered care—care for the total patient within the context of his or her family—and their responsibility for ensuring collaborative care. Other strategies in hospital nursing to confront med-

icine's domination involve taking the relationship with the patient as central to nursing, while relegating the instrumental functions to medicine, and claiming a share of the management role in hospitals.

4.   Laura S. Brown has outlined how lesbian therapists risk the possibility of abusing their power over their clients; her analysis is directly applicable to feminist physicians and nurse-practitioners. Feminists caring for patients like themselves, particularly within the context of a small community, may have overlapping roles: as a practitioner, neighbor, board member, parent at the same school, or community activist, they are visible outside of the clinical setting to their women patients. When overlapping roles are unexamined, it becomes possible for clinicians to slip from social or community connections with patients into intimate relationships with them. As mentioned in chapter 8, another possible kind of abuse when doctor and patient share important characteristics is inappropriate self-disclosure, including disclosures not made for the patient's benefit. To address such problems, Brown advocates a feminist code of ethics that takes into consideration the shared community of feminist practitioners and their patients and acknowledges the use of therapeutic self-disclosure as a legitimate aspect of feminist treatment. Brown suggests that it is the clinician's responsibility to anticipate overlaps, to initiate discussion of how she will handle them, and to manage boundaries to be flexible within the patient's and doctor's contexts. As stated in the Feminist Therapy Code of Ethics of the Feminist Therapy Institute, "The therapist accepts responsibility for monitoring such relationships to prevent potential abuse of or harm to the client" (Brown, 1991a, p. 329).

5.   "Power to empower" and "power to enable" convey similar messages. The word *enable*, however, implies ability to do or accomplish; the word *empower* suggests more robustly how one might feel in the world as well as act in it. The meaning of *enable* has also been contaminated by the codependency movement, which defines it as helping another person along in their addiction. Of course, *empower* and *empowerment* have lost much of their punch since being adopted as buzzwords in the 1990s, but they hold few negative nuances.

6.   Initiating a discussion of racism with a patient is, of course, a complex and sensitive matter. Some patients may not be ready to discuss it or may not want to discuss it with a white person. Some patients may perceive the overture as representing a white person's preoccupation with race; they may not consider a discussion of racism relevant to the clinical interaction. Other patients may feel that to bring up racism is to see them in terms of race rather than as a person. Each of these potential objections must be weighed against the disadvantages of the traditional approach of never mentioning race and pretending it is irrelevant to a patient's life, health, and dealings with health care personnel. White health care professionals participate in racism whether they bring the topic up or not. Given that racism is a part of the daily life of all persons of color and that it takes

an inevitable toll on their health and well-being, it is as relevant—perhaps more so—as other personal characteristics. In the context of an ongoing relationship, a white clinician does risk making a mistake by introducing the issue of racism, but over the long run, failing to introduce it colludes with the dominant ideology in denying that racism denigrates and destroys people.

7.   Empathy does not require the clinician to like the patient or have feelings for the patient, but it is always about a real relationship between two human beings. Some clinicians have ascribed a spiritual or religious quality to their experiences of empathy, a sense of "continuity with an existence that is much larger than we are" (Suchman & Mathews, 1988, p. 126). These clinicians deny that empathy is an interpersonal experience; to express their sense of it as an exemplary experience of human harmony, they call it "transpersonal." But they also describe the condition of being human as essentially separate; they see persons as isolated, suffering, and longing for meaning through connection. This rather masculine understanding of empathy contrasts with the daily experience of relatedness and connectedness in the work of many women clinicians, whose practice of empathy is not spiritual but rather very much of the world.

8. *Flexibility* is another word that lost meaning as it became trendy. It sounds straightforward but is actually a difficult accomplishment. Given its positive connotation (and the corresponding negative connotation of rigidity), clinicians are likely to consider themselves to be flexible, adapting to each patient's needs. However, in studies of doctor-patient conversation, doctors tend to adhere to a single communication style in all their exchanges with patients (Byrne & Long, 1976). One could extrapolate that consistency is likely to be more typical of doctors' interactions than flexibility.

9.   Malterud's model explicitly recognizes the importance of the woman's own experience and language but is less explicit about how the practitioner should think about the patient's explanatory system. How should the clinician think about a patient's explanations when they are very different from medical accounts? Sara Ruddick suggests that a different kind of reasoning challenges the ideal of what has been traditionally called rational thinking (certainly an assumption of the medical model). The rational ideal excludes a different kind of thinking by "placing [it] within a governing theory without recognizing its challenge to the theory's fundamental assumptions" (1987, p. 244). The medical model might "place" a patient's explanation as folk belief, superstition, or phobic worry, without ever taking it seriously.

> To hear difference without "placing" it requires careful listening and a suspension of judgement that the active stance of excluding makes difficult. For the excluded, it is a struggle to articulate as reason a way of reasoning that has been characterized as "irrational" in the dominant "rational" culture. To say that certain forms of reason-

ing prevail hegemonically is to say that they structure the conversations in which "rational" people participate. That is, to adapt to these
forms of conversation is part of being what is called rational. If difference is to emerge, there must first be silence, a willing suspension
of habitual speech, and then a patient struggle requiring of speaker
and listener an attentive respect for different reasonings. . . . To be
heard speaking, to be heard as coherent, sensible, and rational, is a
real human need. It is therefore a matter of care to hear differences
wherever people feel silenced or coerced by forms of reason that are
not theirs. This means attending to any person speaking out of a sense
of exclusion and listening for different reason to the best of one's ability. (Ruddick, 1987, p. 245)

Attending to those who have been excluded and listening "for different
reason" are not strengths of medical thinking. The "clinical model" operates out of a scientific imperative and centers on the values of authority,
activity, objectivity, and rationality (Carmichael, 1985; Carmichael &
Carmichael, 1981). It accepts one correct way of thinking about things and
thereby excludes and silences difference. In contrast, Malterud's method
encourages the clinician to hear difference and to perceive the woman
patient as coherent, sensible, and rational in her own terms (see also
Blaxter, 1983).

10.   Failure to recognize women's overload leads to bizarre misreadings
of clinical cases. For instance, a woman brings her daughter to the doctor
for a physical exam before taking her to a psychologist for the child's
behavior problems. The mother resists making a connection between the
daughter's behavior and her own impending divorce. The doctor interprets
the mother's presentation in terms of domination and control and is unable
to consider the mother's need for survival strategies. Instead, she is portrayed as controlling the agenda and not allowing the doctor to investigate
the divorce because it might be prejudicial against her. In this instance, the
mother's approach is labeled "strategic communication"; "intentionally
designed to influence someone's perception of reality . . . aimed more at
constructing certain perceptions of reality than at displaying truth or sincerity" (Maseide, 1983, p. 250). Anyone who uses such "strategic communication" is a "potential deceiver." Although this single mother is pursuing
psychological help for her child, her unwillingness to discuss her divorce
with a male physician is interpreted as *controlling the doctor!*

Missing in such an analysis is any understanding of the gendered
oppression inherent in the woman's position. She may feel that her abilities
as a mother and a woman are faulty because she is unable to hold a marriage together; that her child's disturbance may represent a failure of mothering; that the (probably married) male doctor is more supportive of her
husband in the divorce struggle than of her. Her unwillingness to discuss
her own past emotional problems is seen as an effort not to compromise

herself instead of the manifestation of stigma or guilt. The absence of the father in seeking help for the daughter is not mentioned. The fact that the woman is taking active steps on her own to help her daughter (discussing it with a friend, taking her to the doctor, pursuing a psychological referral) gets lost in the masculinist portrayal of her as deceptive and controlling. Clearly such an interpretation allows no view of her as a woman struggling to understand her situation and as a single mother facing personal and social sources of denigration. This detailed example clarifies how the assumption of power as domination and the denial of gender as an issue function together to deny the reality of a woman patient.

11.   Thomas E. Quill took this position publicly when he published an account of his care of a woman with leukemia named Diane. After a long relationship, months of treatment, a decision not to undertake experimental treatment, and the certain knowledge of her upcoming and debilitated death, Diane requested the choice of controlling the timing and method of her death. Knowing that she understood what constituted a lethal dose, Quill prescribed an ample quantity of phenobarbital. With the full awareness of Diane's family, he empowered her to choose how and when to die. His action, the source of much controversy in the prestigious *New England Journal of Medicine*, confirmed that even though individuals draw the lines differently, empowerment strategies for terminally ill patients may include "assisted suicide" (Quill, 1991).

12.   During hospital births, women and couples must conform to the hospital's protocols for managing labor and delivery—for example, how rooms are used, the number of family members that can be present, and how anesthesia and medication are used. Hospital staff make it clear to patients how they expect patients to behave (Laslie, 1982). The family-centered maternity care movement of the 1970s encouraged couples to demand alternatives to the hospital protocols. Hospitals responded by incorporating family-centered care into hospital routines, allowing husbands—and sometimes boyfriends, mothers, and grandmothers—to support women during childbirth.

Hospitals then advertised their "homelike atmosphere" to capture more of the obstetrical market. This restructuring substantiates Arney's argument that medicine (in this case, obstetrics) is able to incorporate criticisms from the outside and transform itself accordingly. At the same time, the proliferation of fetal monitors with telemetric observation of both mother and fetus guaranteed that medical control was never threatened. Both patients and medical care providers are under scrutiny; all are being watched (Arney, 1982). Nurses and machines watch patients; doctors and nurses watch each other; the lawyers and the courts, by implication, watch the doctors and nurses. Within this hall of mirrors, no action goes unnoticed.

13.   Feminist birth practice is not free of conflict. Challenges come when patients want to be completely medicated and pain-free and their clinicians believe that fewer interventions are healthier, or when the doctor is a firm

believer in breast-feeding and the patient is adamant about bottle feeding. A woman may beg for pain medication but her controlling boyfriend insists on "no drugs for my baby." There are many clinical moments when a contradiction emerges between feminist values (as espoused by the women's health movement) and individual (or family) desires.

14. Shared gender may be helpful in obtaining an empathic life history account, but it alone is not sufficient (Riessman, 1987). Class, race, and culture (as well as scientific models of explanation in medicine) conspire to superimpose on women's stories explanations and interpretations that confirm social expectations but deny the women's validity.

15. Education for empowerment is a two-way street. A seasoned clinician will often confide that a specific patient with a chronic illness "taught me everything I know" about the illness. The idea that the patient is the teacher is not new, but rarely are patients directly acknowledged or rewarded for this work. In residency programs, in which trainees leave after three years and patients remain, the crucial role that patients play in education could be recognized both when residents leave, as part of saying good-bye, and when new residents begin. Reviewing the lineage of residents whom patients have taught and the contributions they have made as individuals is a small but significant gesture that could empower patients as teachers as they begin the process once again. Some patients may be willing to tell their life story and the story of their illness in an extended narrative to a medical student once or twice a year. In our practice, we have designated such patients "community teachers" and give them a stipend for each interview, as a token of respect.

16. As of 1994, lower doses of thiazide diuretics (one-quarter to one-eighth of what was prescribed in 1970) are still appropriate for single or combined drug therapy of hypertension and are not measurably associated with any increased mortality (Siscovick, Raghunathan, Psaty, Koepsell, Wicklund, Lin, Cobb, et al., 1994).

17. Traditionally, placebos have been inactive treatments (like sugar pills) or tangential treatments (like vitamin shots) that doctors use to help patients feel better. Most doctors felt that patients should not know that a treatment was a placebo. The doctor's authority and the power of suggestion seemed necessary to the artifice. In other words, the practice was deceptive. More recently, Brody (1982) and others have pointed out that the placebo effect works even if patients are aware that the drug is inactive. The placebo treatment process somehow taps the patient's self-healing abilities. Brody attributes the liberation of the healing power to the doctor-patient relationship. Clearly the next step is for patients to claim the placebo effect as their own. How doctors might facilitate this within the doctor-patient relationship remains unexplored.

18. Using such maneuvers is commonly recommended in the family therapy literature in order to gain patient compliance. Techniques such as "joining" and "taking the one-down position" provide the "tactical edge"

the physician needs to gain power. The goal is explicitly framed as getting the patient to do what the doctor wants, not empowering the patient. Rissman and Rissman (1987) give two examples: a health food cook who does not want to take antibiotics, and parents who do not want their child to have ear surgery. They suggest allowing the patient to make the choice as a tactic to get them to do what the doctor wants. The patients' real objections and concerns about taking medications and having surgery are not appreciated as legitimate but rather, by implication, appear uninformed, confused, or somehow less legitimate than the doctor's viewpoint. Such techniques are clearly the antithesis of empowerment.

19. The patients have read these accounts and given permission for them to be published. They chose their own pseudonyms.

Bibliography

Abel, G. G.; Becker, J. V.; Cunningham-Rathner, J.; Mittleman, M.; & Rouleau, J.-L. 1988. Multiple paraphilic diagnoses among sex offenders. *Bulletin of the American Academy of Psychiatry and Law* 16:153–68.

Acker, J.; Barry, K.; & Esseveld, J. 1983. Objectivity and truth: Problems in doing feminist research. *Women's Studies International Forum* 6:423–35.

Adisa, O. P. 1992. Undeclared war: African-American women writers explicating rape. *Women's Studies International Forum* 15:363–74.

Ageton, S. S. 1983. *Sexual assault among adolescents*. Lexington, Mass.: D. C. Heath.

Agich, G. J. 1990. Reassessing autonomy in long-term care. *Hastings Center Report* 20 (6):12–17.

Alcoff, L., & Gray, L. 1993. Survivor discourse: Transgression or recuperation? *Signs: Journal of Women in Culture and Society* 18:260–90.

Aldous, J. 1987. New views on the family life of the elderly and the near-elderly. *Journal of Marriage and the Family* 49:227–34.

———1990. Family development and the life course: Two perspectives on family change. *Journal of Marriage and the Family* 52:571–83.

Alexander, P. C.; Moore, S.; & Alexander, E. R. 1991. What is transmitted in the intergenerational transmission of violence? *Journal of Marriage and the Family* 53:657–68.

Allen, C. V. 1980. *Daddy's Girl*. New York: Wyndham Books.

Allen, K. R., & Pickett, R. S. 1987. Forgotten streams in the family life course: Utilization of qualitative retrospective interviews in the analysis of lifelong single women's family careers. *Journal of Marriage and the Family* 49:517–26.

Allers, C. T.; Benjack, K. J.; White, J.; & Rousey, J. T. 1993. HIV vulnerability and the adult survivor of childhood sexual abuse. *Child Abuse and Neglect* 17:291–98.

Alvino, D. 1986. A caring concept: Providing information to make decisions. *Topics in Clinical Nursing* 8 (2):70–76.

Amaro, H.; Russo, N. F.; & Johnson, J. 1987. Family and work predictors of psychological well-being among Hispanic women professionals. *Psychology of Women Quarterly* 11:505–21.

Amato, P. R. 1986. Marital conflict: The parent-child relationship and child self-esteem. *Family Relations* 35:403–10.

American Board of Family Practice. 1991. *The Physicians' view of middle age*, ABFP Report, part 2. Lexington, Ky.: ABFP.

American Medical Association. 1992. American Medical Association diagnostic and treatment guidelines on domestic violence. *Archives of Family Medicine* 1:39–47.

American Psychiatric Association. 1994. *Diagnostic and statistical manual of mental disorders*. 4th ed. Washington, D.C.: American Psychiatric Association.

Anderson, B., & Anderson, W. 1989. Counselors' reports of their use of self-disclosure with clients. *Journal of Clinical Psychology* 45:302–8.

Angelou, M. 1969. *I know why the caged bird sings*. New York: Bantam Books.

Anglin, M. D.; Hser, Y.-I.; & McGlothlin, W. H. 1987. Sex differences in addict careers. 2. Becoming addicted. *American Journal of Drug and Alcohol Abuse* 13:59–71.

Anson, O. 1989. Marital status and women's health revisited: The importance of a proximate adult. *Journal of Marriage and the Family* 51:185–94.

Archbold, P. G. 1983. Impact of parent-caring on women. *Family Relations* 32:39–45.

Aries, E. J., & Olver, R. R. 1985. Sex differences in the development of a separate sense of self during infancy: Directions for future research. *Psychology of Women Quarterly* 9:515–32.

Armstrong, L. 1978. *Kiss daddy goodnight: A speak-out on incest*. New York: Hawthorne.

Arney, W. 1982. *Power and the profession of obstetrics*. Chicago: University of Chicago Press.

Arney, W. R., & Bergen, B. J. 1984. Power and visibility: The invention of teenage pregnancy. *Social Science and Medicine* 18:11–19.

Arnold, J., & Jeffries, P. 1983. Spouse abuse. In R. B. Taylor (ed.), *Family medicine: Principles and practice* (pp. 1608–14). New York: Springer-Verlag.

Aronson, J. 1992. Women and the care of old people: "But who else is going to do it?" *Gender and Society* 6:8–29.

Auerbach, J.; Blum, L.; Smith, V.; & Williams, C. 1985. Commentary: On Gilligan's *In a Different Voice*. *Feminist Studies* 11:149–61.

Auvil, C., & Silver, B. W. 1984. Therapist self-disclosure: When is appropriate? *Perspectives in Psychiatric Care* 22:57–61.

Bachmann, G. A.; Moeller, T. P.; & Benett, J. 1988. Childhood sexual abuse and the consequences in adult women. *Obstetrics & Gynecology* 71:631–42.

Bagley, C., & Ramsay, R. 1986. Sexual abuse in childhood: Psychosocial outcomes and implications for social work practice. *Journal of Social Work and Human Sexuality* 4:33–47.

Baier, A. 1986. Trust and antitrust. *Ethics* 96:231–60.

Baker, F. 1989 (August 25). Two say they were molested by man cleared in alleged attack on daughter (Concord, N.H.). Associated Press.

Baldwin, M. 1987. Interview with Carl Rogers on the use of the self in therapy. In M. Baldwin & V. Satir (eds.), *The use of self in therapy* (pp. 45–52). New York: Haworth Press.

Baldwin, M., & Satir, V., eds. 1987. *The use of self in therapy*. New York: Haworth Press.

Balint, M. 1961. The other part of medicine. *Lancet* 1:40–43.

———1969. The structure of the training-cum-research-seminars: Its implications for medicine. *Journal of the Royal College of General Practitioners* 17:201–11.

———1972. *The doctor, his patient and the illness*. New York: International Universities Press.

Barnett, R. C., & Baruch, G. K. 1978. Women in the middle years: A critique of research and theory. *Psychology of Women Quarterly* 3:187–97.

Barnett, R. C.; Brennan, R. T.; Raudenbush, S. W.; & Marshall, N. L. 1994. Gender and the relationship between marital-role quality and psychological distress: A study of women and men in dual-earner couples. *Psychology of Women Quarterly* 18:105–27.

Barnett, R. C.; Kibria, N.; Baruch, G. K.; & Pleck, J. H. 1988. *Quality of adult daughters' relationships with their mothers and fathers: Effects of daughters' well-being and psychological distress*. Working paper no. 175. Wellesley, Mass.: Center for Research on Women, Wellesley College.

Baron, R. J. 1981. Bridging clinical distance: An empathic rediscovery of the known. *Journal of Medicine and Philosophy* 6:5–23.

———1985. An introduction to medical phenomenology: I can't hear you while I'm listening. *Annals of Internal Medicine* 103:606–11.

Barrett, M., & Roberts, H. 1978. Doctors and their patients: The social control of women in general practice. In C. Smart & B. Smart (eds.), *Women, sexuality and social control* (pp. 41–52). Boston: Routledge & Kegan Paul.

Barringer, C. E. 1992. The survivor's voice: Breaking the incest taboo. *NWSA Journal* 4 (1):4–22.

Barry, K. 1989. Biography and the search for women's subjectivity. *Women's Studies International Forum* 12:561–77.

Barsky, A. J. 1981. Hidden reasons some patients visit doctors. *Annals of Internal Medicine* 94 (pt. 1):492–98.

Baruch, G. K., & Barnett, R. C. 1986. *Role quality, multiple role involvement and psychological well-being in midlife women*. Working paper no. 149. Wellesley, Mass.: Center for Research on Women, Wellesley College.

Baruch, G. K.; Biener, L.; & Barnett, R. C. 1987. Women and gender in research on work and family stress. *American Psychologist* 42:130–36.

Bass, E., & Davis, L. 1988. *The courage to heal: A guide for women survivors of child sexual abuse*. New York: Harper & Row.

Bass, E., & Thornton, L. 1983. *I never told anyone: Writings by women survivors of child sexual abuse*. New York: Harper & Row.

Bates, A. S.; Fitzgerald, J. F.; Dittus, R. S.; & Wolinsky, F. D. 1994. Risk factors for underimmunization in poor urban infants. *Journal of the American Medical Association* 272:1105–10.

Bates, C. M., & Brodsky, A. M. 1989. *Sex in the therapy hour: A case of professional incest*. New York: Guilford Press.

Bauchner, H. 1988. Education after residency. *Pediatrics* 81:724–25.

Beckman, H. B., & Frankel, R. M. 1984. The effect of physician behavior on the collection of data. *Annals of Internal Medicine* 101:692–96.

Behrman, R. E.; Kliegman, R. M.; Nelson, W. E.; & Vaughan, V. C., eds. 1992. *Nelson textbook of pediatrics*. 14th ed. Philadelphia: W. B. Saunders.

Behrman, R. E., & Vaughan, V. C., eds. 1983. *Nelson textbook of pediatrics*. 12th ed. Philadelphia: W. B. Saunders.

Belenky, M. F.; Clinchy, B. M.; Goldberger, N. R.; & Tarule, J. M. 1986. *Women's ways of knowing: The development of self, voice, and mind*. New York: Basic Books.

Bell, L. G.; Cornwell, C. S.; & Bell, D. C. 1988. Peer relationships of adolescent daughters: A reflection of family relationship patterns. *Family Relations* 37:171–74.

Belsky, J.; Lang, M. E.; & Rovine, M. 1985. Stability and change in marriage across the transition to parenthood: A second study. *Journal of Marriage and the Family* 47:855–65.

Bender, L., & Blau, A. 1937. The reaction of children to sexual relations with adults. *American Journal of Orthopsychiatry* 7:500–518.

Bender, L., & Grugett, A. E. 1952. A follow-up report on children who had atypical sexual experience. *American Journal of Orthopsychiatry* 22:825–37.

Benner, P. 1991. The role of experience, narrative, and community in skilled ethical comportment. *Advances in Nursing Science* 14 (2):1–21.

Benner, P., & Wrubel, J. 1989. *The primacy of caring: Stress and coping in health and illness*. Reading, Mass.: Addison-Wesley.

Ben-Sira, Z. 1976. The function of the professional's affective behaviour in client satisfaction: A revised approach to social interaction theory. *Journal of Health and Social Behaviour* 17 (1):3–11.

————1980. Affective and instrumental components in the physician-patient relationship: An additional dimension of interaction theory. *Journal of Health and Social Behaviour* 21 (2):170–80.

Berger, J., & Mohr, J. 1976. *A fortunate man: The story of a country doctor*. London: Writers and Readers Publishing Cooperative.

Bergman, A. B. 1988. Resident stress. *Pediatrics* 82:260–63.

Berk, R. A.; Berk, S. F.; Loseke, D. R.; & Rauma, D. 1983. Mutual combat and other family violence myths. In D. Finkelhor, R. J. Gelles, G. T. Hotaling, & M. A. Straus (eds.), *The dark side of families: Current family violence research* (pp. 197–212). Beverly Hills, Calif.: Sage.

Bertakis, K. D., & Callahan, E. J. 1992. A comparison of initial and established patient encounters using the Davis Observational Code. *Family Medicine* 24:307–11.

Bertakis, K. D.; Roter, D.; & Putnam, S. M. 1991. The relationship of physicians' medical interview style to patient satisfaction. *Journal of Family Practice* 32:175–81.

Best, R. 1989. *We've all got scars: What boys and girls learn in elementary schools*. Bloomington: Indiana University Press.

Billson, J. M. 1991. The Progressive Verification Method: Toward a feminist methodology for studying women cross-culturally. *Women's Studies International Forum* 14:201–15.

Birns, B. 1985. *The mother-infant tie: Fifty years of theory, science and science fiction.* Work in progress no. 21. Wellesley, Mass.: Stone Center for Developmental Services and Studies.

Blanchard, C. G.; Labrecque, M. S.; Ruckdeschel, J. C.; & Blanchard, E. B. 1990. Physician behaviors, patient perceptions, and patient characteristics as predictors of satisfaction of hospitalized adult cancer patients. *Cancer* 65:186–92.

Blaxter, M. 1983. The causes of disease: Women talking. *Social Science and Medicine* 17:59–69.

Bleser, C., ed. 1988. *Secret and sacred: The diaries of James Henry Hammond, a southern slaveholder.* New York: Oxford University Press.

Blieszner, R., & Shifflett, P. A. 1990. The effects of Alzheimer's disease on close relationships between patients and caregivers. *Family Relations* 39:57–62.

Bloom, H., & Rosenbluth, M. 1989. The use of contracts in the inpatient treatment of the borderline personality disorder. *Psychiatric Quarterly* 60:317–27.

Blum, L.; Homiak, M.; Housman, J.; & Scheman, N. 1973–74. Altruism and women's oppression. *Philosophical Forum* 5:196–221.

Boehm, S. 1989. Patient contracting. *Annual Review of Nursing Research* 7:143–53.

Boeing, M. H., & Mongera, C. O. 1989. Powerlessness in critical care patients. *Dimensions of Critical Care Nursing* 8:274–79.

Boeringer, S. B.; Shehan, C. L.; & Akers, R. L. 1991. Social contexts and social learning in sexual coercion and aggression: Assessing the contribution of fraternity membership. *Family Relations* 40:58–64.

Bograd, M. 1984. Family systems approaches to wife battering: A feminist critique. *American Journal of Orthopsychiatry* 54:558–68.

———1986. A feminist examination of family systems models of violence against women in the family. In M. Ault-Riche (ed.), *Women and family therapy* (pp. 34–50). Rockville, Md.: Aspen.

Borkan, J. M.; Quirk, M.; & Sullivan, M. 1991. The meaning of hip fracture for the healthy elderly. *Social Science and Medicine* 33:947–57.

Boston Women's Health Book Collective. 1971. *Our bodies, ourselves: A book by and for women.* 2nd ed. New York: Simon and Schuster.

Bowker, L. H.; Arbitell, M.; & McFerron, J. R. 1988. On the relationship between wife beating and child abuse. In K. Yllo & M. Bograd (eds.), *Feminist perspectives on wife abuse* (pp. 158–74). Newbury Park, Calif.: Sage.

Boyd, C. J. 1989. Mothers and daughters: A discussion of theory and research. *Journal of Marriage and the Family* 51:291–301.

Boyer, D., & Fine, D. 1992. Sexual abuse as a factor in adolescent pregnancy and child maltreatment. *Family Planning Perspectives* 24 (4):4–11.

Brady, K. 1979. *Father's days: A true story of incest.* New York: Seaview.

Brazelton, T. B., & Cramer, B. G. 1990. *The earliest relationship: Parents, infants, and the drama of early attachment.* Reading, Mass.: Addison-Wesley.

Breines, W., & Gordon, L. 1983. The new scholarship on family violence. *Signs* 8:490–531.

Briere, J. 1987. Predicting self-reported likelihood of battering: Attitudes and childhood experiences. *Journal of Research in Personality* 21:61–69.

———1989. *Therapy for adults molested as children: Beyond survival.* New York: Springer.

Briere, J., & Runtz, M. 1988. Symptomatology associated with childhood sexual victimization in a nonclinical adult sample. *Child Abuse and Neglect* 12:51–59.

Briere, J., & Zaidi, L. Y. 1989. Sexual abuse histories and sequelae in female psychiatric emergency room patients. *American Journal of Psychiatry* 146:1602–6.

Brim, O. G., & Ryff, C. D. 1980. On the properties of life events. In P. B. Baltes & O. G. Brim (eds.), *Life-span development and behavior* (vol. 3, pp. 367–88). New York: Academic Press.

Brody, D. S. 1980. The patient's role in clinical decision-making. *Annals of Internal Medicine* 93:718–22.

Brody, E. M.; Johnsen, P. T.; & Fulcomer, M. C. 1984. What should adult children do for elderly parents? Opinions and preferences of three generations of women. *Journal of Gerontology* 39:736–46.

Brody, H. 1982. The lie that heals: The ethics of giving placebos. *Annals of Internal Medicine* 97:112–18.

———1988. *Stories of sickness.* New Haven, Conn.: Yale University Press.

———1992a (March 6). *Empathy, caring, and vulnerability.* Paper presented at the conference "Empathic Expertise: Gender, Ethics, and the Therapeutic Relationship," Institute for the Medical Humanities, Galveston, Tex.

——— 1992b. *The Healer's Power.* New Haven, Conn.: Yale University Press.

Brooks, L. 1974. Interactive effects of sex and status on self-disclosure. *Journal of Counseling Psychology* 21:469–74.

Broverman, I. K.; Broverman, D. M.; Clarkson, F. E.; Rosenkrantz, P. S.; & Vogel, S. R. 1970. Sex-role stereotypes and clinical judgments of mental health. *Journal of Consulting and Clinical Psychology* 34:1–7.

Brown, J.; Stewart, M.; McCracken, E.; McWhinney, I. R.; & Levenstein, J. 1986. The patient-centered clinical method. 2. Definition and application. *Family Practice* 3:75–79.

Brown, L. 1986. The experience of care: Patient perspectives. *Topics in Clinical Nursing* 8 (2):56–62.

Brown, L. S. 1991a. Ethical issues in feminist therapy: Selected topics. *Psychology of Women Quarterly* 15:323–36.

———1991b. Therapy with an infertile lesbian client. In C. Silverstein (ed.), *Gays, lesbians, and their therapists: Studies in psychotherapy* (pp. 15–30). New York: W. W. Norton.

Browning, D. H., & Boatman, B. 1977. Incest: Children at risk. *American Journal of Psychiatry* 134:69–72.

Broyard, A. 1992. *Intoxicated by my illness and other writings on life and death.* New York: Clarkson Potter.

Bruner, J. S. 1985. *Narrative and paradigmatic modes of thought*. 84th yearbook of the National Society for the Study of Education. Chicago: University of Chicago Press.

Brush, L. D. 1990. Violent acts and injurious outcomes in married couples: Methodological issues in the national survey of families and households. *Gender and Society* 4:56–67.

Bryant, Z. L., & Coleman, M. 1988. The black family as portrayed in introductory marriage and family textbooks. *Family Relations* 37:255–59.

Bryer, J. B.; Nelson, B. A.; Miller, J. B.; & Krol, P. A. 1987. Childhood sexual and physical abuse as factors in adult psychiatric illness. *American Journal of Psychiatry* 144:1426–30.

Burge, S. K. 1989. Violence against women as a health care issue. *Family Medicine* 21:368–73.

Burnam, M. A.; Stein, J. A.; Golding, J. M.; Siegel, J. M.; Sorenson, S. B.; Forsythe, A. B.; & Telles, C. A. 1988. Sexual assault and mental disorders in a community population. *Journal of Consulting and Clinical Psychology* 56:843–50.

Burt, M. R. 1980. Cultural myths and supports for rape. *Journal of Personality and Social Psychology* 38:217–30.

Byrne, P. S., & Long, B. E. L. 1976. *Doctors talking to patients: A study of the verbal behaviour of general practitioners consulting in their surgeries*. London: H. M. Stationery Office.

Caldirola, D.; Gemperle, M. B.; Guzinski, G. M.; Gross, R. J.; & Doerr, H. 1983. Incest and pelvic pain: The social worker as part of a research team. *Health and Social Work* 8:309–19.

Callahan, D. 1984. Autonomy: A moral good, not a moral obsession. *Hastings Center Report* 14 (5):40–42.

Calof, D. L. 1993. A conversation with Pamela Freyd, Ph.D. co-founder and executive director, False Memory Syndrome Foundation, Inc., parts 1 and 2. *Treating Abuse Today* 3 (3):25–39; (4):26–33.

Campbell, E. J. M. 1987. The diagnosing mind. *Lancet* i:849–51.

Campbell, J. 1981. Misogyny and homicide of women. *Advances in Nursing Science* 3:78.

———1984. Abuse of female partners. In J. Campbell, J. Humphreys, (eds.), *Nursing care of victims of family violence* (pp. 75–118). Reston, Va.: Reston Publishing.

———1986. Nursing assessment for risk of homicide with battered women. *Advances in Nursing Science* 8 (4):36–51.

Candib, L. M. 1981. An interview with G. Gayle Stephens, M.D. *Family Medicine* 13:3–6.

———1987. What doctors tell about themselves to patients: Implications for intimacy and reciprocity in the relationship. *Family Medicine* 19:23–30.

Candib, L., & Glenn, M. 1983. Family medicine and family therapy: Comparative development, methods, and roles. *Journal of Family Practice* 16:773–79.

Candib, L. M.; Steinberg, S. L.; Bedinghaus, J.; Martin, M.; Wheeler, R.; Pugnaire, M.; & Wertheimer, R. 1987. Doctors having families: The effect of pregnancy and childbearing on relationships with patients. *Family Medicine* 19:114–19.

Caplan, A. L. 1988. Informed consent and provider-patient relationships in rehabilitation medicine. *Archives of Physical Medicine and Rehabilitation* 69:312–17.

Caputi, J. 1989. The sexual politics of murder. *Gender and Society* 3:437–56.

Card, C. 1990. Caring and evil. *Hypatia* 5:101–8.

Carlson, N. R. 1977 (February 1). *Incest: An analysis of the state of scientific research and clinical analysis.* Unpublished.

Carmichael, L. P. 1976. The family in medicine: Process or entity? *Journal of Family Practice* 3:562–63.

———1985. A different way of doctoring. *Family Medicine* 17:185–87.

Carmichael, L. P., & Carmichael, J. S. 1981. The relational model in family practice. *Marriage and Family Review* 4:123–33.

Carse, A. L. 1991. The "voice of care": Implications for bioethical education. *Journal of Medicine and Philosophy* 16:5–28.

Carter, B., & McGoldrick, M., eds. 1988. *The changing family life cycle: A framework for family therapy.* 2nd ed. New York: Gardner Press.

Cassell, E. J. 1977. The function of medicine. *Hastings Center Report* 7 (6):16–19.

———1985. *The healer's art.* Cambridge, Mass.: MIT Press.

Caudill, W., & Weinstein, H. 1969. Maternal care and infant behavior in Japan and America. *Psychiatry* 32:12–43.

Centers for Disease Control. 1990. Infant mortality by marital status of mother: United States, 1983. *Morbidity and Mortality Weekly Reports* 39:521–23.

———1993. Use of race and ethnicity in public health surveillance: Summary of the CDC/ATSDR workshop. *Morbidity and Mortality Weekly Reports* 42 (RR-10).

Chaikin, A. L., & Derlega, V. J. 1974. Liking for the norm-breaker in self-disclosure. *Journal of Personality* 42:117–29.

Charon, R.; Greene, M.; & Adelman, R. 1994. Women readers, women doctors: A feminist reader response theory for medicine. In E. S. More & M. A. Milligan (eds.), *The empathic practitioner: Empathy, gender, and the therapeutic relationship* (pp. 205–21). New Brunswick, N.J.: Rutgers University Press.

Check, J. V. P., & Malamuth, N. M. 1983. Sex role stereotyping and reactions to depictions of stranger versus acquaintance rape. *Journal of Personality and Social Psychology* 45:344–56.

Chellingsworth, M. C. 1987. Multiple sclerosis. In H. Mandell & H. Spiro (eds.), *When doctors get sick* (pp. 89–93). New York: Plenum Medical.

Chelune, G. N. 1977. Nature and assessment of self-disclosing behavior. In P. McReynolds (ed.), *Advances in Psychological Assessment IV* (pp. 278–320). San Francisco: Jossey-Bass.

———1979. *Self-disclosure: Origins, patterns, and implications of openness in interpersonal relationships.* San Francisco: Jossey-Bass.

Chiriboga, D. A.; Weiler, P. G.; & Nielsen, K. 1988. The stress of caregivers. *Journal of Applied Social Sciences* 13 (1):118–41.

Chodorow, N. 1978. *The reproduction of mothering: Psychoanalysis and the sociology of gender*. Berkeley: University of California Press.

Chow, E. N.-L., & Berheide, C. W. 1988. The interdependence of family and work: A framework for family life education, policy, and practice. *Family Relations* 37:23–28.

Christie-Seely, J., ed. 1984. *Working with the family in primary care: A systems approach to health and illness*. New York: Praeger.

Chudacoff, H. P., & Hareven, T. K. 1979. From the empty nest to family dissolution: Life course transitions into old age. *Journal of Family History* 4:69–83.

Cicirelli, V. G. 1994. Sibling relationships in cross-cultural perspective. *Journal of Marriage and the Family* 56:7–24.

Cleeland, C. S.; Gonin, R.; Hatfield, A. K.; Edmonson, J. H.; Blum, R. H.; Stewart, J. A.; & Pandya, K. J. 1994. Pain and its treatment in outpatients with metastatic cancer. *New England Journal of Medicine* 330:592–96.

Clements, C. D., & Sider, R. C. 1983. Medical ethics' assault upon medical values. *Journal of the American Medical Association* 250:2011–15.

Code, L. 1987. Persons and others. In J. Genova (ed.), *Power, gender, values* (pp. 143–61). Edmonton, Alberta: Academic Printing and Publishing.

———1994. "I know just how you feel": Empathy and the problem of epistemic authority. In E. S. More & M. A. Milligan (eds.), *The empathic practitioner: Empathy, gender, and the therapeutic relationship* (pp. 77–96). New Brunswick, N.J.: Rutgers University Press.

Coleman, D. H., & Straus, M. A. 1986. Marital power, conflict, and violence in a nationally representative sample of American couples. *Violence and Victims* 1 (2):141–57.

Coleman, E. 1982. Family intimacy and chemical abuse: The connection. *Journal of Psychoactive Drugs* 14 (1–2):153–58.

Collins, P. H. 1989. The social construction of black feminist thought. *Signs* 14:745–73.

Comaroff, J. 1976. Communicating information about non-fatal illness: The strategies of a group of general practitioners. *Sociological Review* 24:269–90.

Comas-Diaz, L. 1987. Feminist therapy with mainland Puerto Rican women. *Psychology of Women Quarterly* 11:461–74.

Combrinck-Graham, L. 1988. Adolescent sexuality in the family life spiral. In C. J. Falicov (ed.), *Family transitions: Continuity and change over the life cycle* (pp. 107–31). New York: Guilford Press.

Connidis, I. A. 1992. Life transitions and the adult sibling tie: A qualitative study. *Journal of Marriage and the Family* 54:972–82.

Conrad, P. 1987. The noncompliant patient in search of autonomy. *Hastings Center Report* 17 (4):15–17.

Cook, J. A. 1988. Who "mothers" the chronically mentally ill? *Family Relations* 37:42–49.

Coolidge-Young, J. 1989. Use of clinician self-disclosure within the health care encounter. *Medical Encounter: A Newsletter on the Medical Interview and Related Skills* 6 (3–4):2–3.

Coontz, S. 1992. *The way we never were: American families and the nostalgia trap*. New York: Basic Books.

Cooper, I., & Cormier, B. M. 1982. Inter-generational transmission of incest. *Canadian Journal of Psychiatry* 27:231–35.

Cornwell, J. 1984. *Hard-earned lives: Accounts of health and illness from East London*. New York: Tavistock.

Cotterill, P. 1992. Interviewing women: Issues of friendship, vulnerability, and power. *Women's Studies International Forum* 15:593–606.

Council on Scientific Affairs, American Medical Association. 1992. Violence against women: Relevance for medical practitioners. *Journal of the American Medical Association* 267:3184–89.

Courtois, C. A. 1988. *Healing the incest wound: Adult survivors in therapy*. New York: W. W. Norton.

Cowan, C. P., & Cowan, P. A. 1992. *When partners become parents: The big life change for couples*. New York: Basic Books.

Cowan, F. J. 1991. *Adult abuse, neglect, and exploitation: A medical protocol for health care providers and community service agencies*. Lexington, Ky.: Office of the Attorney General, Commonwealth of Kentucky.

Cowan, G.; Warren, L. W.; & Young, J. L. 1985. Medical perceptions of menopausal symptoms. *Psychology of Women Quarterly* 9:3–14.

Cozby, P. C. 1973. Self-disclosure: A literature review. *Psychological Bulletin* 79:73–91.

Crouch, M. A., & Roberts, L., eds. 1987. *The family in medical practice: A family systems primer*. New York: Springer-Verlag.

Cunningham, J. D., & Antill, J. K. 1984. Changes in masculinity and femininity across the family life cycle: A reexamination. *Developmental Psychology* 20:1135–41.

Curran, W. J. 1982. Breaking off the physician-patient relationship: Another legal hazard. *New England Journal of Medicine* 307:1058–60.

Danis, M., & Churchill, L. R. 1991. Autonomy and the common weal. *Hastings Center Report* 21 (1):25–31.

Dannefer, D. 1984. Adult development and social theory: A paradigmatic reappraisal. *American Sociological Review* 49:100–116.

Danziger, S. K. 1979. Treatment of women in childbirth: Implications for family beginnings. *American Journal of Public Health* 69:895–901.

Davidson, L. R., & Duberman, L. 1982. Friendship: Communication and interactional patterns in same-sex dyads. *Sex Roles* 8:73–91.

Davies, J. M., & Frawley, M. G. 1994. *Treating the survivor of childhood sexual abuse: Psychoanalytic perspective*. New York: Basic Books.

Davis, T. C.; Crouch, M. A.; Long, S. W.; Jackson, R. H.; Bates, P.; George, R. B.; & Bairnsfather, L. E. 1991. Rapid assessment of literacy levels of adult primary care patients. *Family Medicine* 23:433–35.

Davis, T. C.; Crouch, M. A.; Wills, G.; Miller, S.; & Abdehou, D. M. 1990. The gap between patient reading comprehension and the readability of patient education materials. *Journal of Family Practice* 31:533–38.

Davis, T. C.; Long, S. W.; Jackson, R. H.; Mayeaux, E. J.; George, R. B.; Murphy, P. W.; & Crouch, M. A. 1993. Rapid estimate of adult literacy in medicine: A shortened screening instrument. *Family Medicine* 25:391–95.

deGruy, F. V.; Dickinson, L. C.; Dickinson, W. P.; Candib, L. M.; Hobson, F.; & McIntyre, I. (1994, September). *Patterns of Somatization in Primary Care.* Proceedings from the Eighth Annual NIMH International Research Conference on Mental Health Problems in the General Health Care Sector, McLean, VA.

DeLorey, C. 1989. Women at midlife: Women's perceptions, physicians' perceptions. *Journal of Women and Aging* 1:57–69.

Demos, J. 1986. *Past, present, and personal: The family and the life course in American history.* New York: Oxford University Press.

Dietz, C. A., & Craft, J. L. 1980. Family dynamics of incest: A new perspective. *Social Casework: The Journal of Contemporary Social Work* 61:602–9.

DiGiacomo, S. M. 1987. Biomedicine as a cultural system: An anthropologist in the kingdom of the sick. In H. A. Baer (ed.), *Encounters with biomedicine* (pp. 315–46). New York: Gordon and Breach Science Publishers.

Dillon, R. S. 1992. Care and respect. In E. B. Cole & S. Coultrap-McQuin (eds.), *Explorations in Feminist Ethics* (pp. 69–81). Bloomington: Indiana University Press.

Dobash, R. P.; Dobash, R. E.; Wilson, M.; & Daly, M. 1992. The myth of sexual symmetry in marital violence. *Social Problems* 39:71–91.

Dornbusch, S. M.; Carlsmith, J. M.; Bushwall, S. J.; Ritter, P. L.; Leiderman, H.; Hastorf, A. H.; & Gross, R. T. 1985. Single parents, extended households, and the control of adolescents. *Child Development* 56:326–41.

Drass, K. A. 1982. Negotiation and the structure of discourse in medical consultation. *Sociology of Health and Illness* 4 (3):320–41.

Drossman, D. A.; Lesserman, J.; Nachman, G.; Li, Z. M.; Gluck, H.; Toomey, T. C.; & Mitchell, C. M. 1990. Sexual and physical abuse in women with functional or organic gastrointestinal disorders. *Annals of Internal Medicine* 113:828–33.

Du Bois, B. 1983. Passionate scholarship: Notes on values, knowing and method in feminist social science. In G. Bowles & R. D. Klein (eds.), *Theories of Women's Studies* (pp. 105–16). Boston: Routledge & Kegan Paul.

Dugger, K. 1988. Social location and gender-role attitudes: A comparison of black and white women. *Gender and Society* 2:425–48.

Duhl, B. S. 1987. Uses of the self in integrated contextual systems therapy. In M. Baldwin & V. Satir (eds.), *The use of self in therapy* (pp. 71–84). New York: Haworth Press.

Dula, A. K. 1994. The life and death of Miss Mildred: An elderly black woman. *Clinics in Geriatric Medicine* 10 (3):419–30.

Duncan, G. J. 1988. The volatility of family income over the life course. In P. B. Baltes, D. L. Featherman, & R. M. Lerner (eds.), *Life-span development and behavior* (vol. 9, pp. 317–58). Hillsdale, N.J.: Lawrence Erlbaum Associates.

Duncan, G. J., & Rodgers, W. L. 1988. Longitudinal aspects of childhood poverty. *Journal of Marriage and the Family* 50:1007–21.

Dutton, D. G. 1986. Wife assaulter's explanations for assault: The neutralization of self-punishment. *Canadian Journal of Behavioral Science* 18:381–90.

Duvall, E. M. 1988. Family development's first forty years. *Family Relations* 37:127–34.

Dworkin, G. 1976. Autonomy and behavior control. *Hastings Center Report* 6 (1):23–28.

Dye, E., & Roth, S. 1990. Psychotherapists' knowledge about and attitudes toward sexual assault victim clients. *Psychology of Women Quarterly* 14:191–212.

Edelson, J. L., & Brygger, M. P. 1986. Gender differences in reporting of battering incidences. *Family Relations* 35:377–82.

Edwall, G. E., & Hoffman, N. G. 1988. Correlates of incest reported by adolescent girls in treatment for substance abuse. In L. E. A. Walker (ed.), *Handbook of sexual abuse of children: Assessment and treatment issues* (pp. 94–106). New York: Springer.

Edwards, R. 1990. Connecting methods and epistemology: A white woman interviewing black women. *Women's Studies International Forum* 13:477–90.

Ehrenreich, B., & English, D. 1972. *Witches, midwives, and nurses: A history of women healers.* Glass Mountain pamphlet no. 1. Old Westbury, N.Y.: Feminist Press.

Ehrhart, J. K., with Sandler, B. R. 1990. *Rx for success: Improving the climate for women in medical schools and teaching hospitals.* Washington, D.C.: American Association of Colleges.

Elder, G. H. 1981. History and the family: The discovery of complexity. *Journal of Marriage and the Family* 33:489–519.

Elliott, D. M., & Briere, J. 1992. Sexual abuse trauma among professional women: Validating the trauma symptom checklist-40. (TSC-40) *Child Abuse and Neglect* 16:391–98.

Emans, S. J.; Woods, E. R.; Flagg, N. T.; & Freeman, A. 1987. Genital findings in sexually abused, symptomatic and asymptomatic girls. *Pediatrics* 79:778–85.

Ende, J.; Kazis, L.; Ash, A.; & Moskowitz, M. A. 1989. Measuring patients' desire for autonomy: Decision making and information-seeking preferences among medical patients. *Journal of General Internal Medicine* 4:23–30.

Enders-Dragaesser, U. 1988. Women's identity and development within a paradoxical reality. *Women's Studies International Forum* 11:583–90.

Epstein, L., & Feiner, A. H., eds. 1979. *Countertransference.* New York: Aronson.

Erikson, E. H. 1963. *Childhood and society.* 2nd ed. New York: W. W. Norton.

——1968. *Identity: Youth and crisis.* New York: W. W. Norton.

Erikson, E. H., & Erikson, J. M. 1981. On generativity and identity: From a conversation with Erik and Joan Erikson. *Harvard Educational Review* 51:249–69.

Eugene, T. M. 1989. Sometimes I feel like a motherless child: The call and response for a liberational ethic of care by black feminists. In M. M. Brabeck (ed.), *Who cares? Theory, research, and educational implications of the ethic of care* (pp. 45–62). Westport, Conn.: Praeger.

Evans, N. J. 1985. Women's development across the life span. In N. J. Evans (ed.), *Facilitating the development of women* (pp. 9–27). New Directions for Student Services no. 29. San Francisco: Jossey-Bass.

Evers, H. 1985. The frail elderly women: Emergent questions in aging and women's health. In E. Lewin & V. Olesen (eds.), *Women, health, and healing: Toward a new perspective* (pp. 86–112). New York: Tavistock.

Everstine, D. S., & Everstine, L. 1989. *Sexual trauma in children and adolescents: Dynamics and treatment.* New York: Brunner/Mazel.

Falicov, C. J., ed. 1988. *Family transitions: Continuity and change over the life cycle.* New York: Guilford Press.

Falicov, C. J., & Karrer, B. M. 1980. Cultural variations in the family life cycle: The Mexican American family. In B. Carter and M. McGoldrick (eds.), *The family life cycle: A framework for family therapy* (pp. 383–425). New York: Gardner Press.

Family Therapy Networker. 1990. Men nurturing men. Vol. 14.

Farber, M. A. 1990 (June 1). The tormenting of Hilary. *Vanity Fair* 53 (6):120–27.

Faust, D. G. 1982. *James Henry Hammond and the Old South: A design for mastery.* Baton Rouge: Louisiana State University Press.

Featherman, D. L. 1983. Life-span perspectives in social science research. In P. B. Baltes & O. G. Brim (eds.), *Life-span development and behavior* (vol. 5, pp. 1–57). New York: Academic Press.

Feild, H. S. 1978. Attitudes toward rape: A comparative analysis of police, rapists, crisis counselors, and citizens. *Journal of Personality and Social Psychology* 36:156–79.

Feinberg, P. H. 1990. Teaching sketch: Circular questions: Establishing the relational context. *Family Systems Medicine* 8:273–77.

Felitti, V. J. 1991. Long-term medical consequences of incest, rape, and molestation. *Southern Medical Journal* 84:328–31.

Fengler, A. P., & Goodrich, N. 1979. Wives of elderly disabled men: The hidden patients. *The Gerontologist* 19:175–83.

Fenster, S.; Phillips, S. B.; & Rapoport, E. R. G. 1986. *The therapist's pregnancy: Intrusion in the analytic space.* Hillsdale, N.J.: Analytic Press.

Ferree, M. M. 1990. Beyond separate spheres: Feminism and family research. *Journal of Marriage and the Family* 52:866–84.

Fillmore, K. M. 1985. The social victims of drinking. *British Journal of Addictions* 80:307–14.

Finch, J., & Groves, D., eds. 1983. *A labour of love: Women, work and caring.* Boston: Routledge & Kegan Paul.

Finkelhor, D., & Browne, A. 1985. The traumatic impact of child sexual abuse: A conceptualization. *American Journal of Orthopsychiatry* 55:530–41.

Finkelhor, D.; Gelles, R. J.; Hotaling, G. T.; & Straus, M. A., eds. 1983. *The dark side of families: Current family violence research.* Beverly Hills, Calif.: Sage.

Finn, J. 1986. The relationship between sex role attitudes and attitudes supporting marital violence. *Sex Roles* 14:235–45.

Finucane, T. E., & Carrese, J. A. 1990. Racial bias in presentation of cases. *Journal of General Internal Medicine* 5:120–21.

Fischer, L. R. 1986. *Linked lives: Adult daughters and their mothers*. New York: Harper & Row.

Fisher, S. 1983. Doctor talk/patient talk: How treatment decisions are negotiated in doctor-patient communication. In S. Fisher & A. D. Todd (eds.), *The social organization of doctor-patient communication* (pp. 135–57). Washington, D.C.: Center for Applied Linguistics.

Fisher, S. 1990. *In the patient's best interest: Women and the politics of medical decisions*. New Brunswick, N.J.: Rutgers University Press.

Fisher, S., & Todd, A. D., eds. 1983. *The social organization of doctor-patient communication*. Washington, D.C.: Center for Applied Linguistics.

Fonow, M. M.; Richardson, L.; & Wemmerus, V. A. 1992. Feminist rape education: Does it work? *Gender and Society* 6:108–21.

Ford, E.; Cooper, R.; Castaner, A.; Simmons, B.; & Mar, M. 1989. Coronary arteriography and coronary bypass survey among whites and other racial groups relative to hospital-based incidence rates for coronary artery disease: Findings from NHDS. *American Journal of Public Health* 79:437–40.

Forrest, L., & Mikolaitis, N. 1986. The relational component of identity: An expansion of career development theory. *Career Development Quarterly* 35:76–88.

Fox, M.; Gibbs, M.; & Auerbach, D. 1985. Aging and gender dimensions of friendship. *Psychology of Women Quarterly* 9:489–502.

Frankel, R. M. 1983. The laying on of hands: Aspects of the organization of gaze, touch, and talk in a medical encounter. In S. Fisher & A. D. Todd (eds.), *The social organization of doctor-patient communication* (pp. 19–54). Washington, D.C.: Center for Applied Linguistics.

———1984. From sentence to sequence: Understanding the medical encounter through microinteractional analysis. *Discourse Processes* 7:135–70.

———1990. Talking in interviews: A dispreference for patient-initiated questions in physician-patient encounters. In G. Psathas (ed.), *Studies in ethnomethodology and conversation analysis* (pp. 231–62). Washington, D.C.: International Institute for Ethnomethodology and Conversation Analysis and University Press of America.

Frankel, R. M.; Morse, D. S.; Suchman, A.; & Beckman, H. B. 1991. Can I really improve my listening skills with only 15 minutes to see my patients? *HMO Practice* 5 (4):114–20.

Fraser, S. 1987. *My father's house: A memoir of incest and of healing*. New York: Harper & Row.

Freire, P. 1970. *Pedagogy of the oppressed*. New York: Seabury Press.

French, J. R. P., & Raven, B. 1959. The bases of social power. In D. Cartwright (ed.), *Studies in social power* (pp. 150–67). Ann Arbor: University of Michigan.

Fried, S. 1994. *War of remembrance. Philadelphia* (January): 66–71, 149–57.

Friedlander, W. J. 1982. The basis of privacy and autonomy in medical practice. *Social Science and Medicine* 16:1709–18.

Friedman, A. R. 1992. Rape and domestic violence: The experience of refugee women. In E. Cole, O. M. Espin, & E. D. Rothblum (eds.), *Refugee women and their mental health: Shattered societies, shattered lives* (pp. 65–78). New York: Haworth.

Friedman, L. S.; Samet, J. H.; Roberts, M. S.; Hudlin, M.; & Hans, P. 1992. Inquiry about victimization experiences: A survey of patient preferences and physician practices. *Archives of Internal Medicine* 152:1186–90.

Friedman, M. 1987a. Beyond caring: The de-moralization of gender. In M. Hanen & K. Nielsen (eds.), *Science, morality and feminist theory* (pp. 87–110). *Canadian Journal of Philosophy*, supp. vol. 13. Calgary, Alberta: University of Calgary Press.

————1987b. Care and context in moral reasoning. In E. F. Kittay & D. T. Meyers (eds.), *Women and Moral Theory* (pp. 190–204). Totowa, N.J.: Rowman & Littlefield.

Friedman, S. S. 1985. Authority in the feminist classroom: A contradiction in terms? In M. Culley & C. Portuges (eds.), *Gendered subjects: The dynamics of feminist teaching* (pp. 203–8). Boston: Routledge and Kegan Paul.

Friedman, W. J.; Robinson, A. B.; & Friedman, B. L. 1987. Sex differences in moral judgments? A test of Gilligan's theory. *Psychology of Women Quarterly* 11:37–46.

Frieze, I. H., & McHugh, M. C. 1992. Power and influence strategies in violence and nonviolent marriages. *Psychology of Women Quarterly* 16:449–65.

Fromuth, M. E. 1986. The relationship of childhood sexual abuse with later psychological and sexual adjustment in a sample of college women. *Child Abuse and Neglect* 10:5–15.

Furby, L.; Fischhoff, B.; & Morgan, M. 1991. Rape prevention and self-defense: At what price? *Women's Studies International Forum* 14:49–62.

Gabbard, G. O., ed. 1989. Sexual exploitation in professional relationships. Washington, D.C.: American Psychiatric Press.

Gadow, S. A. 1985. Nurse and patient: The caring relationship. In A. H. Bishop & J. R. Scudder (eds.), *Caring, curing, coping: Nurse, physician, patient relationships* (pp. 31–43). University: University of Alabama Press.

Gardiner, J. K. 1987. Self psychology as feminist theory. *Signs* 12:761–80.

Garfield, R. 1989. The vulnerable therapist. *Family Therapy Networker* 13 (1):58–62.

Garrett-Gooding, J., & Senter, R. 1987. Attitudes and acts of sexual aggression on a university campus. *Sociological Inquiry* 57:348–71.

Geiger, S. N. G. 1986. Women's life histories: Method and content. *Signs* 11:334–51.

Gelinas, D. J. 1983. The persisting negative effects of incest. *Psychiatry* 46:312–32.

Gergen, K. J. 1980. The emerging crisis in life-span developmental theory. In P. B. Baltes & O. G. Brim (eds.), *Life-span development and behavior* (vol. 3, pp. 31–63). New York: Academic Press.

Gergen, M. M. 1990. Finished at 40: Women's development within the patriarchy. *Psychology of Women Quarterly* 14:471–93.

Gesell, A. 1940. *The first five years of life: A guide to the study of the preschool child.* New York: Harper & Brothers.

Gibson, C. D., & Kramer, B. M. 1965. Site of care in medical practice. *Medical Care* 3:14–17.

Gidycz, C. A.; Coble, C. N.; Latham, L.; & Layman, M. J. 1993. Sexual assault experience in adulthood and prior victimization experiences. *Psychology of Women Quarterly* 17:151–68.

Gilbert, L. A. 1980. Feminist therapy. In A. M. Brodsky & R. T. Hare-Mustin (eds.), *Women and psychotherapy: An assessment of research and practice* (pp. 245–65). New York: Guilford Press.

Gillick, M. R. 1992. From confrontation to cooperation in the doctor-patient relationship. *Journal of General Internal Medicine* 7:83–86.

Gilligan, C. 1979. Woman's place in man's life cycle. *Harvard Educational Review* 49:431–46.

———1982. *In a different voice: Psychological theory and women's development.* Cambridge, Mass.: Harvard University Press.

———1986. Remapping the moral domain: New images of the self in relationship. In T. C. Heller, M. Sosna, & D. E. Wellbery (eds.), *Reconstructing individualism: Autonomy, individuality, and the self in western thought* (pp. 237–52). Stanford, Calif.: Stanford University Press.

Gilligan, C.; Lyons, N. P.; & Hanmer, T. J., eds. 1990. *Making connections: The relational worlds of adolescent girls at Emma Willard School.* Cambridge, Mass.: Harvard University Press.

Gilligan, C., & Pollak, S. 1988. The vulnerable and invulnerable physician. In C. Gilligan, J. V. Ward, & J. M. Taylor, with B. Bardige (eds.), *Mapping the moral domain: A contribution of women's thinking to psychological theory and education* (pp. 245–62). Cambridge, Mass.: Center for the Study of Gender, Education and Human Development, Harvard University School of Education.

Gilligan, C.; Ward, J. V.; & Taylor, J. M.; with Bardige, B., eds. 1988. *Mapping the moral domain: A contribution of women's thinking to psychological theory and education.* Cambridge, Mass.: Center for the Study of Gender, Education and Human Development, Harvard University School of Education.

Glazer, N. Y. 1990. The home as workshop: Women as amateur nurses and medical care providers. *Gender and Society* 4:479–99.

Gleason, N. A. 1991. Daughters and mothers: College women look at their relationships. In J. V. Jordan et al., *Women's growth in connection: Writings from the Stone Center* (pp. 132–40). New York: Guilford Press.

Glenn, E. N. 1987. Gender and the family. In B. B. Hess & M. M. Ferree (eds.), *Analyzing gender: A handbook of social science research* (pp. 348–80). Beverly Hills, Calif.: Sage.

Glenn, M. L. 1984. *On diagnosis: A systemic approach.* New York: Brunner/Mazel.

Glenn, N. D. 1975. Psychological well-being in the postparental stage: Some evidence from national surveys. *Journal of Marriage and the Family* 37:105–75.

Glick, P. C. 1977. Updating the life cycle of the family. *Journal of Marriage and the Family* 39:5–13.

————1988. Fifty years of family demography: A record of social change. *Journal of Marriage and the Family* 50:861–73.

Gluck, N. R.; Dannefer, E.; & Milea, K. 1980. Women in families. In B. Carter & M. McGoldrick (eds.), *The family life cycle: A framework for family therapy* (pp. 295–327). New York: Gardner Press.

Goetting, A. 1986. The developmental tasks of siblingship over the life cycle. *Journal of Marriage and the Family* 48:703–14.

Goffman, E. 1963. *Stigma: Notes on the management of spoiled identity.* Englewood Cliffs, N.J.: Prentice-Hall.

————1967. *Interaction ritual: Essays on face-to-face behavior.* Garden City, N.Y.: Anchor Books.

Goldner, V. 1988. Generation and gender: Normative and covert hierarchies. *Family Process* 27:17–31.

Goldstein, D. 1983. Spouse abuse. In A. P. Goldstein & L. Krasner (eds.), *Prevention and control of aggression* (pp. 37–65). New York: Pergamon Press.

Goldstein, J. 1990. Desperately seeking science: The creation of knowledge in family practice. *Hastings Center Report* 20 (6):26–32.

Goodrich, T. J., ed. 1991. *Women and power: Perspectives for family therapy.* New York: W. W. Norton.

Goodrich, T. J.; Rampage, C.; Ellman, B.; & Halstead, K., eds. 1988. *Feminist family therapy: A casebook.* New York: W. W. Norton.

Goodwin, J. 1982. *Sexual abuse: Incest victims and their families.* Boston: Wright.

Goodwin, J.; Attias, R.; McCarty, T.; Chandler, S.; & Romanik, R. 1988. Letter to the editor: Reporting by adult psychiatric patients of childhood sexual abuse. *American Journal of Psychiatry* 145:1183.

Gordon, D. R. 1988. Tenacious assumptions in western medicine. In M. Lock & D. R. Gordon (eds.), *Biomedicine reexamined* (pp. 19–56). Boston: Kluwer Academic.

Gordon, L. 1988. *Heroes of their own lives: The politics and history of family violence, Boston 1880–1960.* New York: Penguin.

————1992. Family violence, feminism, and social control. In B. Thorne with M. Yalom (eds.), *Rethinking the family: Some feminist questions.* Revised edition (pp. 262–86). Boston: Northeastern University Press.

Graham, H. 1993. Social division in caring. *Women's Studies International Forum* 16:461–70.

Green, J. A. 1988. Minimizing malpractice risks by role clarification: The confusing transition from tort to contract. *Annals of Internal Medicine* 109:234–41.

Greenfield, S.; Kaplan, S.; & Ware, J. E. 1985. Expanding patient involvement in care: Effects on patient outcomes. *Annals of Internal Medicine* 102:520–28.

Greenfield, S.; Kaplan, S. H.; Ware, J. E.; Yano, E. M.; & Frank, H. J. 1988. Patients' participation in medical care: Effects on blood sugar control and quality of life in diabetes. *Journal of General Internal Medicine* 3:448–57.

Greenspan, M. 1983. *A new approach to women and therapy.* New York: McGraw-Hill.

Greenwood, C. L.; Tangalos, E. G.; & Maruta, T. 1990. Prevalence of sexual abuse, physical abuse, and concurrent traumatic life events in a general medical population. *Mayo Clinic Proceedings* 65:1067–71.

Greil, A. L.; Leitko, T. A.; & Porter, K. L. 1988. Infertility: His and hers. *Gender and Society* 2:172–79.

Griffiths, M. 1992. Autonomy and the fear of dependence. *Women's Studies International Forum* 15:351–62.

Grimshaw, J. 1986. *Philosophy and Feminist Thinking.* Minneapolis: University of Minnesota Press.

Grotevant, H. D., & Cooper, C. R. 1986. Individuation in family relationships: A perspective on individual differences in the development of identity and role-taking skill in adolescence. *Human Development* 29:82–100.

————1988. The role of family experience in career exploration: A lifespan perspective. In P. B. Baltes, D. L. Featherman, & R. M. Lerner (eds.), *Life-span development and behavior* (vol. 8, pp. 231–58). Hillsdale, N.J.: Lawrence Erlbaum Associates.

Groth, A. N. 1982. The incest offender. In S. M. Sgroi (ed.), *Handbook of clinical intervention in child sexual abuse* (pp. 215–39). Lexington, Mass.: Lexington Books.

Guarnaccia, P. J.; Good, B. J.; & Kleinman, A. 1990. A critical review of epidemiological studies of Puerto Rican mental health. *American Journal of Psychiatry* 147:1449–56.

Guinan, M. E. 1993. War crimes of the 90's: Rape as a strategy. *Journal of the American Medical Women's Association* 48:59, 61.

Gutheil, T. G., & Avery, N. C. 1977. Multiple overt incest as family defense against loss. *Family Process* 16:105–16.

Hahn, R. A. 1987. Divisions of labor: Obstetrician, woman, and society in Williams Obstetrics, 1903–1985. *Medical Anthropology Quarterly* 18(3): 256–82.

Hall, E. R.; Howard, J. A.; & Boezio, S. L. 1986. Tolerance of rape: A sexist or antisocial attitude? *Psychology of Women Quarterly* 10:101–17.

Hall, J. A.; Epstein, A. M.; DeCiantis, M. L.; & McNeil, B. J. 1993. Physicians' liking for their patients: More evidence for the role of affect in medical care. *Health Psychology* 12:140–46.

Hall, J. A.; Roter, K. L.; & Katz, N. R. 1988. Meta-analysis of correlates of provider behavior in medical encounters. *Medical Care* 26:657–75.

Hannan, E. L.; Kilburn, Jr., H.; O'Donnell, J. F.; Lukacik, G.; & Shields, E. P. 1991. Interracial access to selected cardiac procedures for patients hospitalized with coronary artery disease in New York State. *Medical Care* 29:430–41.

Harding, S. 1986. *The science question in feminism.* Ithaca, N.Y.: Cornell University Press.

————1987. The curious coincidence of feminine and African moralities: Challenges for feminist theory. In E. F. Kittay & D. T. Meyers (eds.), *Women and moral theory* (pp. 296–315). Totowa, N.J.: Rowman & Littlefield.

Hardwig, J. 1984. Should women think in terms of rights? *Ethics* 94:441–55.

————1990. What about the family? *Hastings Center Report* (March-April): 5–10.

Hare-Mustin, R. T. 1987. The problem of gender in family therapy theory. *Family Process* 26:15–27.

———1988. Family change and gender differences: Implications for theory and practice. *Family Relations* 37:36–41.

Hare-Mustin, R. T., & Maracek, J. 1986. Autonomy and gender: Some questions for therapists. *Psychotherapy* 23:205–12.

Hareven, T. K. 1974. The family as process: The historical study of the family cycle. *Journal of Social History* 7:322–29.

———1981. *Family time and industrial time.* New York: Cambridge University Press.

Harkins, E. B. 1978. Effects of empty nest transition on self-report of psychological and physical well-being. *Journal of Marriage and the Family* 40:549–56.

Harley, S. 1990. For the good of family and race: Gender, work, and domestic roles in the black community, 1880–1930. *Signs* 15:336–49.

Harris, R. L.; Ellicott, A. M.; & Holmes, D. S. 1986. The timing of psychosocial transitions and changes in women's lives: An examination of women aged 45–60. *Journal of Personality and Social Psychology* 51:409–16.

Harter, S.; Alexander, P. C.; & Neimeyer, R. A. 1988. Long-term effects of incestuous child abuse in college women: Social adjustment, social cognition, and family characteristics. *Journal of Consulting and Clinical Psychology* 56:5–8.

Havens, L. L. 1978. Taking a history from the difficult patient. *Lancet* 1:138–40.

Held, V. 1987a. Non-contractual society: A feminist view. In M. Hanen & K. Nielsen (eds.), *Science, morality and feminist theory* (pp. 111–37). *Canadian Journal of Philosophy,* supp. vol. 13. Calgary, Alberta: University of Calgary Press.

———1987b. Feminism and moral theory. In E. F. Kittay & D. T. Meyers (eds.), *Women and moral theory* (pp. 111–28). Totowa, N.J.: Rowman & Littlefield.

Henao, S., & Grose, N. P., eds. 1985. *Principles of family systems in family medicine.* New York: Brunner/Mazel.

Henley, N. 1977. *Body politics: Power, sex, and non-verbal communication.* Englewood Cliffs, N.J.: Prentice-Hall.

Hennen, B. K. 1987. The family life cycle and anticipatory guidance. In D. B. Shires, B. K. Hennen, & D. I. Rice (eds.), *Family medicine: A guidebook for practitioners of the art,* 2nd ed. (pp. 25–31). New York: McGraw-Hill.

Herman, J. L. 1992. *Trauma and recovery.* New York: Basic Books.

Herman, J. L., with Hirschman, L. 1981. *Father-daughter incest.* Cambridge, Mass.: Harvard University Press.

Herman, J. L.; Perry, J. C.; & van der Kolk, B. A. 1989. Childhood trauma in borderline personality disorder. *American Journal of Psychiatry* 146:490–95.

Herman, J. L.; Russell, D.; & Trocki, K. 1986. Long-term effects of incestuous abuse in childhood. *American Journal of Psychiatry* 143:1293–96.

Herxheimer, A. 1991. How much drug in the tablet? *Lancet* 337:346–48.

Higginbotham, E. B. 1992. African-American women's history and the metalanguage of race. *Signs* 17:251–74.

Hilberman, E. 1980. Overview: The "wife beater's wife" reconsidered. *American Journal of Psychiatry* 137:1336–47.

Hilberman, E., & Munson, K. 1977–78. Sixty battered women. *Victimology* 2:460–70.

Hill, R., & Mattessich, P. 1979. Family development theory and life-span development. In P. B. Baltes & O. G. Brim (eds.), *Life-span development and behavior* (vol. 2., pp. 161–204). New York: Academic Press.

Hoagland, S. L. 1990a. *Lesbian ethics: Toward new value.* Palo Alto, Calif.: Institute of Lesbian Studies.

————1990b. Some concerns about Nel Noddings's *Caring. Hypatia* 5:109–14.

Hobbs, C. H., & Wynne, J. M. 1987. Child sexual abuse: An increasing rate of diagnosis. *Lancet* 2:837–41.

Hochschild, A., with Machung, A. 1989. *The second shift: Working parents and the revolution at home.* New York: Viking.

Hoekelman, R. A.; Friedman, S. P.; Nelson, N. M.; & Seidel, H. M., eds. 1992. *Primary pediatric care.* 2nd ed. Boston: Mosby.

Hoff, L. A. 1988. Collaborative feminist research and the myth of objectivity. In K. Yllo & M. Bograd (eds.), *Feminist perspectives on wife abuse* (pp. 269–81). Beverly Hills, Calif.: Sage.

Hoffman-Graff, M. A. 1977. Interviewer use of positive and negative self-disclosure and interviewer-subject sex pairing. *Journal of Counseling Psychology* 24:184–90.

Hondagneu-Sotelo, P. 1992. Overcoming patriarchal constraints: The reconstruction of gender relations among Mexican immigrant women and men. *Gender and Society* 6:393–415.

Hornung, C. A.; McCullough, B. C.; & Sugimoto, T. 1981. Status relationships in marriage: Risk factors in spouse abuse. *Journal of Marriage and the Family* 43:675–92.

Horowitz, A. 1985. Sons and daughters as caregivers to older parents: Differences in role performance and consequences. *The Gerontologist* 25:612–17.

Houston. B. 1990. Caring and exploitation. *Hypatia* 5:115–19.

Hultsch, D. F., & Plemons, J. K. 1979. Life events and life-span development. In P. B. Baltes & O. G. Brim (eds.), *Life-span development and behavior* (vol. 2, pp. 1–36). New York: Academic Press.

Humphries, L. L.; Barclay, G.; & Mohler, S. N. 1986. Perspectives on a case of multiple incestuous relationships. *Journal of the American Medical Women's Association* 41 (2):45–49.

Hunter, K. M. 1991. *Doctors' stories: The narrative structure of medical knowledge.* Princeton, N.J.: Princeton University Press.

Hurley, D. L. 1991. Women, alcohol and incest: An analytical review. *Journal of Studies on Alcohol* 52:253–68.

Huygen, F. J. A. 1982. *Family medicine: The medical life history of families.* New York: Brunner/Mazel.

Illich, I. 1976. *Medical nemesis: The expropriation of health*. New York: Pantheon.

Inui, T. S., & Frankel, R. M. 1992. *Do physicians' caring actions make a difference?* Paper presented to the Caring Physician Seminar of the Center for Advanced Studies of Behavior Science, Stanford University.

Jacobson, A., & Richardson, B. 1987. Assault experiences of 100 psychiatric inpatients: Evidence of the need for routine inquiry. *American Journal of Psychiatry* 144:908–13.

James, J., & Meyerding, J. 1977. Early sexual experience and prostitution. *American Journal of Psychiatry* 134:1381–85.

Jason, J.; Williams, S. L.; Burton, A.; & Rochat, R. 1982. Epidemiologic differences between sexual and physical child abuse. *Journal of the American Medical Association* 247:3344–48.

Jecker, N. S. 1990. The role of intimate others in medical decision making. *The Gerontologist* 30:65–71.

———1993. Privacy beliefs and the violence family: Extending the ethical argument for physician intervention. *Journal of the American Medical Association* 269:776–80.

Jefferys, M., & Sachs, H. 1983. *Rethinking general practice: Dilemmas in primary medical care*. New York: Tavistock.

Jennings, B.; Callahan, D.; & Caplan, A. L. 1988. Ethical challenges of chronic illness. *Hastings Center Report* [special supplement] 18 (1) (February–March):1–16.

Jensen, R. 1995. Pornographic lives. *Violence Against Women* 1 (1):32–54.

Johnson, J. T. 1992. *Mothers of incest survivors: Another side of the story*. Bloomington: Indiana University Press.

Jones, A., & Schecter, S. 1992. *When love goes wrong: What to do when you can't do anything right*. New York: HarperCollins.

Jones, J. 1981. *Bad blood: The Tuskegee syphilis experiment—a tragedy of race and medicine*. New York: Free Press.

Jordan, J. V. 1991a. Empathy and self-boundaries. In J. V. Jordan et al., *Women's growth in connection: Writings from the Stone Center* (pp. 67–80). New York: Guilford Press.

———1991b. The meaning of mutuality. In J. V. Jordan et al. , *Women's growth in connection: Writings from the Stone Center* (pp. 81–96). New York: Guilford Press.

Jordan, J. V.; Kaplan, A. G.; Miller, J. B.; Stiver, I. P.; & Surrey, J. L. 1991. *Women's growth in connection: Writings from the Stone Center*. New York: Guilford Press.

Josselson, R. 1991. *Finding herself: Pathways to identity development in women*. San Francisco: Jossey-Bass.

Jourard, S. M. 1968. *Disclosing man to himself*. New York: Van Nostrand.

———1971. *Self-disclosure: An experimental analysis of the transparent self*. New York: Wiley-Interscience.

Kaminer, W. (1990, February 11). Chances are you're codependent too. *New York Times Book Review* (February 11): 3, 26–27.

Kanin, E. H. 1985. Date rapists: Differential sexual socialization and relative deprivation. *Archives of Sexual Behavior* 14:219–31.

Kaplan, A. G. 1988. How normal is normal development? Some connections between adult development and the roots of abuse and victimization. In M. B. Straus (ed.), *Abuse and victimization across the life span* (pp. 127–39). Baltimore: Johns Hopkins University Press.

Kaplan, A. G., & Klein, R. 1991. The relational self in late adolescent women. In J. V. Jordan et al., *Women's growth in connection: Writings from the Stone Center* (pp. 122–31). New York: Guilford Press.

Kaplan, H. I., & Sadock, B. J. 1985. *Comprehensive textbook of psychiatry*. Baltimore: Williams & Wilkins.

Kaufert, P. 1988. Menopause as process or event: The creation of definitions in biomedicine. In M. Lock & D. R. Gordon (eds.), *Biomedicine examined* (pp. 331–49). Boston: Kluwer Academic Publishers.

Kellam, S. G.; Ensminger, M. E.; & Turner, R. J. 1977. Family structure and the mental health of children. *Archives of General Psychiatry* 34:1012–22.

Kerber, L. K.; Greeno, C. G.; Maccoby, E. E.; Luria, Z.; Stack, C. B.; & Gilligan, C. 1986. On *In a Different Voice*: An interdisciplinary forum. *Signs* 11:304–33.

Kessel, N. 1979. Reassurance. *Lancet* 1:1128–33.

Ketchum, S. A., & Pierce, C. 1981. Rights and responsibilities. *Journal of Medicine and Philosophy* 6:271–79.

Kimmel, D. C. 1978. Adult development and aging: A gay perspective. *Journal of Social Issues* 34:113–30.

Klassen, A. D., & Wilsnack, S. C. 1986. Sexual experience and drinking among women in a U.S. national survey. *Archives of Sexual Behavior* 15:363–92.

Klein, H., & Chao, B. S. 1995. Sexual abuse during childhood and adolescence as predictors of HIV-related sexual risk during adulthood among female sexual partners of injection drug users. *Violence Against Women* 1 (1):55–76.

Klein, R. D. 1983. How to do what we want to do: Thoughts about feminist methodology. In G. Bowles & R. D. Klein (eds.), *Theories of women's studies* (pp. 88–104). Boston: Routledge & Kegan Paul.

Kleinman, A. 1980. *Patients and healers in the context of culture*. Berkeley: University of California Press.

———1988. *The illness narratives: Suffering, healing and the human condition*. New York: Basic Books.

Kleinman, C. S. 1987. Hodgkin's disease. In H. Mandell & H. Spiro (eds.), *When doctors get sick* (pp. 305–16). New York: Plenum Medical.

Kluft, R. P., ed. 1990a. *Incest-related syndromes of adult psychopathology*. Washington, D.C.: American Psychiatric Press.

———1990b. Incest and subsequent revictimization: The case of therapist-patient sexual exploitation, with a description of the sitting duck syndrome. In R. P. Kluft (ed.), *Incest-related syndromes of adult psychopathology* (pp. 263–87). Washington, D.C.: American Psychiatric Press.

———1990c. On the apparent invisibility of incest: A personal reflection on things known and forgotten. In R. P. Kluft (ed.), *Incest-related syndromes of adult psychopathology* (pp. 11–34). Washington, D.C.: American Psychiatric Press.

Knudsen, M. P. 1987. The natural history of palpitations in a family practice. *Journal of Family Practice* 24:357–60.

Kohlberg, L. 1981. *The philosophy of moral development: Moral stages and the idea of justice.* New York: Harper & Row.

Kohut, H. 1984. *How does analysis cure?* Chicago: University of Chicago Press.

Komaromy, M.; Bindman, A. B.; Haber, R. J.; & Sande, M. A. 1993. Sexual harassment in medical training. *New England Journal of Medicine* 328:322–26.

Komter, A. 1989. Hidden power in marriage. *Gender and Society* 3:187–216.

Kooden, H. 1991. Self-disclosure: The gay male therapist as agent of social change. In C. Silverstein (ed.), *Gays, lesbians, and their therapists: Studies in psychotherapy* (pp. 143–54). New York: W. W. Norton.

Korsch, B. M.; Freemon, B.; & Negrete, V. F. 1971. Practical implications of doctor-patient interaction analysis for pediatric practice. *American Journal of Diseases of Children* 121:110–14.

Koss, M. P., & Gaines, J. A. 1993. The prediction of sexual aggression by alcohol use, athletic participation, and fraternity affiliation. *Journal of Interpersonal Violence* 8:94–108.

Koss, M. P.; Gidycz, C. A.; & Wisniewski, N. 1987. The scope of rape: Incidence and prevalence of sexual aggression and victimization in a national sample of higher education students. *Journal of Consulting and Clinical Psychology* 55:162–70.

Koss, M. P., & Heslet, L. 1992. Somatic consequences of violence against women. *Archives of Family Medicine* 1:53–59.

Koss, M. P.; Koss, P. G.; & Woodruff, J. 1991. Deleterious effects of criminal victimization on women's health and medical utilization. *Archives of Internal Medicine* 151:342–47.

Koss, M. P.; Leonard, K. E.; Beezley, D. A.; & Oros, C. J. 1985. Nonstranger sexual aggression: A discriminant analysis of the psychological characteristics of undetected offenders. *Sex Roles* 12:981–92.

Kramer, J. R. 1985. *Family interfaces: Transgenerational patterns.* New York: Brunner/Mazel.

Kurz, D. 1989. Social science perspectives on wife abuse: Current debates and future directions. *Gender and Society* 3:489–505.

Kuykendall, E. H. 1983. Toward an ethic of nurturance: Luce Irigaray on mothering and power. In J. Trebilcot (ed.), *Mothering: Essays in feminist theory* (pp. 261–74). Totowa, N.J.: Rowman & Allanheld.

Kuzel, A. J. 1986. Naturalistic inquiry: An appropriate model for family medicine. *Family Medicine* 18:369–74.

LaCombe, M. A. 1990. Living the patient's story. *Annals of Internal Medicine* 113:890–91.

Ladd, J. 1982. The distinction between rights and responsibilities: A defense. *Linacre Quarterly* 49:121–42.

Lancet. 1986 (November 8). Letters to the editor, p. 1100.

Lancet. 1987a (March 14). Letters to the editor, pp. 620–21.

Lancet. 1987b (December 12). pp. 1396–398.

Landale, N. S., & Hauan, S. M. 1992. The family life course of Puerto Rican children. *Journal of Marriage and the Family* 54:912–24.

Lang, F. 1990. Resident behaviors during observed pelvic examinations. *Family Medicine* 22:153–55.

Lang, J. 1994. Is empathy always nice? Empathy, sympathy and the psychoanalytic situation. In E. S. More & M. A. Milligan (eds.), *The empathic practitioner: Empathy, gender, and the therapeutic relationship* (pp. 98–112). New Brunswick, N.J.: Rutgers University Press.

Laslie, A. E. 1982. Ethical issues in childbirth. *Journal of Medicine and Philosophy* 7:179–95.

Lavine, L. O., & Lombardo, J. P. 1984. Self-disclosure: Intimate and non-intimate disclosures to parents and best friends as a function of BEM sex-role category. *Sex Roles* 11:735–44.

Lazare, A., & Eisenthal, S. 1979. A negotiated approach to the clinical encounter. In A. Lazare (ed.), *Outpatient psychiatry: Diagnosis and treatment* (pp. 141–56). Baltimore: Williams and Wilkins.

Lazarus, E. S. 1988. Theoretical considerations for the study of the doctor-patient relationship: Implications of a perinatal study. *Medical Anthropology Quarterly* 2:34–58.

Leaman, T. 1980. Adult development. In E. M. Rosen, J. P. Geyman, & R. H. Layton (eds.), *Behavioral science in family practice* (pp. 49–66). New York: Appleton-Century-Crofts.

Lear, M. W. 1980. *Heartsounds.* New York: Simon and Schuster.

Lechner, M. E.; Vogel, M. E.; Garcia-Shelton, L. M.; Leichter, J. L.; & Steibel, K. R. 1993. Self-reported medical problems of adult female survivors of childhood sexual abuse. *Journal of Family Practice* 36:633–38.

Lee, T. R.; Mancini, J. A.; & Maxwell, J. W. 1990. Sibling relationships in adulthood: Contact patterns and motivations. *Journal of Marriage and the Family* 52:431–40.

Lent, B. 1986. Diagnosing wife assault. *Canadian Family Physician* 32:547–49.

Lerman, H. 1986. From Freud to feminist personality theory: Getting here from there. *Psychology of Women Quarterly* 10:1–18.

Lerner, R. M., & Ryff, C. D. 1978. Implementation of the life-span view of human development: The sample case of attachment. In P. B. Baltes (ed.), *Lifespan development and behavior* (vol. 1, pp. 381–407). New York: Academic Press.

Levenstein, J. H.; McCracken, E. C.; McWhinney, I. R.; Stewart, M. A.; & Brown, J. B. 1986. The patient-centered clinical method. 1. A model for the doctor-patient interaction in family medicine. *Family Practice* 3:24–30.

Levinson, D. J.; Darrow, C. N.; Klein, E. B.; Levinson, M. H.; & McKee, B. 1978. *Seasons of a man's life.* New York: Alfred A. Knopf.

Lew, M. 1988. *Victims no longer: Men recovering from incest and other sexual child abuse.* New York: Harper & Row.

Lewis, J., & Meredith, B. 1988. *Daughters who care: Daughters caring for mothers at home.* New York: Routledge.

Lichstein, P. R. 1982. The resident leaves the patient: Another look at the doctor-patient relationship. *Annals of Internal Medicine* 96 (part 1):762–65.

Liese, B. S., & Price, J. G. 1990. The family life cycle. In R. E. Rakel (ed.), *Textbook of family practice*, 4th ed. (pp. 41–60). Philadelphia: W. B. Saunders.

Lincoln, Y. S., & Guba, E. G. 1985. *Naturalistic inquiry.* Beverly Hills, Calif.: Sage.

Lindemann, S. K., & Oliver, E. L. 1982. Consciousness, liberation, and health delivery systems. *Journal of Medicine and Philosophy* 7:135–52.

Lipkin, M.; Quill, T.; & Napodano, R. J. 1984. The medical interview: A core curriculum for residencies in internal medicine. *Annals of Internal Medicine* 100:277–84.

Lister, E. D. 1982. Forced silence: A neglected dimension of trauma. *American Journal of Psychiatry* 139:872–76.

Lock, M. 1991. Contested meanings of the menopause. *Lancet* 337:1270–72.

Loewenstein, R. J. 1990. Somatoform disorders in victims of incest and child abuse. In R. P. Kluft (ed.), *Incest-related syndromes of adult psychopathology* (pp. 75–111). Washington, D.C.: American Psychiatric Press.

Loftus, E. F. 1993. The reality of repressed memories. *American Psychologist* 48:518–37.

Loftus, E. F.; Polonsky, S.; & Fullilove, M. T. 1994. Memories of childhood sexual abuse: Remembering and repressing. *Psychology of Women Quarterly* 18:67–84.

Lombardo, J. P.; Franco, R.; Wolf, T. M.; & Fantasia, S. C. 1976. Interest in entering helping activities and self-disclosure to three targets on the Jourard Self-disclosure Scale. *Perceptual Motor Skills* 42:299–302.

Loomis, C. P. 1936. The study of the life cycle of families. *Rural Sociology* 1:180–99.

Lopata, H. Z. 1987. Women's family roles in life course perspective. In B. B. Hess & M. M. Ferree (eds.), *Analyzing gender: A handbook of social science research* (pp. 381–407). Beverly Hills, Calif.: Sage.

—————1993. The interweave of public and private: Women's challenge to American society. *Journal of Marriage and the Family* 55:176–90.

Lorber, J. 1984. *Women physicians: Careers, status and power.* New York: Tavistock.

—————1991. Can women physicians ever be true equals in the American medical profession? *Current Research on Occupations and Professions* 6:25–37.

LoVerde, M. E.; Prochazka, A. V.; & Byyny, R. L. 1989. Research consent forms: Continued unreadability and increasing length. *Journal of General Internal Medicine* 4:410–12.

Luepnitz, D. A. 1988. *The family interpreted: Feminist theory in clinical practice.* New York: Basic Books.

Lustig, N.; Dresser, N. W.; Spellman, S. W.; & Murray, T. B. 1966. Incest: A family group survival pattern. *Archives of General Psychiatry* 14:31–40.

Macaulay, A. C. 1992. Saying good-bye: Termination of the doctor-patient relationship. *Family Medicine* 24:64–65.

MacFarlane, K.; Waterman, J.; with Conerly, S.; Damon, L.; Durfee, M.; &

Long, S. 1986. *Sexual abuse of young children: Evaluation and treatment.* New York: Guilford Press.

Machotka, P.; Pittman, F. S.; & Flomenhaft, K. 1967. Incest as a family affair. *Family Process* 6:98–116.

Mahler, M.; Pine, F.; & Bergman, A. 1975. *The psychological birth of the human infant: Symbiosis and individuation.* New York: Basic Books.

Makepeace, J. M. 1986. Gender differences in courtship victimization. *Family Relations* 35:383–88.

Malamuth, N. M.; Sockloskie, R. J.; Koss, M. P.; & Tanaka, J. S. 1991. Characteristics of aggressors against women: Testing a model using a national sample of college students. *Journal of Counseling and Clinical Psychology* 59:670–81.

Malcolm, J. 1984. *In the Freud archives.* New York: Alfred A. Knopf.

Malterud, K. 1987a. Illness and disease in female patients. 1. Pitfalls and inadequacies of primary health care classification systems: A theoretical review. *Scandinavian Journal of Primary Health Care* 5:205–9.

———1987b. Illness and disease in female patients. 2. A study of consultation techniques to improve the exploration of illness in general practice. *Scandinavian Journal of Primary Health Care* 5:211–16.

———1990. *The encounter between the general practitioner and the female patients: A clinical method.* Thesis summary. Bergen, Norway.

———1994. Key questions: A strategy for modifying clinical communication: Transforming tacit skills into a clinical method. *Scandinavian Journal of Primary Health Care* 12:121–27.

Mandell, H., & Spiro, H., eds. 1987. *When doctors get sick.* New York: Plenum Medical.

Mark, E. W., & Alper, T. G. 1985. Women, men, and intimacy motivation. *Psychology of Women Quarterly* 9 (1):81–88.

Martin, J. 1988. Maternal and paternal abuse of children: Theoretical and research perspectives. In K. Yllo & M. Bograd (eds.), *Feminist perspectives on wife abuse* (pp. 293–304). Newbury Park, Calif.: Sage.

Martin, P. Y., & Hummer, R. A. 1989. Fraternities and rape on campus. *Gender and Society* 3:457–73.

Maseide, P. 1983. Analytical aspects of clinical reasoning: A discussion of models for medical problem solving. In S. Fisher & A. D. Todd (eds.), *The social organization of doctor-patient communication* (pp. 241–65). Washington, D.C.: Center for Applied Linguistics.

Mass, B. 1976. *Population target: The political economy of population control in Latin America.* Toronto, Ont.: Charters Publishing.

Masson, J. M. 1984. *The assault on truth: Freud's suppression of the seduction theory.* New York: Farrar, Straus and Giroux.

Mathews, B. 1988. The role of therapist self-disclosure in psychotherapy: A survey of therapists. *American Journal of Psychotherapy* 42:521–31.

Mathews, D. A., & Feinstein, A. R. 1988. A review of systems for the personal aspects of patient care. *American Journal of Medical Sciences* 295 (3):159–71.

May, L., & Strikwerda, R. 1994. Men in groups: Collective responsibility for rape. *Hypatia* 9:134–51.

May, W. F. 1975. Code, covenant, contract, or philanthropy. *Hastings Center Report* 5 (6):29–38.

———1983. *The physician's covenant: Images of the healer in medical ethics.* Philadelphia: Westminster Press.

Mayeroff, M. 1965. On caring. *International Philosophical Quarterly* 5:462–74.

———1971. *On caring.* New York: Harper & Row.

Maynard, C.; Fisher, L. D.; Passamani, E. R.; & Pullum, T. 1986. Blacks in the Coronary Artery Surgery Study (CASS): Race and clinical decision making. *American Journal of Public Health* 76:1446–48.

Maynard, D. W. 1989. Notes on the delivery and reception of diagnostic news regarding mental disabilities. In D. T. Helm, W. T. Anderson, A. J. Meehan, & A. W. Rawls (eds.), *The interactional order: New directions in the study of social order* (pp. 54–67). New York: Irvington.

———1991. Bearing bad news in clinical settings. In B. Dervin (ed.), *Progress in communication sciences* (vol. 10, pp. 143–72). Norwood, N.J.: Ablex.

McAdoo, H. P. 1980. Black mothers and the extended family support network. In L. F. Rodgers-Rose (ed.), *The Black Woman* (pp. 125–44). Beverly Hills, Calif.: Sage.

———1988. *Changes in the formation and structure of black families: The impact on black women.* Working paper no. 182. Wellesley, Mass.: Center for Research on Women, Wellesley College.

McCann, J. 1990. Use of the colposcope in childhood sexual abuse examinations. *Pediatric Clinics of North America* 37 (4):863–80.

McCann, J.; Voris, J.; & Simon, M. 1988. Labial adhesions and posterior fourchette injuries in childhood sexual abuse. *American Journal of Diseases of Children* 142:659–63.

McCray, C. A. 1980. The black woman and family roles. In L. F. Rodgers-Rose (ed.), *The black woman* (pp. 67–78). Beverly Hills, Calif.: Sage.

McCullough, P. 1980. Launching children and moving on. In B. Carter & M. McGoldrick (eds.), *The family life cycle: A framework for family therapy* (pp. 171–95). New York: Gardner Press.

McFarlane, J.; Parker, B.; Soeken, K.; & Bullock, L. 1992. Assessing for abuse during pregnancy: Severity and frequency of injuries and associated entry into prenatal care. *Journal of the American Medical Association* 267: 3176–78.

McFarlane, K.; Waterman, J.; with Conerly, S.; Damon, L.; Durfee, M.; & Long, S. (1986). *Sexual abuse of young children: Evaluation and treatment.* New York: Guilford Press.

McGoldrick, M. 1988. Women and the family life cycle. In B. Carter & M. McGoldrick (eds.), *The changing family life cycle: A framework for family therapy*, 2nd ed. (pp. 29–68). New York: Gardner Press.

———1989a. Sisters. In M. McGoldrick, C. M. Anderson, & F. Walsh (eds.), *Women in families: A framework for family therapy* (pp. 244–66). New York: W. W. Norton.

————1989b. Women through the family life cycle. In M. McGoldrick, C. M. Anderson, & F. Walsh (eds.), *Women in families: A framework for family therapy* (pp. 200–226). New York: W. W. Norton.

McGoldrick, M.; Anderson, C. M.; & Walsh, F., eds. 1989. *Women in families: A framework for family therapy.* New York: W. W. Norton.

McGoldrick, M., & Gerson, R. 1985. *Genograms in family assessment.* New York: W. W. Norton.

McGoldrick, M.; Pearce, J. K.; & Giordano, J., eds. 1982. *Ethnicity and family therapy.* New York: Guilford Press.

McIntyre, K. 1981. Role of mothers in father-daughter incest: A feminist analysis. *Social Work* 26: 462–66.

McKegney, C. P. 1993. Surviving survivors: Coping with caring for patients who have been victimized. *Primary Care* 20 (2):481–94.

McKibben, L.; De Vos, E.; & Newberger, E. H. 1989. Victimization of mothers of abused children: A controlled study. *Pediatrics* 84:531–35.

McLanahan, S., & Booth, K. 1989. Mother-only families: Problems, prospects, and politics. *Journal of Marriage and the Family* 51:557–80.

McLanahan, S. S.; Sorensen, A.; & Watson, D. 1989. Sex differences in poverty, 1950–1980. *Signs* 15:102–22.

McLeer, S. V., & Anwar, R. 1989. A study of battered women presenting in an emergency department. *American Journal of Public Health* 79:65–66.

————1992. The abused assaulted adult. In G. R. Schwartz, C. G. Cayten, M. A. Mangelsen, & T. Mayer (eds.), *Principles and practice of emergency medicine* (pp. 2701–12). Philadelphia: Lea & Febiger.

McLeer, S. V.; Anwar, R. A. H.; Herman, S.; & Maquiling, K. 1989. Education is not enough: A systems failure in protecting battered women. *Annals of Emergency Medicine* 18:651–53.

McNaron, T., & Yarrow, M. 1982. *Voices in the night: Women speaking about incest.* Minneapolis: Cleis Press.

McWhinney, I. R. 1977. The naturalist tradition in family practice. *Journal of Family Practice* 5:375–78.

Medalie, J. H., ed. 1978. *Family medicine: Principles and applications.* Baltimore: Williams and Wilkins.

————1979. The family life cycle and its implications for family practice. *Journal of Family Practice* 9:47–56.

————1984. Male midlife development. *Journal of Family Practice* 19:211–17.

————1992. The interaction between the child and the family. In R. E. Behrman, R. M. Kliegman, W. E. Nelson, & V. C. Vaughan (eds.), *Nelson textbook of pediatrics*, 14th ed. (pp. 101–4). Philadelphia: W. B. Saunders.

Meyer, M. J. 1992. Patients' duties. *Journal of Medicine and Philosophy* 17:541–55.

Midmer, D. K. 1992. Does family-centered maternity care empower women? The development of the woman-centered childbirth model. *Family Medicine* 24:216–21.

Mies, M. 1983. Towards a methodology for feminist research. In G. Bowles & R. D. Klein (eds.), *Theories of women's studies* (pp. 117–39). Boston: Routledge & Kegan Paul.

Miller, G. D., & Baldwin, D. C. 1987. Implications of the wounded-healer paradigm for the use of the self in therapy. In M. Baldwin & V. Satir (eds.), *The use of self in therapy* (pp. 139–51). New York: Haworth Press.

Miller, J. B. 1976. *Toward a new psychology of women*. Boston: Beacon Press.

———1986. *What do we mean by relationships?* Work in progress no. 22. Wellesley, Mass.: Stone Center for Developmental Services and Studies.

———1991. Women and power. In J. V. Jordan et al., *Women's growth in connection: Writings from the Stone Center* (pp. 197–205). New York: Guilford Press.

Miller, L. J. 1990. The formal treatment contract in the inpatient management of borderline personality disorder. *Hospital and Community Psychiatry* 41:985–87.

Miller, M. L.; Moen, P.; & Dempster-McClain, D. 1991. Motherhood, multiple roles, and maternal well-being. *Gender and Society* 5:565–82.

Mills, T. 1984. Victimization and self-esteem: On equating husband abuse and wife abuse. *Victimology* 9:254–61.

———1985. The assault on the self: Stages in coping with battering husbands. *Qualitative Sociology* 8:103–23.

Mills, T.; Rieker, P. P.; & Carmen, E. H. 1984. Hospitalization experiences of victims of abuse. *Victimology* 9:436–49.

Mirkin, M. P., ed. 1990. *Social and political context of family therapy*. Needham Heights, Mass.: Allyn & Bacon.

Mishler, E. G. 1984. *The discourse of medicine: Dialectics of medical interviews*. Norwood, N.J.: Ablex.

Mishler, E. G.; Clark, J. A.; Ingelfinger, J.; & Simon, M. P. 1989. The language of attentive patient care. *Journal of General Internal Medicine* 4:325–35.

Mitchell, V., & Helson, R. 1990. Women's prime of life: Is it the 50s? *Psychology of Women Quarterly* 14:451–70.

Moen, P.; Dempster-McClain, D.; & Williams, R. M. 1989. Social integration and longevity: An event history analysis of women's roles and resilience. *American Sociological Review* 54:635–47.

Moen, P.; Downey, G.; & Bolger, N. 1990. Labor-force reentry among U.S. homemakers in midlife: A life-course analysis. *Gender and Society* 4:230–43.

Moore, R. D.; Stanton, D.; Gopalan, R.; & Chaisson, R. E. 1994. Racial differences in the use of drug therapy for HIV disease in an urban community. *New England Journal of Medicine* 330:763–68.

More, E. 1994. "Empathy" enters the profession of medicine. In M. Milligan & E. More (eds.), *The empathic practitioner: Empathy, gender, and the therapeutic relationship* (pp. 19–39). New Brunswick, N.J.: Rutgers University Press.

Morison, R. S. 1984. The biological limits on autonomy. *Hastings Center Report* 14 (5):43–49.

Moros, D. A.; Rhodes, R.; Baumrin, B.; & Strain, J. J. 1991. Chronic illness and the physician-patient relationship: A response to the Hastings Center's

"Ethical Challenges of Chronic Illness." *Journal of Medicine and Philosophy* 16:161–81.

Morris, M. 1982. *If I should die before I wake.* Los Angeles: J. P. Tarcher.

Morrison, J. 1989. Childhood sexual histories of women with somatization disorder. *American Journal of Psychiatry* 146:239–41.

Moscarello, R.; Margittai, K. J.; & Rossi, M. 1994. Differences in abuse reported by female and male Canadian medical students. *Canadian Medical Association Journal* 150:357–63.

Mosher, D. L., & Anderson, R. D. 1986. Macho personality, sexual aggression, and reactions to guided imagery of realistic rape. *Journal of Research in Personality* 20:77–94.

Moskowitz, A. J.; Kuipers, B. J.; & Kassirer, J. P. 1988. Dealing with uncertainty, risks, and tradeoffs in clinical decisions: A cognitive science approach. *Annals of Internal Medicine* 108:435–49.

Motenko, A. K. 1989. The frustrations, gratifications, and well-being of dementia caregivers. *The Gerontologist* 29:166–72.

Muehlenhard, C. L.; Friedman, D. E.; & Thomas, C. M. 1985. Is date rape justifiable? The effects of dating activity, who initiated, who paid, and men's attitudes toward women. *Psychology of Women Quarterly* 9:297–309.

Mukand, J., ed. 1990. *Vital lines: Contemporary fiction about medicine.* New York: Ballantine.

Mullen, P. E.; Romans-Clarkson, S. E.; Walton, V. A.; & Herbison, G. P. 1988. Impact of sexual and physical abuse on women's mental health. *Lancet* 1:841–45.

Mullett, S. 1987. Only connect: The place of self-knowledge in ethics. In M. Hanen & K. Nielsen (eds.), *Science, morality and feminist theory* (pp. 309–38). *Canadian Journal of Philosophy*, supp. vol. 13. Calgary, Alberta: University of Calgary Press.

Mullings, L. 1990 (May 8). *The underserved: Facts and fictions.* Plenary presentation at the 23rd annual spring conference of the Society of Teachers of Family Medicine, Seattle.

Muram, D. 1989. Child sexual abuse: Genital tract findings in prepubertal girls. 1. The unaided medical examination. *American Journal of Obstetrics and Gynecology* 160:P328–33.

Myer, M. H. 1984–85. A new look at mothers of incest victims. *Journal of Social Work and Human Sexuality* 3:47–58.

Naples, N. A. 1992. Activist mothering: Cross-generational continuity in the community work of women from low-income neighborhoods. *Gender and Society* 6: 441–63.

Nava, M. 1988. Cleveland and the press: Outrage and anxiety in the reporting of child sexual abuse. *Feminist Review* (no. 28): 103–21.

Neugarten, B. L.; Wood, B.; Kraines, R. J.; & Loomis, B. 1968. Women's attitudes toward the menopause. In B. L. Neugarten (ed.), *Middle age and aging* (pp. 195–200). Chicago: University of Chicago Press.

Newsweek. 1990. Little girl lost and found. (March 13): 115:78–80.

Nightingale, S. D.; Yarnold, P. R.; & Greenberg, M. S. 1991. Sympathy, empathy, and the physician resource utilization. *Journal of General Internal Medicine* 6:420–23.

Noddings, N. 1984. *Caring: A feminine approach to ethics and moral education*. Berkeley: University of California Press.

North, R .L., & Rothenberg, K. H. 1993. Partner notification and threat of domestic violence against women with HIV infection. *New England Journal of Medicine* 329:1194–96.

Nouwen, H. J. 1979. *The wounded healer*. New York: Image Books.

Novack, D. H. 1987. Therapeutic aspects of the clinical encounter. *Journal of General Internal Medicine* 2:346–55.

Oakley, A. 1980. *Becoming a mother*. New York: Schocken.

———1981. Interviewing women: A contradiction in terms. In H. Roberts (ed.), *Doing feminist research* (pp. 30–61). Boston: Routledge & Kegan Paul.

Oboler, S. K., & LaForce, F. M. 1989. The periodic physical examination in asymptomatic adults. *Annals of Internal Medicine* 110:214–26.

Olafson, E.; Corwin, D. L.; & Summit, R. C. 1993. Modern history of child sexual abuse awareness: Cycles of discovery and suppression. *Child Abuse and Neglect* 17:7–24.

Osherson, S. 1986. *Finding our fathers: How a man's life is shaped by his relationship with his father*. New York: Free Press.

Osler, W. 1932. *Aequanimitas*. Philadelphia: P. Blakiston's Son & Co.

Paget, M. A. 1983. On the work of talk: Studies in misunderstandings. In S. Fisher & A. D. Todd (eds.), *The social organization of doctor-patient communication* (pp. 55–74). Washington, D.C.: Center for Applied Linguistics.

Palombo, J. 1987. Spontaneous self-disclosures in psychotherapy. *Clinical Social Work Journal* 15:107–20.

Paradis, G. 1984. Psychological problems in adults: Violence in the family. In J. Christie-Seely (ed.), *Working with the family in primary care: A systems approach to health and illness* (pp. 411–21). New York: Praeger.

Paradise, J. E. 1990. The medical evaluation of the sexually abused child. *Pediatric Clinics of North America* 37 (4):839–62.

Pauker, S. H., & Kopelman, R. I. 1992. How sure is sure enough? *New England Journal of Medicine* 326:688–91.

Pavalko, E. K., & Elder, G. H. 1993. Women behind the men: Variations in wives' support of husbands' careers. *Gender and Society* 7:548–67.

Peabody, F. W. 1927. The care of the patient. *Journal of the American Medical Association* 88:877–82.

Peck, T. A. 1986. Women's self-definition in adulthood: From a different model? *Psychology of Women Quarterly* 10:274–84.

Pellegrino, E. D. 1982. Being ill and being healed: Some reflections on the grounding of medical morality. In V. Kestenbaum (ed.), *The humanity of the ill: Phenomenological perspectives* (pp. 157–66). Knoxville: University of Tennessee Press.

———1985. The caring ethic: The relation of physician to patient. In

A. H. Bishop & J. R. Scudder (eds.), *Caring, curing, coping: Nurse, physician, patient relationships* (pp. 8–30). University: University of Alabama Press.

Pendleton, D. A., & Bochner, S. 1980. The communication of medical information in general practice consultations as a function of patients' social class. *Social Science and Medicine* 14A:669–73.

Penn, P. 1983. Coalitions and binding interactions in families with chronic illness. *Family Systems Medicine* 1 (2):37–47.

Perlman, G. 1991. The question of therapist self-disclosure in the treatment of a married gay man. In C. Silverstein (ed.), *Gays, lesbians, and their therapists: Studies in psychotherapy* (pp. 201–9). New York: W. W. Norton.

Peters, S. D.; Wyatt, G. E.; & Finkelhor, D. 1986. Prevalence. In D. Finkelhor & Associates, *A sourcebook on child sexual abuse* (pp. 15–59). Beverly Hills, Calif.: Sage.

Petersen, B. 1991. *Dancing with daddy.* New York: Bantam.

Phillips, S. P., & Schneider, M. S. 1993. Special article: Sexual harassment of female doctors by patients. *New England Journal of Medicine* 329:1936–39.

Pittman, F. S. 1985. Evaluating the family in crisis. In S. Henao & N. P. Grose (eds.), *Principles of family systems in family medicine* (pp. 347–71). New York: Brunner/Mazel.

Platt, F. W., & McMath, J. C. 1979. Clinical hypocompetence: The interview. *Annals of Internal Medicine* 91:898–902.

Pope, S. K.; Whiteside, L.; Brooks-Gunn, J.; Kelleher, K. J.; Rickert, V. I.; Bradly, R. H.; & Casey, P. H. 1993. Low-birth-weight infants born to adolescent mothers. *Journal of the American Medical Association* 269:1396–1400.

Porter, M. 1988. Mothers and daughters: Linking women's life histories in Grand Bank, Newfoundland, Canada. *Women's Studies International Forum* 11:545–58.

Pratt, C. C.; Schmall, V. L.; Wright, S.; & Cleland, M. 1985. Burden and coping strategies of caregivers to Alzheimer's patients. *Family Relations* 34:27–33.

Presser, H. B. 1980. Puerto Rico: Recent trends in fertility and sterilization. *Family Planning Perspectives* 12 (2):102–6.

Ptacek, J. 1988. Why do men batter their wives? In K. Yllo & M. Bograd (eds.), *Feminist perspectives on wife abuse* (pp. 133–57). Newbury Park, Calif.: Sage.

Puka, B. 1990. The liberation of caring; A different voice for Gilligan's *Different Voice. Hypatia* 5:58–82.

Putnam, F. W.; Guroff, J. J.; Silberman, E. K.; Barban, L.; & Post, R. M. 1986. The clinical phenomenology of multiple personality disorder: Review of 100 cases. *Journal of Clinical Psychiatry* 47:285–93.

Quill, T. E. 1983. Partnerships in patient care: A contractual approach. *Annals of Internal Medicine* 98:228–34.

———1991. Death and dignity: A case of individualized decision-making. *New England Journal of Medicine* 324:691–94.

Radley, A. R. 1984. The embodiment of social relations in coronary heart disease. *Social Science and Medicine* 19:1227–34.

Rakel, R. E., ed. 1990. *Textbook of family practice.* 4th ed. Philadelphia: W. B. Saunders.

Ramirez de Arellano, A. B., & Seipp, C. 1983. *Colonialism, Catholicism, and contraception*. Chapel Hill: University of North Carolina Press.

Ramsay, C. N., ed. 1989. *Family systems in medicine*. New York: Guilford Press.

Randall, M. 1987. *This is about incest*. Ithaca, N.Y.: Firebrand Books.

Randall, T. 1991. Response to letter to the editor. *Journal of the American Medical Association* 265:460–61.

Ransom, D. C. 1983. Random notes: The legacy of the Peckham Experiment. *Family Systems Medicine* 1 (4):104–7.

————1985. The evolution from an individual to a family approach. In S. Henao & N. P. Grose (eds.), *Principles of family systems in family medicine* (pp. 5–23). New York: Brunner/Mazel.

Ransom, D. C., & Grace, N. T. 1979. Family therapy. In G. M. Rosen, J. P. Geyman, & R. H. Layton (eds.), *Behavioral science in family practice* (pp. 247–63). New York: Appleton-Century-Crofts.

Ransom, D. C., & Vandervoort, H. E. 1973. The development of family medicine: Problematic trends. *Journal of the American Medical Association* 225:1098–1102.

Rath, G. D.; Jarratt, L. G.; & Leonardson, G. 1989. Rates of domestic violence against adult women by men partners. *Journal of the American Board of Family Practice* 2:227–33.

Raymond, C. A. 1988. Studies question how much role menopause plays in some women's emotional distress. *Journal of the American Medical Association* 289:3522–23.

Raymond, J. G. 1982. Medicine as patriarchal religion. *Journal of Medicine and Philosophy* 7:197–216.

Realini, J. P.; Ortiz, E.; Turnbull, J. M.; & Couchman, G. R. 1984. Family dynamics: A case of incest. *Journal of Family Practice* 18:529–41.

Reinharz, S. 1983. Experiential analysis: A contribution to feminist research. In G. Bowles & R. D. Klein (eds.), *Theories of women's studies* (pp. 162–91). Boston: Routledge & Kegan Paul.

Reinke, B. J.; Holmes, D. S.; & Harris, R. L. 1985. The timing of psychosocial changes in women's lives. *Journal of Personality and Social Psychology* 48:1353–64.

Renvoize, J. 1982. *Incest: A family pattern*. London: Routledge & Kegan Paul.

Reverby, S. M. 1987. *Ordered to care: The dilemma of American nursing, 1850–1945*. New York: Cambridge University Press.

Ribbens, J. 1989. Interviewing: An "unnatural situation"? *Women's Studies International Forum* 12:579–92.

Richardson, H. B. 1945/1983. The family equilibrium. Chap. 4 of *Patients have families*. New York: Commonwealth Fund. Reprinted in *Family Systems Medicine* 1 (1):62–74.

Richardson, V., & Sands, R. G. 1985. Developmental patterns of women returning to school ages 30 through 49. *Gerontology and Geriatrics Education* 5:29–41.

Rieker, P. P., & Carmen, E. H. 1986. The victim-to-patient process: The disconfirmation and transformation of abuse. *American Journal of Orthopsychiatry* 56:360–70.

Riessman, C. K. 1987. When gender is not enough: Women interviewing women. *Gender and Society* 1:172–207.

Rissman, R., & Rissman, B. Z. 1987. Compliance. *Family Systems Medicine* 5:446–67.

Roberts, H. 1981. Women and their doctors: Power and powerlessness in the research process. In H. Roberts (ed.), *Doing feminist research* (pp. 7–29). Boston: Routledge & Kegan Paul.

Robinson, I. 1990. Personal narratives, social careers and medical courses: Analysing life trajectories in autobiographies of people with multiple sclerosis. *Social Science and Medicine* 30:1173–86.

Rogers, C. R. 1961. *On becoming a person: A therapist's view of psychotherapy.* Boston: Houghton Mifflin.

Romero, G. J.; Castro, F. G.; & Cervantes, R. C. 1988. Latinas without work: Family, occupational, and economic stress following unemployment. *Psychology of Women Quarterly* 12:281–97.

Roscoe, B., & Benaske, N. 1985. Courtship violence experienced by abused wives: Similarities in patterns of abuse. *Family Relations* 34:419–24.

Rose, K., & Saunders, D. G. 1986. Nurses' and physicians' attitudes about women abuse: The effects of gender and professional role. *Health Care for Women International* 7:427–38.

Rosen, K. H., & Stith, S. M. 1993. Intervention strategies for treating women in violent dating relationships. *Family Relations* 42:427–33.

Rosen, R. H. 1980. Adolescent pregnancy decision-making: Are parents important? *Adolescence* 15:43–54.

Rosenfeld, A. A. 1979. Incidence of a history of incest among 18 female psychiatric patients. *American Journal of Psychiatry* 136:791–95.

Rosenfeld, A., & Sarles, R. M. 1992. Sexual abuse of children. In R. A. Hoeckelman, S. P. Friedman, N. M. Nelson, & H. M. Seidel (eds.), *Primary pediatric care*, 2nd ed. (pp. 600–608). St Louis: Mosby Year Book.

Rosenfeld, J. A. 1992. Maternal work outside the home and its effect on women and their families. *Journal of the American Medical Women's Association* 47:47–53.

Ross, C. E.; Mirowsky, J.; & Goldsteen, K. 1990. The impact of family on health: The decade in review. *Journal of Marriage and the Family* 52:1059–78.

Rost, K.; Roter, D.; Bertakis, K.; & Quill, T. 1990. Physician-patient familiarity and patient recall of medication changes. The Collaborative Study Group of the SGIM Task Force on the Doctor and Patient. *Family Medicine* 22:453–57.

Roter, D. L.; Hall, J. A.; & Katz, N. R. 1988. Patient-physician communication: A descriptive summary of the literature. *Patient Education and Counseling* 12:99–119.

Roter, D. L.; Lipkin, M.; & Korsgaard, A. 1991. Sex differences in patients' and physicians' communication during primary care medical visits. *Medical Care* 29:1083–93.

Roth, P. A., & Harrison, J. K. 1991. Orchestrating social change: An imperative in care of the chronically ill. *Journal of Medicine and Philosophy* 16:343–59.

Rothenberg, P. 1990. The construction, deconstruction, and reconstruction of difference. *Hypatia* 5:42–57.

Rothfield, P. 1987. Contradictions in teaching feminism. *Women's Studies International Forum* 10:525–27.

Rubin, L. B. 1979. *Women of a certain age: The midlife search for self.* New York: Harper & Row.

Ruddick, S. 1983. Maternal thinking. In J. Trebilcot (ed.), *Mothering: Essays in feminist theory* (pp. 213–30). Totowa, N.J.: Rowman & Allanheld.

———1987. Remarks on the sexual politics of reason. In E. F. Kittay & D. T. Meyers (eds.), *Women and moral theory* (pp. 237–60). Totowa, N.J.: Rowman & Littlefield.

Rudolph, A. M.; Hoffman, J. I. E.; Rudolph, C. D.; & Sagan, P. 1991. *Rudolph's pediatrics.* 19th ed. Norwalk, Conn.: Appleton & Lange.

Russell, D. E. H. 1986. *The secret trauma: Incest in the lives of girls and women.* New York: Basic Books.

———1995. The making of a whore. *Violence Against Women* 1 (1):77–98.

Rutter, P. 1989. *Sex in the forbidden zone: When men in power—therapists, doctors, clergy, teachers and others—betray women's trust.* Los Angeles: Jeremy P. Tarcher.

Ruzek, S. B. 1978. *The women's health movement: Feminist alternatives to medical control.* New York: Praeger.

Sahler, O. J. Z., & Kreipe, R. E. 1991. Psychological development in normal adolescents. In W. R. Hendee (ed.), *The health of adolescents: Understanding and facilitating biological, behavioral, and social development* (pp. 58–88). San Francisco: Jossey-Bass.

Sanday, P. R. 1981. The socio-cultural context of rape: A cross-cultural study. *Journal of Social Issues* 37:5–27.

———1990. *Fraternity gang rape: Sex, brotherhood, and privilege on campus.* New York: New York University Press.

Sandelowski, M. J. 1990. Failures of volition: Female agency and infertility in historical perspective. *Signs* 15:475–99.

Sapira, J. D. 1972. Reassurance therapy: What to say to symptomatic patients with benign diseases. *Annals of Internal Medicine* 77:603–4.

Sarton, M. 1973. *As we are now.* New York: Norton.

Saunders, D. G., & Kindy, P. 1993. Predictors of physicians' responses to woman abuse: The role of gender, background, and brief training. *Journal of General Internal Medicine* 8:606–9.

Saunders, E. A., & Arnold, F. 1991. *Borderline personality disorder and childhood sexual abuse: Revisions in clinical thinking and treatment approach.* Work in progress no. 51. Wellesley, Mass.: Stone Center for Developmental Services and Studies.

Scannell, J. G. 1986–87. The care of the patient: The man and the patient behind an epigram. *Harvard Medical Alumni Bulletin* (Winter): 60 (4):45–49.

Schafer, R. 1959. Generative empathy in the treatment situation. *Psychoanalytic Quarterly* 28:342–73.

Scheman, N. 1983. Individualism and the objects of psychology. In S. Harding & M. B. Hintikka (eds.), *Discovering reality* (pp. 225–44). Boston: D. Reidel.

Schensul, S. L.; Borrero, M.; Barrera, V.; Backstrand, J.; & Guarnaccia, P. 1982. A model of fertility control in a Puerto Rican community. *Urban Anthropology* 11 (1):81–99.

Schmitt, R. 1990. Murderous objectivity: Marxism and the Holocaust. In R. Gottlieb (ed.), *Thinking the unthinkable: Meanings of the Holocaust* (pp. 64–87). New York: Paulist Press.

———1995. *Beyond separateness: The social nature of human beings—their autonomy, knowledge, and power*. Boulder, CO: Westview Press.

Schon, D. A. 1983. *The reflective practitioner: How professionals think in action*. New York: Basic Books.

Schulz, R., & Visintainer, P. 1990. Psychiatric and physical morbidity effects of caregiving. *Journal of Gerontology*. Also published by the School of Applied Social Sciences, Case Western Reserve University, working paper no. 9.

Schwartz, C. G., & Kahne, M. J. 1983. Medical help as negotiated achievement. *Psychiatry* 46:333–49.

Schweickart, P. P. 1990. Reading, teaching, and the ethic of care. In S. L. Gabriel & I. Smithson (eds.), *Gender in the classroom: Power and pedagogy* (pp. 78–95). Chicago: University of Illinois Press.

Scully, D. 1980. *Men who control women's health: The miseducation of obstetrician-gynecologists*. Boston: Houghton Mifflin.

———1988. Convicted rapists' perceptions of self and victim: Role taking and emotions. *Gender and Society* 2:200–213.

———1990. *Understanding sexual violence: A study of convicted rapists*. Boston: Unwin Hyman.

Scully, D., & Bart, P. 1973. A funny thing happened on my way to the orifice; Woman in gynaecology textbooks. *American Journal of Sociology* 78:1045–50.

Scutt, J. A. 1988. The privatization of justice: Power differentials, inequality, and the palliative of counselling and mediation. *Women's Studies International Forum* 11:503–20.

Seaver, R. L. 1987. Myocardial infarction. In H. Mandell & H. Spiro (eds.), *When doctors get sick* (pp. 29–38). New York: Plenum Medical.

Sedney, M. A., & Brooks, B. 1984. Factors associated with a history of childhood sexual experience in a nonclinical female population. *Journal of the American Academy of Child Psychiatry* 23:215–18.

Sgroi, S. M. 1982. *Handbook of clinical intervention in child sexual abuse*. Lexington, Mass.: Lexington Books.

Shadley, M. L. 1987. Are all therapists alike? Use of self in family therapy: A multidimensional perspective. In M. Baldwin & V. Satir (eds.), *The use of self in therapy* (pp. 127–37). New York: Haworth Press.

Shanas, E. 1980. Older people and their families: The new pioneers. *Journal of Marriage and the Family* 42:9–15.

Shapiro, J. 1993. The use of narrative in the doctor-patient relationship. *Family Systems Medicine* 11:47–53.

Shapiro, M. C.; Najman, J. M.; Chang, A.; Keeping, J. D.; Morrison, J.; & Western, J. S. 1983. Information control and the exercise of power in the obstetrical encounter. *Social Science and Medicine* 17:139–46.

Shapiro, S. 1987. Self-mutilation and self-blame in incest victims. *American Journal of Psychotherapy* 41:46–54.

Shearer, S. L., & Herbert, C. A. 1987. Long-term effects of unresolved sexual trauma. *American Family Physician* 36:169–75.

Sheehan, N. W., & Nuttall, P. 1988. Conflict, emotion, and personal strain among family caregivers. *Family Relations* 37:92–98.

Sherwin, S. 1989. Feminist and medical ethics: Two different approaches to contextual ethics. *Hypatia* 4:57–72.

———1992. *Patient no longer: Feminist ethics and health care*. Philadelphia: Temple University Press.

Shields, N. M., & Hanneke, C. R. 1988. Battered wives' reactions to marital rape. In K. Yllo & M. Bograd (eds.), *Feminist perspectives on wife abuse* (pp. 132–50). Newbury Park, Calif.: Sage.

Shuy, R. W. 1983. Three types of interference to an effective exchange of information in the medical interview. In S. Fisher & A. D. Todd (eds.), *The social organization of doctor-patient communication* (pp. 189–202). Washington, D.C.: Center for Applied Linguistics.

Siegler, M. 1981. Searching for moral certainty in medicine: A proposal for a new model of the doctor-patient encounter. *Bulletin of the New York Academy of Medicine* 57:56–69.

Silverstein, C., ed. 1991. *Gays, lesbians, and their therapists: Studies in psychotherapy*. New York: W. W. Norton.

Simons, R. L., & Whitbeck, L. B. 1991. Sexual abuse as a precursor to prostitution and victimization among adolescent and adult homeless women. *Journal of Family Issues* 12:361–79.

Singer, M. 1987. Cure, care and control: An ectopic encounter with biomedical obstetrics. In H. A. Baer (ed.), *Encounters with biomedicine: Case studies in medical anthropology* (pp. 249–65). New York: Gordon and Breach Science Publishers.

Siscovick, D. S.; Raghunathan, T. E.; Psaty, B. M.; Koepsell, T. D.; Wicklund, K. G.; Lin, X.; Cobb, L.; Rautaharju, P. M.; Copass, M. K.; & Wagner, E. H. 1994. Diuretic therapy for hypertension and the risk of primary cardiac arrest. *New England Journal of Medicine* 330:1852–57.

Sluzki, C. 1974. On training to "think interactionally." *Social Science and Medicine* 8:483–85.

Smiley, J. 1991. *A thousand acres*. New York: Fawcett Columbine.

Smilkstein, G.; Aspy, C. N.; & Quiggins, P. A. 1994. Conjugal conflict and violence: A review and theoretical paradigm. *Family Medicine* 26:111–16.

Smith, R. C, & Hoppe, R. B. 1991. The patient's story: Integrating the patient- and physician-centered approaches to interviewing. *Annals of Internal Medicine* 115:470–77.

Snow, C., & Willard, D. 1989. *I'm dying to take care of you: Nurses and code-*

pendence—breaking the cycles. Redmond, Wash.: Professional Counselor Books.

Sollie, D. L., & Fischer, J. L. 1985. Sex-role orientation, intimacy of topic, and target person differences in self-disclosure among women. *Sex Roles* 12:917–25.

Spain, J. 1980. Counseling adolescents in reproductive health care settings. 1980–0–722–743/783. Washington, D.C.: U.S. Department of Health and Human Services, Bureau of Community Health Service, U.S. Government Printing Office.

Spencer, M. J., & Dunklee, P. 1986. Sexual abuse of boys. *Pediatrics* 78:133–38.

Spenner, K. I. 1988. Occupations, work settings and the course of adult development. In P. B. Baltes, D. L. Featherman, & R. M. Lerner (eds.), *Life-span development and behavior* (vol. 9, pp. 243–85). Hillsdale, N.J.: Lawrence Erlbaum Associates.

Springs, F. E., & Friedrich, W. N. 1992. Health risk behaviors and medical sequelae of childhood sexual abuse. *Mayo Clinic Proceedings* 67:527–32.

Stacey, J. 1988. Can there be a feminist ethnography? *Women's Studies International Forum* 11:21–27.

Stack, C. B. 1974. *All our kin: Strategies for survival in a black community.* New York: Harper & Row.

Stark, E., & Flitcraft, A. 1988. Women and children at risk: A feminist perspective on child abuse. *International Journal of Health Services* 18:97–118.

Stark, E.; Flitcraft, A.; Zuckerman, D.; Grey, A.; Robison, J.; & Frazier, W. 1981. *Wife abuse in the medical setting: An introduction for health personnel.* Domestic Violence Monograph Series. Rockville, Md.: National Clearing House on Domestic Violence.

Stein, H. F. 1985. *The psychodynamics of medical practice: Unconscious factors in patient care.* Berkeley: University of California Press, 1985.

Stephens, G. G. 1980. What kind of research in family practice? *Family Medicine Teacher* 12 (2):8–9, 21–26.

———1982. *The intellectual basis of family practice.* Tucson, Ariz.: Winter Publishing.

———1985a. On seeing and hearing in medicine. *Continuing Education for the Family Physician* 20:754–56.

———1985b. Clinical biographies: Issues in longitudinal care. *Continuing Education for the Family Physician* 20:260–75.

———1986. Careers of illness: Problems in the diagnosis of chronic illness. *Perspectives in Biology and Medicine* 29:464–74.

———1989. Family medicine as counterculture. *Family Medicine* 21:103–9.

Stern, C. R. 1984. The etiology of multiple personalities. *Psychiatric Clinics of North America* 7 (no. 1):149–59.

Stern, D. N. 1985. *The interpersonal world of the infant: A view from psychoanalysis and developmental psychology.* New York: Basic Books.

Stern, L. 1990. Conceptions of separation and connection in female adolescents. In C. Gilligan, N. P. Lyons, & T. J. Hanmer (eds.), *Making connections: The relational worlds of adolescent girls at Emma Willard School* (pp.

73–87). Cambridge, Mass.: Harvard University Press.

Stiles, W. B.; Putnam, S. M.; & Jacob, M. C. 1982. Verbal exchange structure of initial medical interviews. *Health Psychology* 1:315–36.

Stimson, G. V. 1977. Social care and the role of the general practitioner. *Social Science and Medicine* 11:485–90.

Stiver, I. P. 1991a. Beyond the Oedipus complex: Mothers and daughters. In J. V. Jordan et al., *Women's growth in connection: Writings from the Stone Center* (pp. 97–121). New York: Guilford Press.

————1991b. The meaning of care: Reframing treatment models. In J. V. Jordan et al., *Women's growth in connection: Writings from the Stone Center* (pp. 250–67). New York: Guilford Press.

————1991c. The meanings of "dependency" in female-male relationships. In J. V. Jordan et al., *Women's growth in connection: Writings from the Stone Center* (pp. 143–61). New York: Guilford Press.

Stoeckle, J. D. 1992. Cooperation without contract. *Journal of General Internal Medicine* 7:117–18.

Stoller, E. P. 1983. Parental caregiving by adult children. *Journal of Marriage and the Family* 45:851–58.

Stone, R.; Cafferata, G. L.; & Sangl, J. 1987. Caregivers of the frail elderly: A national profile. *The Gerontologist* 27:616–26.

Stone, R. I., & Short, P. F. 1990. The competing demands of employment and informal caregiving to disabled elders. *Medical Care* 28:513–26.

Stoudemire, A., ed. 1990. *Human behavior: An introduction for medical students.* Philadelphia: J. B. Lippincott.

Straus, M. A. 1977. Wife-beating: How common, and why? *Victimology* 2:443–58.

————1980. Victims and aggressors in marital violence. *American Behavioral Scientist* 23:681–704.

————1986. Domestic violence and homicide antecedents. *Bulletin of the New York Academy of Medicine* 62:446–65.

Stricker, G., & Fisher, M. 1990. *Self-disclosure in the therapeutic relationship.* New York: Plenum.

Strull, W. M.; Lo, B.; & Charles, G. 1984. Do patients want to participate in medical decision making? *Journal of the American Medical Association* 252:2990–94.

Suchman, A. L., & Matthews, D. A. 1988. What makes the patient-doctor relationship therapeutic? Exploring the connexional dimension of medical care. *Annals of Internal Medicine* 108:125–30.

Sugg, N. K., & Inui, T. 1992. Primary care physicians' response to domestic violence: Opening Pandora's box. *Journal of the American Medical Association* 267:3157–60.

Summit, R. C. 1983. The child sexual abuse accommodation syndrome. *Child Abuse and Neglect* 7:177–93.

Surrey, J. L. 1991a. Relationship and empowerment. In J. V. Jordan et al., *Women's growth in connection: Writings from the Stone Center* (pp. 162–80). New York: Guilford Press.

————1991b. The relational self in women: Clinical implications. In J. V.

Jordan et al., *Women's growth in connection: Writings from the Stone Center* (pp. 35–43). New York: Guilford Press.

————1991c. The "self-in-relation": A theory of women's development. In J. V. Jordan et al., *Women's Growth in Connection: Writings from the Stone Center* (pp. 51–66). New York: Guilford Press.

Swanson, L., & Biaggio, M. K. 1985. Therapeutic perspectives on father-daughter incest. *American Journal of Psychiatry* 142:667–74.

Swanson-Kauffman, K. M. 1986. Caring in the instance of unexpected early pregnancy loss. *Topics in Clinical Nursing* 8 (2):37–46.

Swift, C. 1986. *Surviving: Women's strength through connection.* Wellesley, Mass.: Stone Center for Developmental Services and Studies.

————1987. *Women and violence: Breaking the connection.* Work in progress no. 27. Wellesley, Mass.: Stone Center for Developmental Services and Studies.

Szasz, T. S., & Hollender, M. H. 1956. A contribution to the philosophy of medicine: The basic models of the doctor-patient relationship. *Archives of Internal Medicine* 97:585–92.

Taussig, M. T. 1980. Reification and the consciousness of the patient. *Social Science and Medicine* 14B:3–13.

Tavris, C. 1993. Beware the incest-survivor machine. *New York Times Book Review* (January 3): 1, 16–17.

Taylor, D. A., & Hinds, M. 1985. Disclosure reciprocity and liking as a function of gender and personalism. *Sex Roles* 12:1137–53.

Taylor, R. B., ed. 1983. *Family medicine: Principles and practice.* 2nd ed. New York: Springer-Verlag.

————, ed. 1988. *Family medicine: Principles and practice.* 3rd ed. New York: Springer-Verlag.

Terkelsen, K. G. 1980. Toward a theory of the family life cycle. In E. A. Carter & M. McGoldrick (eds.), *The family life cycle: A framework for family therapy* (pp. 21–52). New York: Gardner.

Thomas, A., & Chess, S. 1977. *Temperament and development.* New York: Brunner/Mazel.

Thomas, S. B., & Quinn, S. C. 1991. The Tuskegee syphilis study 1932 to 1972: Implications for HIV education and AIDS risk reduction programs in the black community. *American Journal of Public Health* 81:1498–1505.

Thomasma, D. C. 1983. Beyond medical paternalism and patient autonomy: A model of physician conscience for the physician-patient relationship. *Annals of Internal Medicine* 98:243–48.

Tilelli, J. A.; Durek, D.; & Jaffe, A. C. 1980. Sexual abuse of children: Clinical findings and implications for management. *New England Journal of Medicine* 302:319–23.

Todd, A. D. 1983. A diagnosis of doctor-patient discourse in the prescription of contraception. In S. Fisher & A. D. Todd (eds.), *The social organization of doctor-patient communication* (pp. 161–87). Washington, D.C.: Center for Applied Linguistics.

Todd, K. H; Samaroo, N.; & Hoffman, J. R. 1993. Ethnicity as a risk factor for inadequate emergency department analgesia. *Journal of the American Medical Association* 269:1537–39.

Treichler, P. A.; Frankel, R. M.; Kramarae, C.; Zoppi, K.; & Beckman, H. B. 1984. Problems and problems: Power relationships in a medical encounter. In C. Kramarae, M. Schulz, & W. M. O'Barr (eds.), *Language and power* (pp. 62–88). Newbury Park, Calif.: Sage.

Trepper, T. S., & Barrett, M. J. 1989. *Systemic treatment of incest: A therapeutic handbook.* New York: Brunner/Mazel.

Tronto, J. C. 1987. Beyond gender difference to a theory of care. *Signs* 12:644–63.

Truesdell, D. L.; McNeil, J. S.; & Deschner, J. P. 1986. Incidence of wife abuse in incestuous families. *Social Work* 31:138–40.

Turner, C. 1984. *Psychosocial barriers to black women's career development.* Work in progress no. 84.04. Wellesley, Mass.: Stone Center for Developmental Services and Studies.

U.S. Bureau of the Census. 1994. *Statistical abstract of the United States 1994.* 114th ed. Washington, D.C.: U.S. Government Printing Office.

Vaillant, G. E. 1977. *Adaptation to life.* Boston: Little, Brown.

Vaillant, G. E., & Vaillant, C. O. 1990. Natural history of male psychological health. 12. A 45-year study of predictors of successful aging at age 65. *American Journal of Psychiatry* 147:31–37.

————1993. Is the U-curve of marital satisfaction an illusion? A 40-year study of marriage. *Journal of Marriage and the Family* 55:230–39.

van der Kolk, B. A. 1989. The compulsion to repeat the trauma: Re-enactment, revictimization, and masochism. *Psychiatric Clinics of North America* 12:389–411.

Vanderpool, J. P. 1977. New visions of adulthood. *Continuing Education for the Family Physician* 7:94–102, 107–9.

Vaughan, V. C., & McKay, R. J., eds. 1975. *Nelson textbook of pediatrics.* 10th ed. Philadelphia: W. B. Saunders.

Veatch, R. M. 1984. Autonomy's temporary triumph. *Hastings Center Report* 14 (5):38–40.

Ventres, W., & Gordon, P. 1990. Communication strategies in caring for the underserved. *Journal of Health Care for the Poor and Underserved* 1:305–14.

Waitzkin, H. 1984a. Doctor-patient communication: Clinical implications of social science research. *Journal of the American Medical Association* 252:2441–46.

————1984b. The micropolitics of medicine: A contextual analysis. *International Journal of Health Services* 14:339–78.

————1989. A critical theory of medical discourse: Ideology, social control, and the processing of social context in medical encounters. *Journal of Health and Social Behavior* 30:220–39.

Waitzkin, H., & Stoeckle, J. D. 1972. The communication of information about illness: Clinical, sociological, and methodological considerations. *Advances in Psychosomatic Medicine* 8:180–215.

Walker, A. J.; Martin, S. S. K.; & Thompson, L. 1988. Feminist programs for families. *Family Relations* 37:17–22.

Walker, A. J., & Pratt, C. C. 1991. Daughters' help to mothers: Intergenerational aid versus caregiving. *Journal of Marriage and the Family* 53:3–12.

Walker, A. J.; Pratt, C. C.; Shin, H.-Y.; & Jones, L. L. 1990. Motives for parental caregiving and relationship quality. *Family Relations* 39:51–56.

Walker, A. J.; Pratt, C. C.; & Wood, B. 1993. Perceived frequency of role conflict and relationship quality for caregiving daughters. *Psychology of Women Quarterly* 17:207–21.

Walker, A. J.; Shin, H.-Y.; & Bird, D. N. 1990. Perceptions of relationship change and caregiver satisfaction. *Family Relations* 39:147–52.

Walker, A. J., & Thompson, L. 1984. Feminism and family studies. *Journal of Family Studies* 5:545–70.

Walker, A. J.; Thompson, L.; & Morgan, C. S. 1987. Two generations of mothers and daughters: Role position and interdependence. *Psychology of Women Quarterly* 11:195–208.

Walker, E.; Katon, W.; Harrop-Griffiths, J.; Holm, L.; Russo, J.; & Hickok, L. R. 1988. Relationship of chronic pelvic pain to psychiatric diagnoses and childhood sexual abuse. *American Journal of Psychiatry* 145:75–80.

Walker, E. A.; Torkelson, N.; Katon, W. J.; & Koss, M. P. 1993. The prevalence rate of sexual trauma in a primary care clinic. *Journal of the American Board of Family Practice* 6:465–71.

Walker, L. 1984. Sex differences in the development of moral reasoning: A critical review. *Child Development* 55:667–91.

Walker, L. E. 1979. *The battered woman*. New York: Harper & Row.

———1987. Inadequacies of the masochistic personality disorder diagnosis for women. *Journal of Personality Disorders* 1:183–89.

———1988. *Handbook on sexual abuse of children: Assessment and treatment issues*. New York: Springer.

Walker, L. E. A., & Browne, A. 1985. Gender and victimization by intimates. *Journal of Personality* 53:179–95.

Walker, M. U. 1989. Moral understandings: Alternative "epistemology" for a feminist ethics. *Hypatia* 4:15–28.

Walsh, B. W., & Rosen, P. M. 1988. *Self-mutilation: Theory, research and treatment*. New York: Guilford Press.

Walsh, R. T. 1989. Do research reports in mainstream feminist psychology journals reflect feminist values? *Psychology of Women Quarterly* 13:433–44.

Walter, C. A. 1988. The dilemma of the female physician in the feminist health center. *Journal of the American Medical Women's Association* 43:45–50.

Walters, M. 1990. The codependent Cinderella who loves too much . . . fights back. *Family Therapy Networker* 14 (4):53–57.

Walters, M.; Carter, B.; Papp, P.; & Silverstein, O. 1988. *The invisible web: Gender patterns in family relationships*. New York: Guilford Press.

Ward, J. V. 1990. Racial identity formation and transformation. In C. Gilligan, N. P. Lyons, & T. J. Hanmer (eds), *Making connections: The relational worlds of adolescent girls at Emma Willard School* (pp. 215–32). Cambridge, Mass.: Harvard University Press.

Ward, S. K.; Chapman, K.; Cohn, E.; White, S.; & Williams, K. 1991. Acquaintance rape and the college social scene. *Family Relations* 40:65–71.

Warshaw, C. 1989. Limitations of the medical model in the care of battered women. *Gender and Society* 3:506–17.

————1993. Domestic violence: Challenges to medical practice. *Journal of Women's Health* 2 (1):73–80.

Wasserman, R. C.; Inui, T. S.; Barriatua, R. D.; Carter, W. B.; & Lippincott, P. 1984. Pediatric clinicians' support for parents makes a difference: An outcome-based analysis of clinician-parent interaction. *Pediatrics* 74:1047–53.

Wattenberg, E. 1985. In a different light: A feminist perspective on the role of mothers in father-daughter incest. *Child Welfare* 64:203–11.

Weeks, R. B. 1976. The sexually exploited child. *Southern Medical Journal* 69:848–50.

Weiss, B. D.; Hart, G.; McGee, D. L.; & D'Estelle, S. 1992. Health status of illiterate adults: Relation between literacy and health status among persons with low literacy skills. *Journal of the American Board of Family Practice* 5:257–64.

Weitzman, L. 1985. *The divorce revolution: The unexpected social and economic consequences for women and children in America.* New York: Free Press.

Wendell, S. 1990. Oppression and victimization: Choice and responsibility. *Hypatia* 5 (1):15–46.

Wenneker, M. B., & Epstein, A. M. 1989. Racial inequalities in the use of procedures for patients with ischemic heart disease in Massachusetts. *Journal of the American Medical Association* 261:253–57.

Wenston, S. R., & Jarratt, K. D. 1988. Self-in-relation theory and latency-age boys. *Social Casework: The Journal of Contemporary Social Work* 69:231–37.

West, C. 1983. "Ask me no questions . . . " An analysis of queries and replies in physician-patient dialogues. In S. Fisher & A. D. Todd (eds.), *The social organization of doctor-patient communication* (pp. 75–106). Washington, D.C.: Center for Applied Linguistics.

————1984. *Routine complications: Troubles with talk between doctors and patients.* Bloomington: Indiana University Press.

Westcott, M. 1979. Feminist criticism of the social sciences. *Harvard Educational Review* 49 (4):422–30.

Westerlund, E. 1986. Freud on sexual trauma: An historical review of seduction and betrayal. *Psychology of Women Quarterly* 10:297–310.

Wheeler, R.; Candib, L. M.; & Martin, M. 1990. Part-time doctors: Reduced working hours for primary care physicians. *Journal of the American Medical Women's Association* 45:47–54.

Whitbeck, C. 1983. A different reality: Feminist ontology. In C. C. Gould (ed.), *Beyond domination: New perspectives on women and philosophy* (pp. 64–88). Totowa, N.J.: Rowman & Allanheld.

White, K. L. 1986. Ciencia y caridad. *Family Medicine* 18:379–83.

Wikstrand, J.; Warnold, I.; Tuomilehto, J.; Olsson, G.; Barber, H. J.; Eliasson, K.; Elmfeldt, D.; Jastrup, B.; Karatzas, N. B.; Leer, J.; Marchetta, F.; Ragnarsson, J.; Robitaille, N.-M.; Valkova, L.; Wesseling, H.; & Berglund, G. 1991. Metoprolol versus thiazide diuretics in hypertension: Morbidity results from the MAPHY study. *Hypertension* 17:579–88.

Wilbush, J. 1981. Climacteric symptom formation: Donovan's contribution. *Maturitas* 3:99–105.

Willis, S. E., & Horner, R. D. 1987. Attitudes, experience, and knowledge of family physicians regarding child sexual abuse. *Journal of Family Practice* 25:516–19.

Wilson, J. L.; Clements, W.; Cadoret, R. J.; Pease, J.; & Lammer, E. 1978. The dynamics of incest: Presentation of one family in acute crisis. *Journal of Family Practice* 7:363–67.

Wisechild, L. M. 1988. *The obsidian mirror: An adult healing from incest.* Seattle: Seal Press.

Withorn, A. 1984. *Serving the people: Social services and social change.* New York: Columbia University Press.

Wrightsman, L. S. 1988. *Personality development in adulthood.* Newbury Park, Calif.: Sage.

Wyatt, G. E. 1985. The sexual abuse of Afro-American and white-American women in childhood. *Child Abuse and Neglect* 9:507–19.

Wyatt, G. W.; Guthrie, D.; & Notgrass, C. M. 1992. Differential effects of women's child sexual abuse and subsequent revictimization. *Journal of Consulting and Clinical Psychology* 60:167–73.

Yanay, N., & Birns, B. 1990. Autonomy as emotion: The phenomenology of independence in academic women. *Women's Studies International Forum* 13:249–60.

Yorukoglu, A., & Kemph, J. P. 1966. Children not severely damaged by incest with a parent. *Journal of the American Academy of Child Psychiatry* 5:111–24.

Zarit, S. H.; Reever, K. E.; & Bach-Peterson, J. 1980. Relatives of the impaired elderly: Correlates of feelings of burden. *The Gerontologist* 20:649–55.

Zdanuk, J. M.; Harris, C. C.; & Wisian, N. L. 1987. Adolescent pregnancy and incest: The nurse's role as counselor. *Journal of Obstetric, Gynecologic, & Neonatal Nursing* 16 (2):99–104.

Zeitlin, H. 1987. Investigation of the sexually abused child. *Lancet* 2:842–45.

Zierler, S.; Feingold, L.; Laufer, D.; Velentgas, P.; Kantrowitz-Gordon, I.; & Mayer, K. 1991. Adult survivors of childhood sexual abuse and subsequent risk of HIV infection. *American Journal of Public Health* 81:572–75.

Zinn, M. B. 1990. Family, feminism, and race in America. *Gender and Society* 4:68–82.

Zola, I. K. 1972. The concept of trouble and sources of medical assistance—to whom one can turn, with what and why. *Social Science and Medicine* 6:673–79.

INDEX